Dental Biomaterials

World Scientific Series:
From Biomaterials Towards Medical Devices

ISSN: 2529-816X

Series Editors:

Roger Guilard
Université de Bourgogne
UFR Sciences et Techniques
Faculté des Sciences Mirande
ICMUB – UMR CNRS 6302
9 Avenue Alain Savary, BP 47870
21078 Dijon Cedex, France
Email: roger.guilard@u-bourgogne.fr

Karl M Kadish
Department of Chemistry
University of Houston
Houston, TX 77204-5003, USA
Email: kkadish@uh.edu

Vol. 1 *Drug Delivery Systems*
edited by Pieter Stroeve (UC Davis) & Morteza Mahmoudi (Tehran University of Medical Sciences, Iran & Harvard Medical School, USA)

Vol. 2 *Dental Biomaterials*
edited by Edward Sacher (École Polytechnique de Montréal, Canada) & Rodrigo França (University of Manitoba, Canada)

Forthcoming

Biomaterials and Bioengineered Device Research for Ligament Reconstruction
edited by Véronique Migonney ((Université Paris 13, France) & L'Hocine Yahia (École Polytechnique de Montréal, Canada)

Biomaterials and Bioengineered Device Research for Joint Prostheses
edited by L'Hocine Yahia (École Polytechnique de Montréal, Canada) & Véronique Migonney (Université Paris 13, France)

Biomaterials and Bioengineered Device Research for Cardiovascular Applications
edited by Laurence Bordenave (Université de Bordeaux, France)

World Scientific Series in
From Biomaterials Towards Medical Devices – Vol. 2

Dental Biomaterials

editors

Edward Sacher
École Polytechnique de Montréal, Canada

Rodrigo França
University of Manitoba, Canada

Series Editors

Roger Guilard
Université de Bourgogne, France

Karl M. Kadish
University of Houston, USA

World Scientific

NEW JERSEY • LONDON • SINGAPORE • BEIJING • SHANGHAI • HONG KONG • TAIPEI • CHENNAI • TOKYO

Published by

World Scientific Publishing Co. Pte. Ltd.
5 Toh Tuck Link, Singapore 596224
USA office: 27 Warren Street, Suite 401-402, Hackensack, NJ 07601
UK office: 57 Shelton Street, Covent Garden, London WC2H 9HE

Library of Congress Cataloging-in-Publication Data
Names: Sacher, Edward, 1934– editor. | França, Rodrigo (Dentist), editor.
Title: Dental biomaterials / edited by Edward Sacher and Rodrigo França.
Other titles: Dental biomaterials (Sacher) | World Scientific series: from biomaterials towards medical devices ; vol. 2.
Description: New Jersey : World Scientific Publishing, 2018. | Series: World scientific series : from biomaterials towards medical devices ; volume 2 | Includes bibliographical references and index.
Identifiers: LCCN 2018033218 | ISBN 9789813225671 (hardcover : alk. paper)
Subjects: | MESH: Dental Materials
Classification: LCC RK652.5 | NLM WU 190 | DDC 617.6/95--dc23
LC record available at https://lccn.loc.gov/2018033218

British Library Cataloguing-in-Publication Data
A catalogue record for this book is available from the British Library.

For any available supplementary material, please visit
https://www.worldscientific.com/worldscibooks/10.1142/10589#t=suppl

Typeset by Stallion Press
Email: enquiries@stallionpress.com

Preface

The development of the science of dental biomaterials has always been a driving force of dentistry. The first controlled testing of dental amalgam by Dr. Greene V. Black in 1900, the introduction of the acid etching technique by Dr. Michael Buonocore in 1955, and the formulation of polymeric dental filling by Dr. Rafael Bowen in 1962 are just a few examples of the impact of dental biomaterials in restorative dentistry. In the same way, in the 21st century, the flourishing of nanotechnology and tissue engineering offer opportunities to innovate new biomaterials to promote oral rehabilitation. In dentistry, we are presently living in a transitional era, where, in dental offices, most practitioners restore cavities as was done fifty years ago, while, in dental biomaterials laboratories, new approaches, such as the dental bioengineering of tissues, are being tested. As a consequence, a transformational wave is forming on the horizon.

The conception and production of dental biomaterials are not easy tasks. In the past, the evolution of dental materials was based on an idea, conceived and exploited by a "hero dentist", while today, this progress depends on teams of experts in several areas of expertise, such as biomedical engineering, dentistry, chemistry, biology, and materials science. The particularity of the oral environment makes dental biomaterials different from those used in other parts of the body. As an example, the color and the coefficient of thermal expansion of a ceramic used in a hip prosthesis are not major issues, while they are so for a ceramic used as a dental veneer. Such complexity requires a new kind of professionals: Dental biomaterials researchers with broad, deep, and multidisciplinary knowledge.

This book was developed in preparation for this new reality. We invited experts from universities in Brazil, Canada, Switzerland, and the United States to present information in advanced recent topics, as aids to novice researchers in the dental biomaterials field. We have done this in the following way. Chapters 1–3 provide fundamental information on dental biomaterials characterizations. Chapter 4 focuses on biomaterials aimed at preventing oral diseases, and Chapter 5 discusses the toxicity of mercury. Chapters 6–8 present comprehensive studies of ceramic materials and their failure modes. Direct restorative materials are discussed in Chapters 9–11. Chapter 12 focuses on the important topic of polymerization contraction stresses occurring in resin-based composites. Chapters 13 and 14 discuss the use of polymers in prosthodontics, and Chapter 15 furnishes information in the new fields of 3D printing and bioprinting in dentistry.

Finally, it is important to recognize that this book was only made possible thanks to the willingness of all the authors to contribute their expertises, as well as to the funding agencies that made much of the work reported in these chapters possible. It is our hope that the knowledge contained herein will help in furnishing further innovations in the field of dental biomaterials.

About the Editors

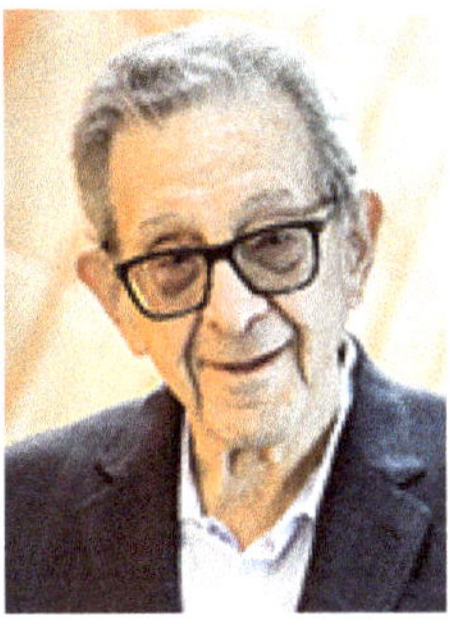

Edward Sacher was born in New York City and educated in its school system. He received a BS in chemistry from the City College of New York and a PhD in physical chemistry from the Pennsylvania State University. After postdoctoral fellowships at Ohio State University and the University of Ottawa, he joined the Film Department of the DuPont Experimental Station. This was followed by a position at the IBM Materials Laboratory. Subsequently, he joined the Department of Engineering Physics of Montréal's École Polytechnique, where he is presently a Professor. He is the Associate Director of the regional Surface Laboratory, where he carries out research on the physico-chemical properties of nanoparticles.

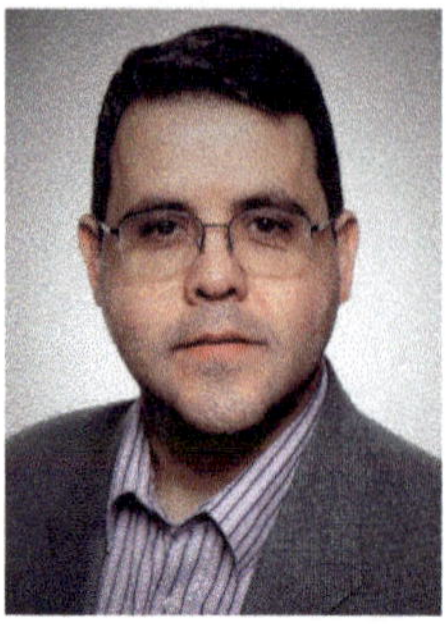

Rodrigo França received his DDS degree in 1988 from the University of Itaúna, Brazil, and his MSc and PhD, in Dental Materials, from the University of São Paulo, Brazil. Subsequently, he obtained a second PhD, in Biomedical Engineering, at Montréal's École Polytechnique. He worked as a general practitioner for 18 years. He has taught dental materials, at both undergraduate and graduate levels, for the past 20 years. Currently, he is an Associate Professor and Head of the Dental Materials Division in the College of Dentistry, University of Manitoba, Canada, and Director of its Dental Biomaterials Research Laboratory; he also has a cross-appointment in the Department of Oral Biology. He is a core member of the Biomedical Engineering graduate program, a member of the Manitoba Institute of Materials, the Academy of Dental Materials, the Canadian and International Associations of Dental Research, and the Canadian Biomaterials Society. His research focuses on physicochemical characterization of the surface of dental biomaterials, at the nanolevel. The results of his research team have been presented at several international dental meetings and published in prestigious peer-reviewed journals.

Contents

Chapter 1

Surface Analysis Techniques for Dental Materials

Edward Sacher*,‡ and Rodrigo França†,§

*Regroupement Québecois de Matériaux de Pointe, Département de Génie Physique, École Polytechnique de Montréal, C.P. 6079, Montréal, Québec H3C 3A7, Canada

†Department of Restorative Dentistry, Dental Biomaterials Research Laboratory, College of Dentistry, University of Manitoba, 780 Bannatyne Av, Winnipeg, Manitoba R3E 0W2, Canada

‡Edward.sacher@polymtl.ca

§Rodrigo.franca@umanitoba.ca

For many years, dental materials researchers have made significant efforts to understand the chemical and mechanical behaviors of restorative materials, implants, etc., to assure positive interaction with oral tissues. The main focus of these studies has been on bulk properties. However, all reactions between dental materials and the host tissues occur at the interface between their two surfaces. Bulk and surface physicochemical compositions may be quite different. Consequently, meticulous surface characterizations should be carried out on dental materials to better comprehend their behaviors in such situations.

1. Introduction

Information on the chemistry, crystal structure, size, roughness, etc., of a surface is often needed by the dental researcher. There are techniques available today that will provide such information. However, these techniques are often in the domain of chemists and physicists, whose primary interests lie outside the area of dental research; dental researchers, who have little background in the physics, chemistry, or mathematics of such techniques, may be loath to use them for that reason, despite the potential benefits. It is the purpose of this chapter to acquaint them with several of the more common surface characterization techniques, and what they will be able to achieve by using them.

This chapter is designed to inform the dental researcher what information any given technique is capable of offering *when carried out by a surface scientist competent in that technique*. While it is not necessary for the dental researcher to have expertise in physics, chemistry, and mathematics, they are the major pillars on which biomaterial surface research is constructed, and there is no reason why the dental researcher should not avail himself of such aid.

1.1. *Surface and Interfaces*

A *surface* is the boundary layer of a solid or liquid; in equilibrium, when exposed to air or vapor; the surface is generally pictured as having length and width, but no depth. In fact, all real surfaces have some minimal depth. This is because, in the interior, an atom is surrounded uniformly, with the interaction energy of that atom (A in Figure 1) and its neighbors uniformly distributed; however, at the surface (B in Figure 1), the energy distribution is not uniform, due to the lack of structural uniformity (i.e. neighbors lying below, but not above, the surface atoms). This generally results in slight structural changes at the surface. Since structural interactions extend beyond nearest neighbors, the energy distribution at the surface does not change abruptly over one monolayer, but over several, creating a surface with some depth, over which conditions change more gradually.

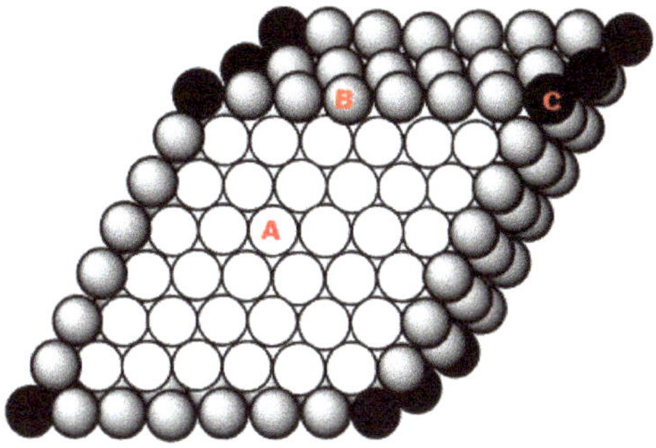

Figure 1. Cross-section representation of the atomic arrangement of a biomaterial. Bulk atoms (A) are in equilibrium, while surface atoms (B and C) have an additional surface free energy

An *interface* is a boundary between two condensed phases in equilibrium: solid–solid, solid–liquid, or two immiscible liquids. The importance of the interface is due to the fact that this is where all reactions between the biomaterial and the biological environment occur. In dentistry, phenomena such as osseointegration and dentin adhesion occur, at the molecular level, at the interface. At this level, all materials exposed to air adsorb gases, which form a thin superficial layer. In the same way, dental materials, when immersed in biological fluids (saliva, blood, etc.), are immediately covered by biomolecules, such as water, sugars, and proteins. Such adsorption is driven by the thermodynamic need to reduce the surface free energy.

1.2. *Surface Energy*

In order to create a surface, energy must be applied to a volume, by breaking bonds and interrupting interactions; that is, the formation of a surface is energetically unfavorable. For *liquids*, the surface energy density (energy per unit area of surface) is identically equal to the surface tension (force necessary to open a unit length of crack to form the surface). For *solids*, unless there is some drastic chemical or physical change that occurs on surface development, they are *essentially* equal.

Thermodynamics informs us that, in three dimensions, physical or chemical reactions will occur spontaneously when the change in *Gibbs* free energy is negative. In a similar fashion, in two dimensions (i.e. at a surface), reactions will occur spontaneously when the change in *Helmholtz* free energy, which is directly related to the surface tension, is negative. This is why, for example, iron rusts: the oxidation that occurs leads to a surface product having a lower surface tension than does the unoxidized surface.

1.3. *Forces at Interfaces*

Interatomic forces within materials, and across their interfaces, can be both polar and non-polar (dispersive). Also, they can be strong or weak. Polar interactions involve permanent dipoles (or multipoles) across an interface, while dispersive interactions involve instantaneous dipoles (i.e. van der Waals interactions). Polar interactions are by far the stronger of the two. Both types of interaction are invariably present, even in highly polar or highly dispersive materials.

In the case of non-crosslinked polymeric filler materials, polar groups are often able to reorient to some extent. For the most used dental adhesive monomers, hydroxyethyl methacrylate (HEMA), this permits the adhesive surface to exhibit a low surface energy to air (polar groups oriented to provide a highly dispersive surface) and a low interfacial energy in water (polar groups oriented to provide a highly polar surface).

1.4. *Reactions at Surfaces: Adsorption*

Adsorption is the exposure to, and adhesion of, species from the surrounding medium to the surface. In the formation of rust, water vapor and oxygen from the surrounding atmosphere adsorb onto the metal surface within a very short time following exposure, subsequently reacting to form a mixed hydrated oxide/hydroxide which, when enough $Fe_2O_3 \cdot H_2O$ is formed, becomes red rust.

Two areas of importance to the dental profession, which bear on adsorption, are adhesion and biocompatibility.[1] Common examples of adsorption in dentistry are the wettability and adsorption of saliva on enamel[2] or a denture acrylic base[3] and the passivation layer formed in titanium implants[4] or basic alloys (NiCr and CoCr).

The adsorption of biomolecules and proteins on surfaces has been noted as a major factor for understanding the biocompatibility of biomaterials.[5,6] Indeed, what distinguishes a biomaterial from other materials used in engineering is the fact that the body reacts tolerantly to them and negatively to the others.[7] All of these biochemical reactions take place at the biomaterial surface, and the adsorption of biomolecules and proteins leads to a hierarchical bioreaction process that can result either in the healing or in the necrosis of the tissue.[8]

To understand protein adsorption, surface characterization methods have been used to provide quantitative details about the atomistic level of the interfaces.[9] The effects of surface-driven forces, including hydrophobic and electrostatic interactions, are fundamentals to protein adsorption and desorption.

In dentistry, protein adsorption has been studied to improve the osseointegration of dental implants,[10] understanding biofilm attachment on tooth structure,[11] and remineralization.[12]

2. Characterization Techniques

These techniques fall into two broad categories, physicochemical and morphological. Physicochemical techniques elucidate the physical and chemical properties of a material, such as its crystal structure and chemical groups, while morphological techniques reveal the size, roughness, and shape of a material. A schematic representation of the techniques is given in Table 1.

There are many different characterization techniques; however, only a few provide insights into the outermost atomic layers. The techniques we have chosen to discuss are those readily found in research laboratories, whose use entails reasonable costs and whose data are readily interpretable by those in the field. Some deal with elements at the surface, while others offer necessary information on molecules. They run the gamut from qualitative to quantitative analyses, wherein qualitative methods give information on only the presence of elements or compounds, while quantitative methods measure their amounts. Further, they vary in sensitivity, ranging from

Table 1. Surface analyses techniques

		Ion spectroscopies		Electron spectroscopies				Vibrational spectroscopies	Diffraction methods
	Contact angle	TOF-SIMS	LA-ICP-MS	XPS	AES	EDX	WDS	ATR-FTIR Raman	XRD[a]
Depth probed	<1 nm	2–5 nm	Bulk	10 nm	1 nm	4 μm		0.5–2 μm	5 nm
Surface energy	Yes	No	No	No	No	No	No	No	No
Composition		+++	++	+++++	++	+++	+++	++	+++
Quantitative	No	No	E[b]	E & M	E	semi	E	M[c]	M
Qualitative	No	E & M	E	E & M		E	E	M	M
Destructive	No	Yes	Yes	No	No	No	No	No	No
UHV required	No	Yes	No	Yes	Yes	Yes	Yes	No	No
Spatial resolution		+++		++	++++	+	+		+++
Trace detection		ppb	ppt	0.1%	0.1%	1%	ppm	0.1%	0.1%
Depth profiling	No	Yes	Yes	Yes		No		Yes	
Mapping	No	Yes	Yes	Yes	Yes	Yes	Yes	Yes	Yes
Elements detected		All		> He	< Zr	> Be		Org	Crystalline

Notes: [a]Using the in-plane XRD technique.
[b]E: Elemental level.
[c]M: Molecular level.

parts per hundred (i.e. percent) to parts per billion (ppb) or parts per trillion (ppt). Many of the techniques to be described operate under high vacuum (UHV), whose main purpose is to extend the mean free path (i.e. the average distance between molecular collisions) of the information-carrying particles (e.g. electrons), so that they may be properly treated before detection. However, using UHV can be a challenge when working with porous materials, such as dentin.

The depth probed varies with the technique. Some techniques can provide information on the outermost monolayer or two (<1 nm), while others probe several nanometers. However, methods can sometimes be applied to increase or decrease the probe depth of these techniques; e.g. changing the XPS take-off angle or progressively etching the surface. In addition, spatial resolution can vary, from <1 nm to several micrometers, and this feature is especially important if chemical mapping is required.

No single technique provides complete answers to surface analytical questions, and therefore several complementary techniques must be used in approaching a problem. Special attention should also be paid to sample preservation. Some techniques can destroy the sample by radiation or sputtering. Destructive techniques should always be preceded by all the non-destructive techniques.

2.1. *Physicochemical Techniques*

2.1.1. *Contact Angle (CA)*

The surface energy of a non-distortable solid is determined indirectly, using liquids whose surface tensions are known. A sessile drop of such a liquid, placed on a flat, smooth solid surface, forms a contact angle, θ, with that surface. In the plane of that surface, the Young–Dupré equation describes the equilibrium at any point along the circumference of the drop:

$$\gamma\,(\textit{at the solid-liquid interface}) + [\cos\theta \times \gamma\,(\textit{at the liquid-vapor interface})] = \gamma\,(\textit{at the solid-vapor interface}).$$

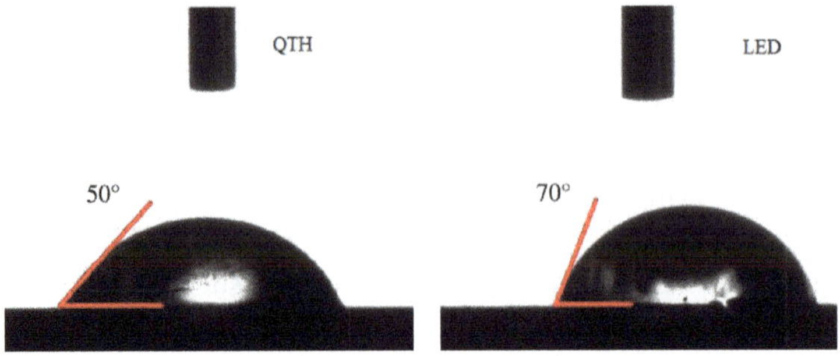

Figure 2. Example of the effect of the light curing source on the surface energy of self-etch resin cement. Two samples of the same self-etch resin cement were cured using a Quartz-Tungsten-Halogen light (QTH) or a Light-Emitting Diode light (LED)

When the surface is wet by the liquid (i.e. $\theta = 0$), γ (at the liquid–vapor interface) is equal to zero, and γ (at the solid–liquid interface) is equal to γ (at the solid–vapor interface). That is, in order to wet a solid surface, the surface tension of the liquid must be equal to, or less than, that of the surface. Wetting assures extensive contact, and is desirable for good adhesion.

CA measurement is the least expensive and simplest technique used to probe the surface. It is also the only one able to directly determine solid surface thermodynamics, such as surface free energy, enthalpy, and entropy. However, they do not provide sample surface composition and are more applicable to low-energy solids, such as polymers, as seen in Figure 2. It is important to note that the Young–Dupré equation applies only to smooth, homogeneous surfaces; rough surfaces require the Wenzel or Cassie–Baxter equations.[12,13,14]

In dentistry, CA is commonly used for determining the hydrophilicity of impression materials[15,16] and dental bonding agents.[17,18] Some water-drop CA values of dental materials are shown in Table 2. New techniques, such as microdroplet approaches, and further detail information can be obtained in specialized reviews.[19,20]

2.1.2. *X-ray Photoelectron Spectroscopy (XPS)*

This technique, also called Electron Spectroscopy for Chemical Analysis (ESCA), uses a probe beam of mono-energetic X-rays to

Table 2. Contact angle of water drop for some dental biomaterials

Biomaterial	CA(θ)
Addition silicone[a]	53
Amalgam[a]	77
Condensation silicone[a]	98
Glass Ionomer cement[b]	65
Polyether[b]	49
Resin-based composite[b]	35
Universal bonding agent[b]	39

Sources: [a]Adapted from Ref. [3]; [b]unpublished data.

irradiate a sample. The X-rays interact with electrons in various orbitals of energy lower than that of the X-rays, causing them to be emitted. The X-rays are photons; quantum mechanics tells us that photons cannot be fragmented. That is, on reacting, they are totally destroyed, with some of their energy overcoming the energy that binds the electron in its orbital, some of the energy overcoming the potential energy of the surface (the work function), and the remainder is given to the emitted electron as kinetic energy (Figure 3). The spectrometer measures the kinetic energy of the emitted electron, which, depending on the magnitude of the energy and the angle of the detector to the sample, can come from depths between 0.8 and 10 nm. Knowing the energy of the X-ray photon, and correcting the energy scale to account for the work function (a simple process), gives the binding energy, the energy in which XPS spectra are presented.

Each element has a specific binding energy ***range*** for each electron orbital (see Table 3 and Figure 4); the electron density around each emitting atom additionally influences the exact binding energy, so that the C1s peak for, e.g. an alcohol falls at ~286.5 eV while that for a carbonyl falls ~1 eV higher (Figure 5). One may, as a result of these effects, qualitatively distinguish ionic valences, as well as polar organic structures (e.g. oxidation products, how many halides are bonded to a single carbon, etc.).

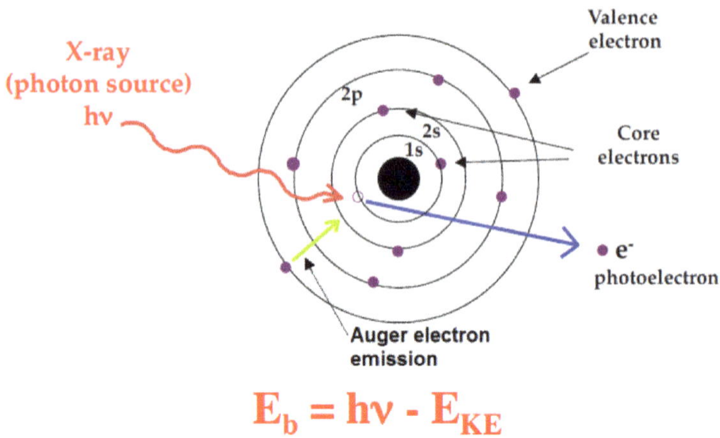

Figure 3. Photoemission on X-ray irradiation. E_b = binding energy with which the electron is held in the atom; h = Planck constant (6.62×10^{-34} J s), ν = frequency (Hz) of the radiation; E_{KE} = kinetic energy of the photoelectron

Table 3. Binding energy of XPS peaks of elements frequently encountered in dentistry

Elements	XPS peak	Binding energy (eV)
Calcium	$Ca2p_{3/2}$	347
Carbon	C1s	285
Fluorine	F1s	684
Oxygen	O1s	532
Phosphate	$P2p_{3/2}$	133
Silicon	$Si2p_{3/2}$	102
Titanium	$Ti2p_{3/2}$	458
Zirconium	$Zr3d_{5/2}$	182

Further, because the quantum mechanical effects that govern photon interactions differ only slightly across any given spectrum, the component peak areas contributing to that spectrum are in the same ratios as are the components in the material being tested. That is, the ratio of the C1s spectral component peaks (e.g. hydroxyl, carbonyl,

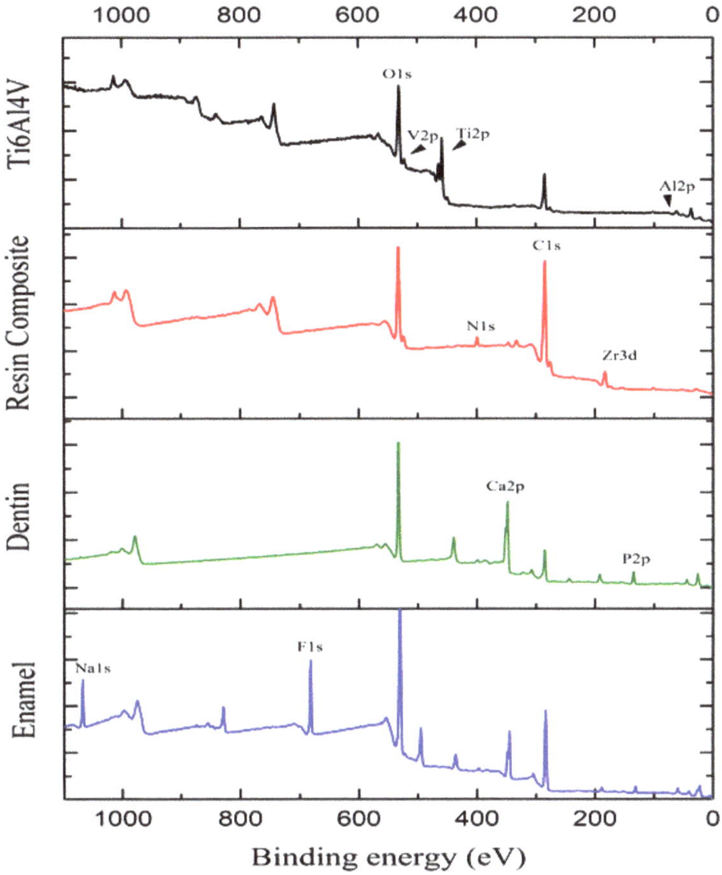

Figure 4. XPS survey spectra of dental enamel, dentin, resin-based composite (Filtek Supreme, 3M, St. Paul, MN, USA), and a dental implant (Astra, Dentsply, SW)

carboxylic acid, etc.) in a given spectrum are in the same ratio as the chemical groups in the material being tested. Moreover, the existence of peak sensitivity factors for each element permits the evaluation of the relative ratios of all the peaks in all the spectra being considered. That is, to within a few percent, an XPS analysis is both qualitative and quantitative. Newer instruments can be used to chemically map a surface, using one of these peak components.

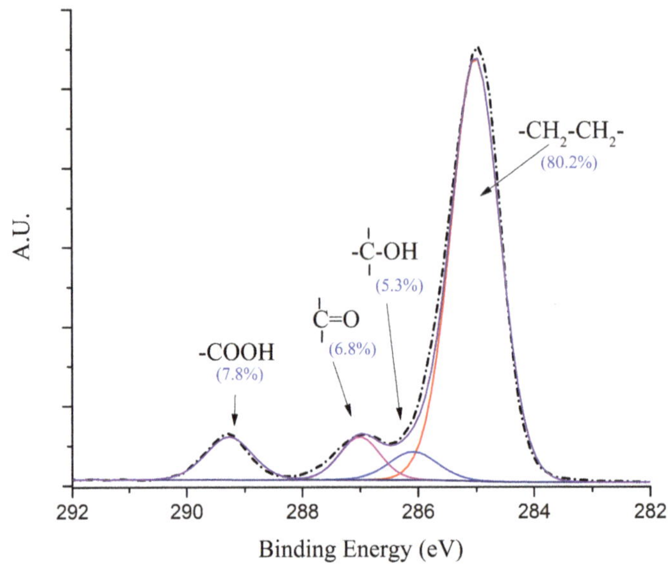

Figure 5. The C1s XPS high-resolution peak deconvolution of a self-etch bonding agent (iBond Self-etch, Heraeus Kulzer, Gr)

Some limitations of this technique include the impossibility to detect H and He, the necessity for UHV (that challenges the analysis of porous surface, such as dentin), and the fact that some spectra overlap others. There are relatively few examples of surface analyses using XPS in dentistry. Some studies, in areas such as bonding agents,[21,22] pulp-capping materials,[23] fluoride gels,[24] and dental implants[4,25] show the potential of this technique. In medicine, XPS is used largely to characterize biomaterials,[26,27] nanoparticles for drug delivery,[28–30] and for infection control.[31]

2.1.3. *Auger Electron Spectroscopy (AES)*

As seen in Figure 3, the emitted photoelectron in the XPS process leaves a hole in its atomic orbital. An electron from the outer layer can fall into the inner layer to occupy the hole, and the excess energy can be emitted as an X-ray photon (X-ray fluorescence, XRF) or emitted as another electron in an outer layer (Auger electron). The detection of this electron is called AES. In an AES spectrometer, the initial hole is formed using an electron beam.

AES is a surface technique, probing ~0.2 to ~1.0 nm. This technique has infrequently been used to provide limited relevant qualitative and quantitative information on the elemental composition and chemical environment of the surface, but is plagued by the often opposing chemical shifts of the three electrons involved in the Auger process. When possible, the use of XPS is simpler and, involving only one electron, is easier to interpret. A distinct advantage of AES lies in the fact that it can be incorporated into a scanning electron microscopy (SEM), using the monoenergetic electron beam to cause the emission of the first electron. Such an electron beam can probe very small sites, and is useful in the study of grain boundaries in metals and alloys. Since the electron beam can be rastered, it is possible to study the surface distribution of elements. AES has been used to probe dental implants[32] and corrosion at dental alloy surfaces,[33] and to assess the interaction of biofilms and restorative material.[34]

2.1.4. *Energy-Dispersive X-ray Spectroscopy (EDX)*

EDX is probably the most often used technique for dental biomaterial chemical characterization. As it is normally installed on an SEM, EDX can be used during SEM examination, providing qualitative elemental analysis of a sample in a few minutes. Another convenience is the fact that it can be used to analyze a broad range of materials and sample sizes.

As mentioned in the section on AES, an atom can reduce its energy by emitting secondary X-rays (X-ray fluorescence). These are detected and displayed, as seen in Figure 6.

Although EDX does not provide quantitative analyses, it may be used as a semi-quantitative method if a known standard, similar to the sample, is available.

Because the probe depth is >1 μm, EDX is not a surface technique. However, it has been used to probe bulk chemical composition, contrasting it with the surface composition obtained by XPS.[23,26] Mapping may be carried out, using the EDS raster mode.

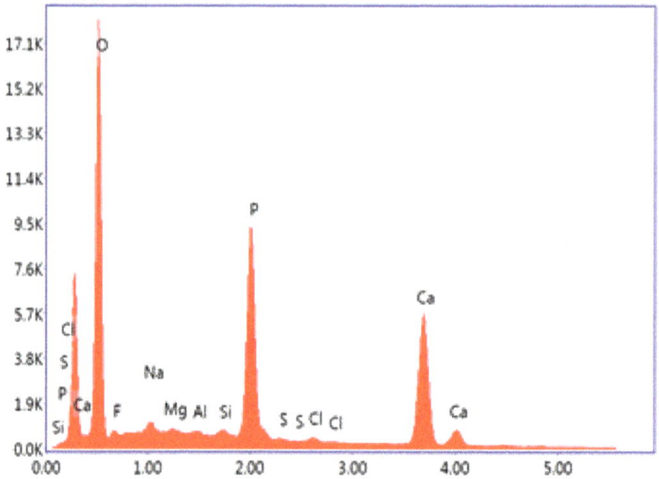

Figure 6. EDX spectra of dental enamel

Other limitations of EDX include the fact that it cannot detect H, He, or lithium (an important component of some dental ceramics), some elements are difficult to be detected due to peak overlap (e.g. titanium and vanadium), and the EDX beam can decompose polymer film samples, such as adhesives.

2.1.5. *Wavelength-Dispersive Spectrometry (WDS)*

This technique, also known as wavelength-dispersive X-ray fluorescence spectrometry (WDSXRF) or X-ray microprobe, was primarily used for X-ray spectral characterization.[35] The major difference between WDS and EDS is that WDS can provide quantitative results of the elements present at the sample.

As with EDS, WDS is not a surface technique, and it cannot detect element < Be, but can provide better bulk information than EDS due to its greater spectral resolution (~5 eV, compared to ~100 eV). Despite these advantages, WDS is less used than EDS, probably because it is slower in producing spectra (hours, compared to seconds), and because the larger size of the equipment (especially for multichannel systems) does not fit easily into SEM systems, as does EDS.

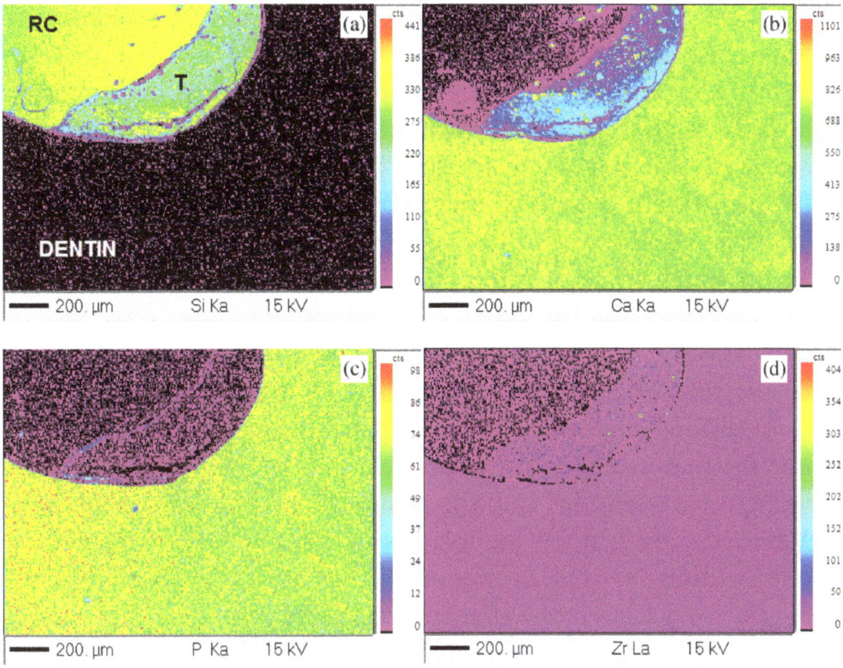

Figure 7. WDS mapping of a pulp-capping material (Theracal, Bisco, IL, USA). Theracal (T) was applied at the pulpal floor of the cavity and restored with resin-based composite (RC). In a, silicon content is displayed; in b, calcium; in c, phosphorus, and in d, zircon

In dentistry, WDS has been used for the analyses of ceramics,[36] protein attachment,[37] and fractographic analyses.[38] It has also been used to map ion release from pulp-capping materials, as seen in Figure 7.

2.1.6. *Time-Of-Flight Secondary Ion Mass Spectrometry (TOF-SIMS)*

Mass spectrometry (MS) is a well-know, well-established technique that measures the masses of charged atoms or molecular fragments, in atomic mass units (or Daltons, D). The use of a primary ion beam (e.g. isotopically pure Bi^+, Cs^+, etc.) to produce the atoms or fragments by an ejection process called sputtering, makes possible the measurement of these secondary ions, and is referred to as secondary ion mass spectrometry (SIMS).

A problem with this technique, for those interested in characterizing surfaces, is that SIMS instruments use high-energy primary beams to characterize depth profiles; this is referred to as dynamic SIMS. Such beams quickly sputter away the surface one may wish to characterize. A variation of this technique uses much less energetic beams, in which an exceedingly small fraction of the surface layer is sputtered away during the length of the experiment; this is referred to as static SIMS. The sputtered atoms are detected in a drift tube, in which the time of flight of a fragment is used to establish its mass; thus, TOF-SIMS. Distinct advantages of the use of a drift tube include the high mass sensitivity possible (0.001 D), the capability of detecting trace quantities, and the possibility of chemical mapping.

While only the first few monolayers are sputtered, those fragments include neutrals, as well as fragments that are both positively and negatively charged; it is the charged fragments that are detected (see Figure 8). Although the use of calibration standards gives quantitative results in fields such as the semiconductor industry, there is a general lack of knowledge of the efficiency of the sputtering process in producing fragments, as well as the fractions of those fragments that are positively or negatively charged; because of this, TOF-SIMS is generally used as a qualitative technique. That is, while the technique is capable of detecting trace ions in the ppb range, the detected intensities of the various fragments cannot be used to quantify the species present in the sample. Nonetheless, TOF-SIMS is useful as a confirmatory technique, as well as in detecting the onset of a chemical reaction.

2.1.7. *Laser Ablation Inductively Coupled Plasma Mass Spectrometry (LA-ICP-MS)*

This technique is exceptional in detecting trace elements in solid samples. In fact, the detection limits obtained by LA-ICP-MS can approach one part per trillion. In this technique, a Nd:YAG laser is focused at the surface, vaporizing the probed area; these fragments

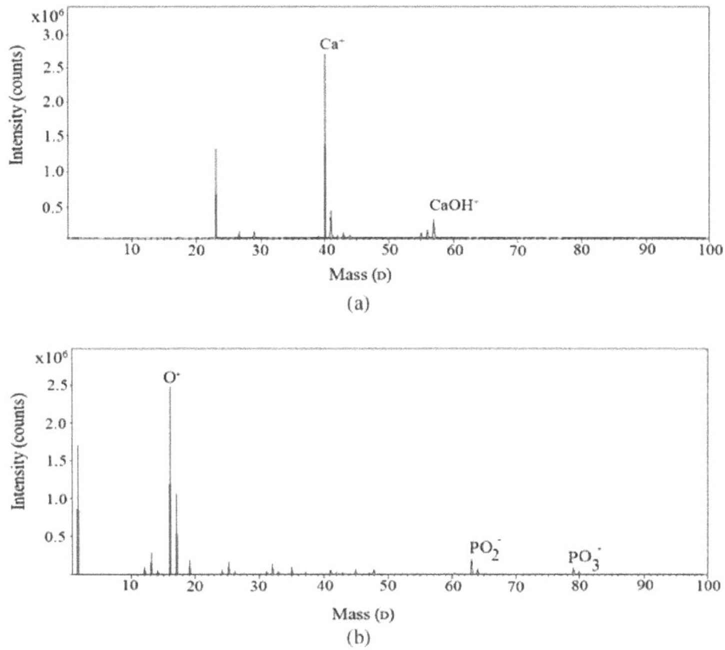

Figure 8. TOF-SIMS spectra for a biphasic calcium phosphate bioceramic (Boneceramic, Straumann, Gr). Part a displays positive ions and part b, negative ions

are transported into a high-energy plasma of an ICP mass spectrometer, and the detected masses are used to detect the composition of the sample.[39]

While this technique is more frequently used for bulk characterization (laser beam size 10–100 μm), LA-ICP-MS offers the possibility of making an elemental map during depth profiling, which can help to understand differences between surface and bulk compositions. A femtosecond laser pulsing technique is now available, which can reduce the beam size to <100 nm.[40]

Being one the most powerful techniques for trace element detection, LA-ICP-MS is frequently used in toxicological studies. An interesting report used this technique on human enamel and dentin, to detect an individual's chronological nutrition record.[41] Another paper assessed the amount of trace titanium in perio-implant oral mucosa.[42]

2.1.8. *Vibrational Spectroscopies: Infrared (FTIR) and Raman*

Beyond the red region of the visible portion of the electromagnetic spectrum lies the infrared (IR) region, appearing at frequencies from ~500 to 4,000 cm^{-1}, where cm^{-1} is referred to as wavenumbers. This is the region in which molecules vibrate, with each vibrational peak representing the motions of an irreducible vibration (i.e. a vibration not composed of a combination of several other vibrations). Further, because the energy (frequency) of the vibration depends on the reduced mass of the atoms participating, each vibration appears at a specific frequency, over a short frequency range; the reason for the short frequency range is that the rest of the molecule attached to the chemical group that is vibrating at that particular frequency offers some slight participation.

The vibrations that are seen include stretching, deformation, wagging, etc., each at its appropriate frequency. Since, e.g. the stretching frequency of one group may fall at, or near, the deformation frequency of another, the group responsible is identified by confirming that all its vibrations appear at their appropriate frequencies in the spectrum. The information gained from a vibrational spectrum identifies the chemical groups present on the sample. For a pure material, the existence and positions of the component peaks serve to identify it, when matched against spectra found in various databases. For an impure material, one will at least know which chemical groups are present. As generally used with solids, vibrational spectroscopy is qualitative, with a sensitivity of ~5%.

Two techniques, based on different physical processes, are used to obtain vibrational spectra: IR and Raman spectroscopies. Because they are based on different processes, the selection rules, concerning which vibrational peaks are seen with that technique, are different. Thus, some peaks appear in both types of spectra, and others, in one or the other. Spectral mapping is possible.

Photoacoustic IR is an interesting application of IR spectroscopy, which is potentially very important to the dental researcher because opaque materials may be sampled. It uses a special airtight photoacoustic cell, generally filled with helium (He) or other inert gas, at atmospheric pressure; the cell is inserted into the sample chamber of the spectrometer. A light source (photo-) provides the energy that provokes the vibration; when the vibration relaxes, a small fraction of a second later, it heats the trapped He, raising its pressure slightly, and is detected by a sensitive miniature microphone (-acoustic) within the cell. A plot of the pressure change as a function of frequency gives the photoacoustic spectrum, essentially identical to the IR spectrum. A distinct advantage of photoacoustic IR is that its probe depth is less than 100 nm, while the probe depth of its IR competitors are much bigger than that.

The spectrometers presently used are IR interferometers, which give interferograms. The mathematical Fourier transform (FT) of an IR interferogram gives the IR spectrum; the process is known as FTIR spectroscopy, and, in the case of Raman, FT Raman spectroscopy.

Attenuated total reflectance (ATR)-FTIR is very often used in dentistry. This involves relatively simple sample preparation, since the sample (film or solid material) can be placed directly on the ATR crystal and probed by the IR radiation passing through the crystal. The sampling depth is ~5 μm, which means ATR cannot probe the surface at nanolevel. However, this type of crystal material can reduce the absorption at the interface, diminishing the probe depth; e.g. using a diamond crystal, the penetration depth is reduced to 2 mm, and using a germanium crystal, ~0.6 μm.[43] ATR-FTIR (or Raman) is used in dentistry for assessing the degree of conversion of polymeric materials, such as resin-based composites and bonding agents. The correlation of the values of the aliphatic C=C peak at ~1,638 cm^{-1} and the aromatic C–C peak at ~1,608 cm^{-1}, before and after curing, makes it possible to estimate the degree of polymerization of a polymer.[44,45]

Figure 9 shows an ATR-FTIR spectrum of a universal dental adhesive. In this spectrum (as in most of organic materials), we can define two regions: 4,000–1,500 cm^{-1}, the functional groups region, and 1,500–400 cm^{-1}, the fingerprint region. Peaks in the first group are used to confirm the presence of specifics types of bonds,

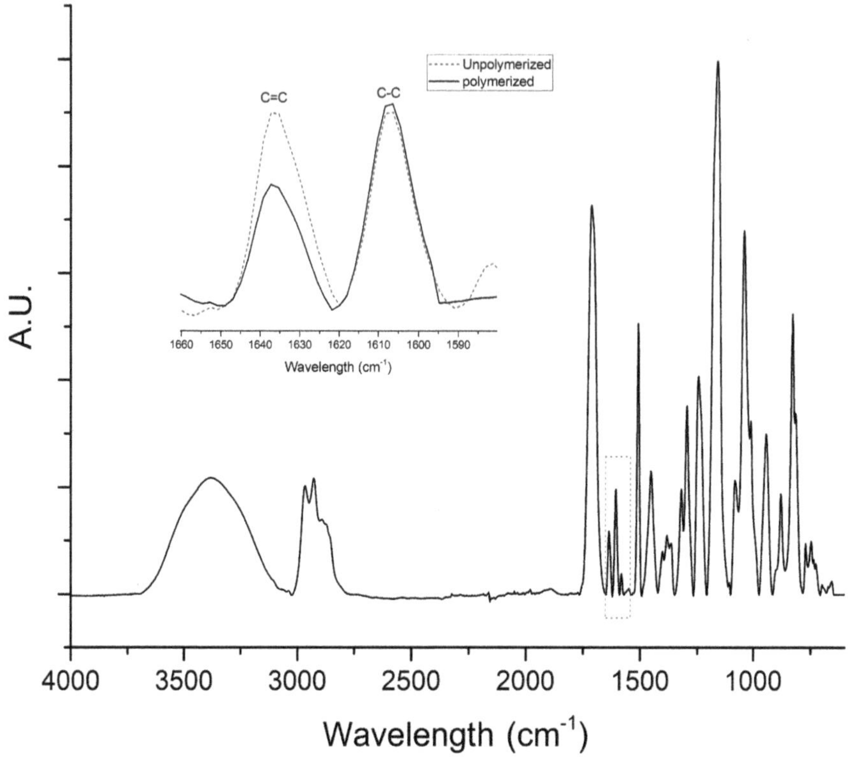

Figure 9. FTIR spectrum of a universal bonding agent (All-Bond Universal, BISCO, IL, USA). The inset shows the range between 1,660 and 1,590 cm^{-1}, with two bands, C=C and C–C, which can be used to determine the degree of conversion of acrylic-based polymers, when compared before and after curing

and peaks in the second region indicate a unique pattern from each organic compound. The interpretation of FTIR spectra can be carried out by comparison of each peak/band position with the large amount of information available in the literature. Table 4 provides a selection of frequently used functional groups of dental materials.

For materials containing many compounds, the spectral interpretation can be a challenge, because peaks may overlap. As an example, the ATR-FTIR spectra of some pulp-capping materials are shown in Figure 10.[23]

Table 4. FTIR frequencies of some functional group vibrational modes often found in dental materials

Functional group	Vibrational mode	Wavelength (cm^{-1})
Hydrocarbons:		
Methyl($-CH_3$)	C–H stretching	2,870 (sym); 2,960 (asym)
Methylene ($-CH_2-$)	C–H stretching	2,860 (sym); 2,930 (asym)
Vinyl ($C{=}CH_2$)	Vinyl bending	910, 990
Vinyl (C=C)	C=C stretching	1,600–1,680
Aromatic C	Monosubstitution	730–770, 680–720
Oxygen groups:		
Aliphatic alcohols (CO→H)	OH stretch (free)	3,600–3,640
Phenols (C–O↓H)	OH stretch (H-bonded)	3,200–3,400
Carboxylic acids (C–C→O)	C–O–H bend	1,300–1,400
aliphatic (C=→O)	C–C–O stretch (dimer)	1,200–1,320
aromatic (C=→O)	C=O stretch (dimer)	1,710
Aldehydes aliphatic	C=O stretch	1,690
Esters aliphatic	C=O stretch	1,730
	C=O stretch	1,745
Amines (aromatic):		
Primary Ar-NH_2	N→H stretch	3,500
Secondary Ar_2NH	N→H stretch	3,400
Tertiary Ar_3N	No NH	
Heteroatom compounds:		
Halogenated compounds:	Aliphatic halide	720–1,400
Phosphorus compounds:	C→F	530–800
Silicon compounds:	C→Cl	
	Phosphates esters	1,250–1,290
	P=→O	720–850
	P→O	800–1,000
	Si→F	2,100–2,200
	Si→H	700–820
	Si→C	1,000–1,100
	Si→O→Si	820–920
	Si→OH	

Source: Adapted from Ref. [43].

2.1.9. *X-ray Diffraction (XRD)*

XRD is used to establish the identity or phase of a solid material through the determination of the diffraction pattern of its crystal

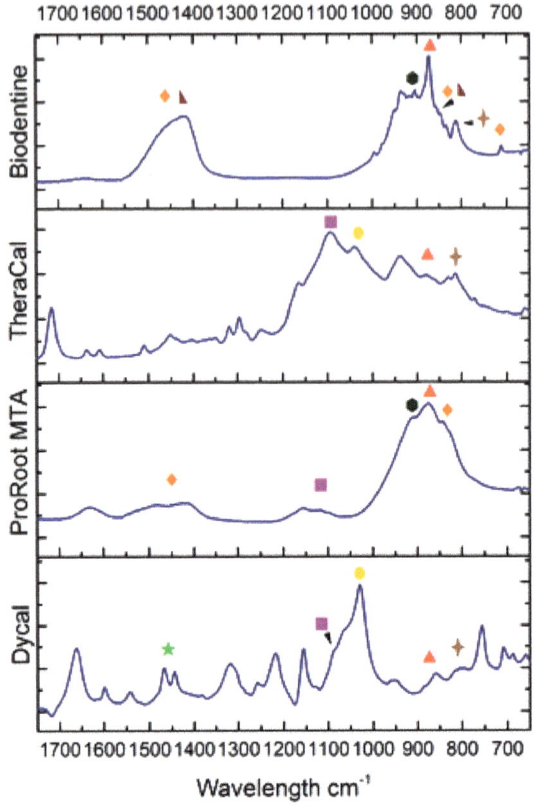

Figure 10. FTIR spectra for four pulp capping materials. Symbols represent calcium compounds: ◆ $CaCO_3$ (Aragonite), ◣ $CaCO_3$ (Calcite), ⬢ Ca_3SiO_5, ▲ Ca_2SiO_4, • $Ca_{10}(PO_4)_6(OH)_2$, ■ $CaSO_4$, + $Ca_2Mg_5Si_8O_{22}(OH)_2$, ★ $Ca(OH)_2$. Adapted from [Ref. 26]

structure. A crystalline sample is rotated with respect to a mono-energetic X-ray beam, using small steps of angle change over a limited range of angles. The diffractogram, having diffraction peaks at specific angles, is normally referred to as a 2θ scan. It is then compared to a database of spectra; the one that is generally used is still referred to as the Joint Committee on Powder Diffraction Standards (JCPDS) data set, despite the fact that the organization renamed itself as the International Centre for Diffraction Data (ICDD) almost 40 years ago. It can be used to identify a pure material, a mixture of materials and, because different phases have different crystal structures, it can distinguish one phase from another.

XRD can function as a surface technique when used in in-plane diffraction. In this technique, the incident and diffracted beams are nearly parallel to the sample surface.[46] In this way, the probed depth can be as small as 5 nm; further, by changing the incident angle, a depth profile can be carried out. XRD can be used to measure crystal size, using the Scherrer formula[47]:

$$\tau = \frac{K\lambda}{\beta\cos\theta},$$

where t is the crystal size (its diameter, if spherical), λ is the wavelength of the incident wave, θ is the Bragg angle of diffraction, H is the width at half peak height, and k usually takes the value 0.89. For accuracy, a known silicon pattern is used, using the XRD peaks near to ~40°.[26]

XRD is extensively used in dentistry to detect phases of titanium implants,[48] dental ceramics,[49] and bioceramics for bone growing[26,50] (see Figure 11).

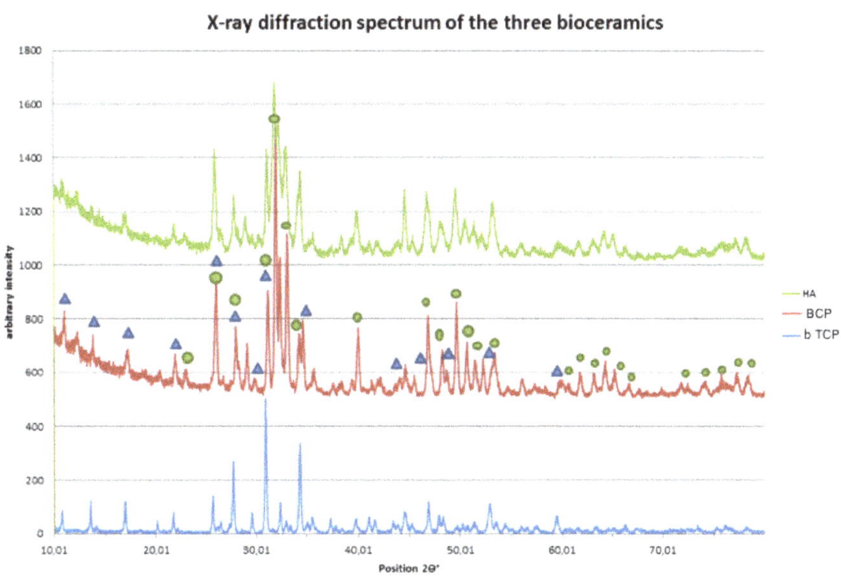

Figure 11. XRD spectra from three bioceramics for bone growing. Adapted from [Ref. 26]

2.2. *Morphological Techniques*

2.2.1. *Electron Microscopies*

Because electrons have shorter wavelengths than visible light, microscopes using an electron probe beam give images having resolution several orders of magnitude higher than that by optical microscopes (~0.1 nm, compared to ~200 nm, all under optimal conditions). There are two basic electron microscopy variants, transmission electron microscopy (TEM) and scanning electron microscopy (SEM). Since the TEM electron beam is transmitted through the sample to obtain an image, it results in an image of the sample volume; for this reason, special, very careful thinning (~100 nm) is required to obtain photomicrographs by this technique, as shown in Figure 12. The use of biological samples is problematic because special techniques are needed to avoid sample drying in the high instrument vacuum. A distinct advantage of the technique, for samples for which drying is not a concern, is that a diffraction pattern may be obtained at any point on the scan, permitting the determination of the crystal structure at that point.

In the case of SEM, the electron beam is rastered across the sample, and the secondary electrons emitted are used to produce the photomicrograph, as shown in Figure 13. It is about an order of magnitude lower in resolution than TEM and, because the source of the secondary electrons is the sample surface, it gives an image of that surface, rather than of the volume. While SEM does not require sample thinning, precautions similar to those for TEM are required, when sample drying is a problem. A variation of SEM, environmental SEM (ESEM), uses differential pumping to accommodate samples in various working atmospheres. Another variation, scanning transmission electron microscopy (STEM), rasters an electron beam that is transmitted through the sample; a distinct advantage of this variation is its ability to obtain high angle annular dark field (HAADF) images, which sense differences in atomic mass, and can distinguish image locations having atoms of different masses.

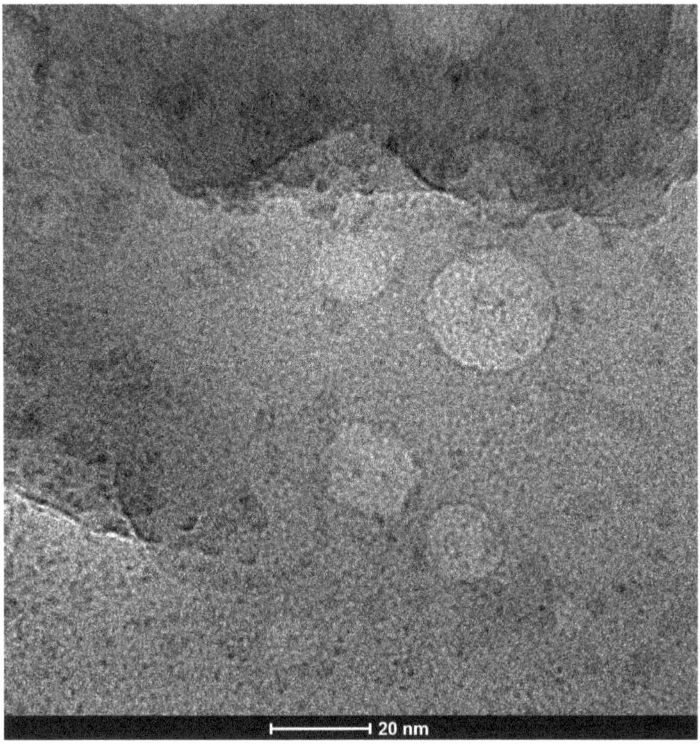

Figure 12. TEM image of a lithium disilicate CAD-CAM ceramic [Unpublished data]

2.2.2. *Atomic Force Microscopy (AFM)*

AFM is a variant of surface probe microscopy, in which a sharp tip is rastered across a surface while a piezoelectric element measures its height displacement. It gives a topographical image of the surface, with a height resolution of less than 1 nm. The lateral resolution is lower, depending on the surface roughness and the curvature of the microscope tip. Several operational modes can be employed, depending on the sample and the information requirements. These include contact mode (where the tip remains in contact with the sample), non-contact mode (where the repulsive interaction between tip and

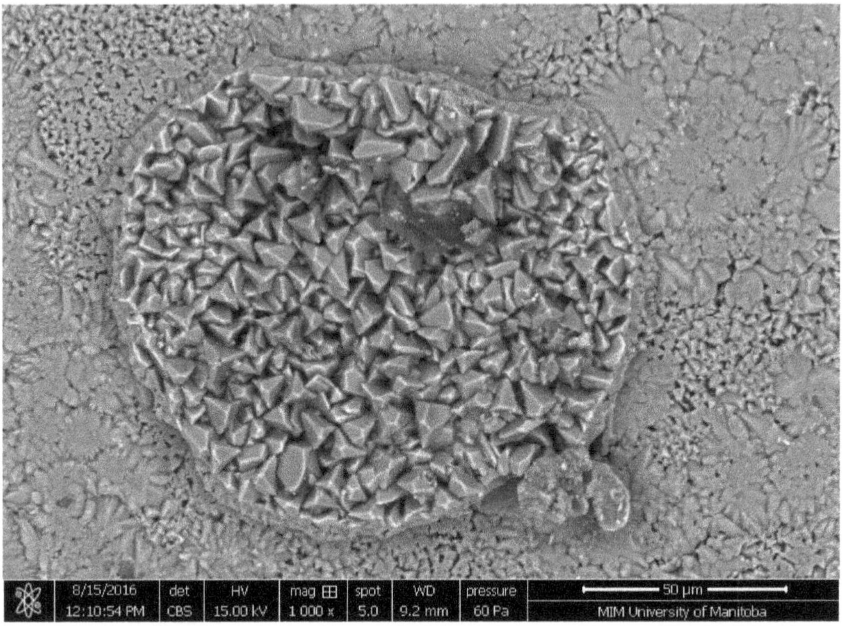

Figure 13. SEM image in backscattering mode of a pulp-capping materials. Topography, crystallinity, and distinction of phases can be assessed [Unpublished data]

sample is measured), and tapping mode (where the tip intermittently contacts the surface at a high frequency).

The information obtainable include roughness, dynamic mechanical properties, magnetic properties, frictional coefficients, etc. A new AFM technique, recently commercialized (Anasys NanoIR2), provides IR data on a 0.1 μm scale. As mentioned before, surface roughness is crucial for understanding adhesion phenomenon, AFM can provide a profile of the surface at nanometric scale. For instance, Figure 15 displays a 2D histogram of depth found in the samples shown in Figure 14.

3. Final Recommendations

Now that the reader is aware of the potential information that can be obtained from skilled surface analysis, we emphasize the following, as the ***order in which such studies should be carried out***:

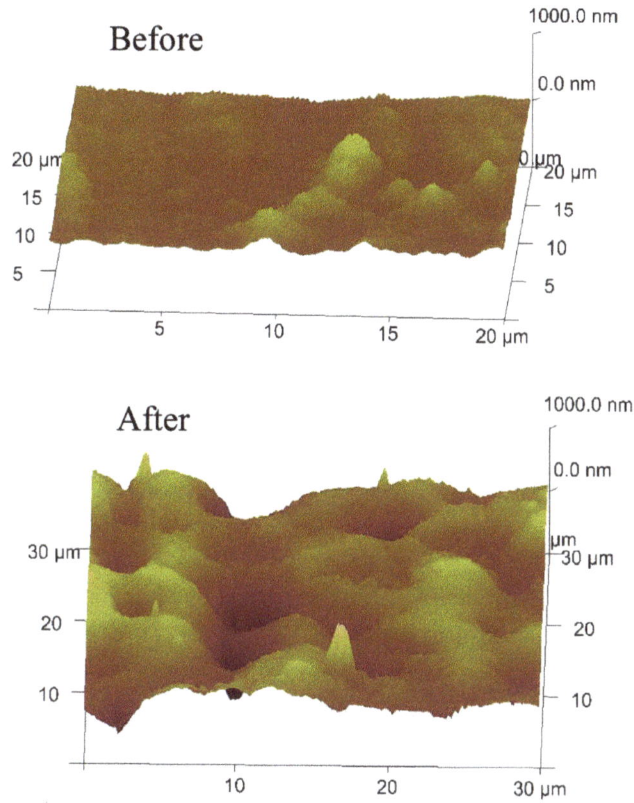

Figure 14. Tapping-mode AFM images showing the effect of bleaching treatment on the enamel surface. The bleaching agent used was 7.5% hydrogen peroxide (Poladay, SDI, Sydney, Au), 15 min once a day for 2 weeks [Unpublished data]

(1) The dental researcher should first meet with the surface scientist to discuss exactly what information is sought, whether the technique chosen is capable of offering such information, and the time and cost of the study. The advice of the surface scientist is extremely important to the success of the study.

(2) The samples should be prepared specifically for the study, in the surface scientist's laboratory, under his supervision, immediately prior to insertion into the instrument.

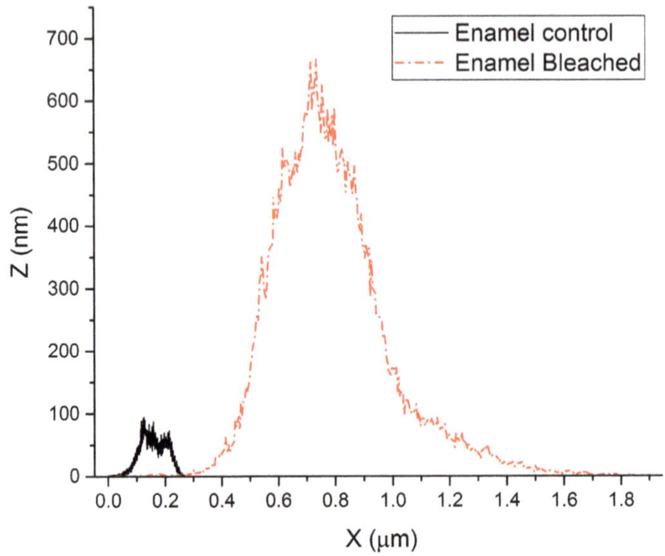

Figure 15. 2D histogram (XZ) of the surface roughness of the samples from Figure 14 [Unpublished data]

(3) The dental researcher should participate in the data acquisition, in order to assure that the correct data are acquired and that time is not wasted.
(4) The dental researcher should participate in the data analysis, to give his views of how the data should be analyzed, and whether further analysis, in a different direction, is warranted.

References

1. Stangel, I.; Ellis, T. H.; Sacher, E. *Dent. Clin. N. Am.* **2007**, *51*, 677.
2. Zhang, Y. F.; Zheng, J.; Zheng, L.; Zhou, Z. R. *J. Mech. Behav. Biomed.* **2015**, *42*, 257.
3. Sakaguchi, R.; Ferracane, J.; Powers, J.; *Craig's Restorative Dental Materials*, 14 ed. Mosby, 352 p.
4. Silverstein, J.; Barreto, O.; França, R. *Eur. J. Orthod.* **2016**, *38*, 146.
5. Shen, M.; Horbett, T. A. *J. Biomed. Mater. Res.* **2001**, *57*, 336.

6. Wei, Y.; Thyparambil, A. A.; Latour, R. A. *Collois. Surf. B* **2013**, *110*, 363.
7. Williams, D. F. *Biomaterials*, **2008**, *28*, 2941.
8. Ratner, B. D. In: *Biomaterials Science, An Introduction to Materials in Medicine*, 3rd ed. Ratner, B. D.; Hoffman, A. S.; Schoen, F. J.; Lemons, J. E., eds. (Oxford, UK: Elsevier, **2013**).
9. Horbett, T.; Brash, J. L.; Norde, W. In: *Proteins and Interfaces III, State of the Art* (Washington, USA: American Chemical Society, **2012**).
10. Fraioli, R.; Rechenmacher, F.; Neubauer, S.; Manero, J. M.; Gil, J.; Kessler, H.; Mas-Moruno, C. *Collois. Surf. B.* **2015**, *128*, 191.
11. Spencer, P.; Ye, Q.; Misra, A.; Gonçalves; S. E. P.; Laurence, J. S. *J. Dent. Res.* **2014**, *93*, 1243.
12. Kwok, D. Y.; Neumann, A. W. In: *Surface Characterization Methods, Surfactant Science Series*, Vol. 87, Miling, A. J., ed. (New York, USA: Marcel Dekker Inc., **1999**), p. 37.
13. Wenzel, R. N. *Ind. Eng. Chem.* **1936**, *28*, 988.
14. Baxer, S.; Cassie, A. B. D. J. *Tex. Inst.* **1945**, *36*, 67.
15. Choi, Y. R.; Kim, K. N.; Kim, K. M.; *J. Prosthet. Dent.* **2014**, *112*, 981.
16. Rupp, F.; Geis-Grestorfer, J. *Int. J. Prosthodont.* **2010**, *23*, 552.
17. Li, F.; Liu, X.; Zhang, L.; Kang, J.; Chen, J. *J. Adhes. Dent.* **2012**, *14*, 113.
18. Amaral, R.; Ozcan, M.; Bottino, M. A.; Valandro, L. F. *J. Adhes. Dent.* **2011**, *13*, 551.
19. Jung, Y. C.; Bhushan, B. J. *Microsc.* **2008**, *229*, 127.
20. Wei, Q. F. *Mater. Charact.* **2004**, *52*, 231.
21. Stangel, I.; Young, C.; Sacher, E.; Hanley, S. *J. Adhes.* **1994**, *47*, 133.
22. Roberston, L.; Gong, V.; Pesun, I.; França, R. *J. Dent. Res.* **2013**, *92*, 1874.
23. Gong, V.; França, R. *J. Dent.* **2017**, *58*, 11.
24. Bubnowicz, L.; Gong, V.; França, R. *Clin. Oral Invest.* **2013**, *17* (3), 1101.
25. Brinkman, B.; Silverstein, J.; Barreto, O.; França, R. *J. Dent. Res.* **2014**, *93*, 303.
26. França, R.; Samani, T. D.; Bayade, G.; Yahia, L'H.; Sacher, E. *J. Colloid Interface Sci.* **2014**, *420*, 182.

27. França, R.; Mbeh, D.; Canh, L. T.; Mateescu, M.; Yahia, L'H.; Sacher, E. *J. Biomed. Mater. Res. B* **2013**, *101B*, 1444.
28. França, R.; Zhang, X. F.; Veres, T.; Yahia, L'H.; Sacher, E. *J. Colloid Interface Sci.* **2012**, *389*, 292.
29. Mbeh, D. A.; França, R.; Merhi, Y.; Zhang, X. F.; Veres, T.; Sacher, E.; Yahia, L'H. *J. Biomed. Mater. Res. Part A* **2012**, *100*, 1637.
30. Poulin, S.; França, R.; Moreau-Bélanger, L.; Sacher, E. *J. Phys. Chem. C* **2010**, *114*, 10711.
31. Franca, R.; Alfa, M.; Olson, N.; Yahia, L.; Sacher, E. *J. Orthop. Res.* **2017**, *35*, 240.
32. Ong, J. L.; Lucas, L. C. *Biomaterials* **1998**, *19*, 455.
33. Takemoto, S.; Hattori, M.; Yoshinari, M.; Kawada, E.; Asami, K.; Oda, Y. *Dent. Mater.* **2009**, *25*, 467.
34. Skjorland, K. K. *Acta. Odontol. Scand.* **1982**, *40*, 129.
35. Goldstein, J. L.; Newbury, D. E.; Echlin, P.; Joy, D. C.; Romig Jr., A. D.; Lyman, C. E.; Fiori, C.; Lifshin, E. In: *Scanning Electron Microscopy and X-Ray Microanalysis* (New York: Plenum Press, **1981**).
36. Spyropoulou, P.; Kamposiora, P.; Eliades, G.; Papavasiliou, G.; Razzoog, M. E.; Thompson, J. Y.; Smith, R. L.; Bayne, S. C. *J. Prosthet. Dent* **2016**, *116*, 269.
37. Bai, Z.; Byrne, T.; Filiaggi, M. J.; Sanderson, R.; Chevrier, V.; Stoffy-Egli, P.; Dahn, J. R. *Surf. Sci.* **2008**, *602*, 795.
38. Madani, A. S.; Astaneh, P. A.; Nakhaei, M.; Bagheri, H. G.; Moosavi, H.; Alavi, S.; Najjaran, N. T. *J. Prosthodont.* **2015**, *24*, 225.
39. Houk, R. S. *Anal. Chem.* **1986**, *58*, 97A.
40. LaHaye, N. L.; Kurian, J.; Diwakar, P. K.; Alff, L.; Harilal, S. S. *Nat. Sci. Rep.* **2015**, *5*, 13121.
41. Kang, D.; Amarasiriwardena, D.; Goodman, A. H. *Anal. Bioanal. Chem.* **2004**, *378*, 1608.
42. He, X.; Reichl, F. X.; Wang, Y.; Michalke, B.; Milz, S.; Yang, Y.; Stolper, P.; Lindemaier, G.; Graw, M.; Hickel, R.; Högg. C. *Dent. Mater.* **2016**, *32*, 1042.
43. Robinson, J. W.; Frame, E. M. S.; Frame II, G. M. In: *Undergraduate Instrumental Analysis* (Florida: CRC Press, **2014**).
44. Araujo, L. O. F.; Barreto, O.; Mendonça, A. A. M.; França, R. *Appl. Adhes. Sci.* **2015**, 3, 26.

45. Robertson, L.; Phaneuf, M.; Haimeur, A.; Pesun, I.; França, R. *Dent. J.* **2016**, *4*, 37.
46. http://www.panalytical.com/Technology-background/Inplane-diffraction-3.htm (consulted in June **2016**).
47. Patterson, A. L. *Phys. Rev.* **1939**, *56*, 978.
48. Jamesh, M.; Narayanan, T. S.; Sankara, N.; Chu, P. K. *Mater. Chem. Phys.* **2013**, *138*, 565.
49. Kohorst, P.; Borchers, L.; Strempel, J.; Stiesch, M.; Hassel, T.; Bach, F. W.; Hubsch, C. *Acta Biomater.* **2012**, *8*, 1213.
50. Zhang, Y.; Venugopal, J. R.; El-Turki, A.; Ramakrishna, S.; Su, B.; Lim, C. T. *Biomaterials* **2008**, *29*, 4314.

Chapter 2

Nanoindentation Techniques in Dental Biomaterials

Mohammad Aramfard* and Chuang Deng†

Department of Mechanical Engineering, University of Manitoba, 15 Gillson Street, Winnipeg, MB, R3T 5V6, Canada

**aramfarm@myumanitoba.ca*
†*chuang.deng@umanitoba.ca*

Since tooth tissues and those artificially made to mimic them are generally small and microscopically heterogeneous, conventional mechanical characterization methods for testing bulk materials are usually not applicable. Nanoindentation, which is a technique to extract various mechanical properties of materials at small volume by impressing a nanometer-scale probe into the surface, thus becomes a crucial tool for characterizing dental biomaterials. In this chapter, the basic principles of nanoindentation, the practical instrumentation of nanoindentation, the adaptation of nanoindentation techniques for testing biomaterials, and some specific applications of nanoindentation in dental materials are briefly introduced and discussed.

1. The Basic Principles of Nanoindentation

1.1. *Overview*

It has been long recognized by the materials science community that the surface contacts between materials are highly dependent on their mechanical properties. The theory of contact mechanics and many experimental techniques based on surface indentation and impression have thus been developed to extract the mechanical properties of various types of materials. Due to its inexpensive and relatively non-destructive nature, indentation is perhaps the simplest, most direct, and most commonly applied means of testing the mechanical properties of materials.

Traditional indentation techniques include Vickers, Rockwell, Brinell, and Knoop hardness tests, depending on the shape of the indenter and the range of hardness result. With the rapid development of nanoscience and nanotechnology, nanoindentation, an indentation with sub-micrometer probe and penetration depth, was developed in the mid-1970s and has now become commonplace for the measurement of mechanical properties at small volumes. Hardness, which is an important mechanical property of materials to tell if a material is "hard" or "soft", is defined based on the contact mechanics and can be directly measured from nanoindentation. Surprisingly, the same setup that is used to measure the hardness can be used to measure the Young modulus based on some assumptions and calculations which are discussed in Section 1.2.

Although the most common use of nanoindentation is for the measurement of hardness and elastic modulus since its introduction in the 1970s, considerable progress has been made in nanoindentation techniques so that it can be used to perform other mechanical tests such as wear, creep, scratch, and compressive tests. In the meantime, nanoindentation has also been improved in such a way that various types of materials, including dental biomaterials under *in vivo* conditions, can be tested. In the following sections, the basic theory, principles, and general techniques of nanoindentation will be briefly introduced.

1.2. *Contact Mechanics*

The main assumptions of nanoindentation come from contact mechanics, which studies bodies in contact. The problem of punching an elastic semi-infinite medium (the half-space) by an elastic sphere (the indenter) was first studied by Hertz,[1,2] as shown in Figure 1.

The contact radius *a* can be obtained by Eq. (1) and is strongly dependent on the elastic properties of the two materials in contact, the geometry of the indenter, and the load applied:

$$a^3 = \frac{3}{4}\frac{PR}{E^*}, \tag{1}$$

where P is the load on the sphere, R is the radius of curvature, and E^* is the sum of the reduced Young moduli of the indenter and the half-space as defined in Eq. (2):

$$\frac{1}{E^*} = \frac{(1-\nu_{\text{ind}}^2)}{E_{\text{ind}}} + \frac{(1-\nu_{\text{hlf}}^2)}{E_{\text{hlf}}}, \tag{2}$$

in which ν is the Poisson ratio. The amount of displacement of the surface under the indenter is computed as

$$h = \frac{1}{E^*}\frac{3}{2}\frac{P}{4a}\left(2 - \frac{r^2}{a^2}\right), \quad r \le a. \tag{3}$$

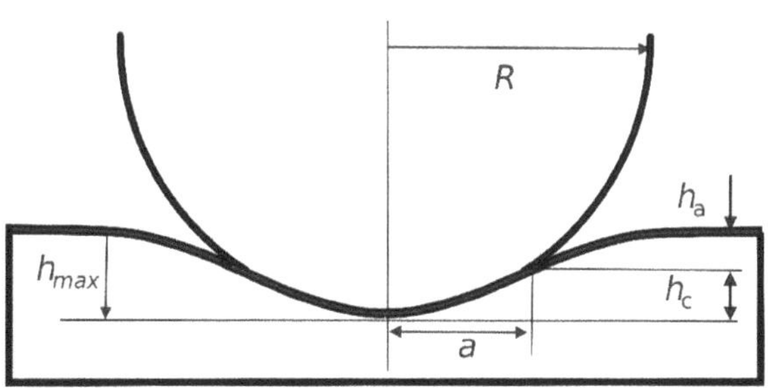

Figure 1. The contact between an elastic sphere and an elastic half-space under the influence of pressure *P*. Adapted from Ref. [3]

For the case of contact between two non-rigid spheres of radii R_1 and R_2, assuming $R = (1/R_1 + 1/R_2)^{-1}$, the relationship between the indentation depth h and the pressure P is given by

$$P = \frac{4}{3} E^* \sqrt{R} h^{3/2}. \tag{4}$$

The mean contact pressure P_m is defined as the ratio of the applied load to the contact area, which helps to relate the load to mechanical stress:

$$P_m = \frac{P}{\pi a^2}. \tag{5}$$

Substituting Eq. (5) into Eq. (1), one can get

$$P_m = \left(\frac{4E^*}{3\pi}\right)\frac{a}{R}. \tag{6}$$

Equation (6) has a significant physical meaning in that it relates a stress to a strain ratio of a/R, so it has an understanding similar to tensile test.

Figure 2 shows a conical indenter with cone angle α penetrating the half-space. The maximum depth of the penetration depends on the load, the reduced moduli of the system, and the cone angle as in Eq. (7):

$$P = \frac{2}{\pi} E^* \tan\alpha \, h_{max}^2. \tag{7}$$

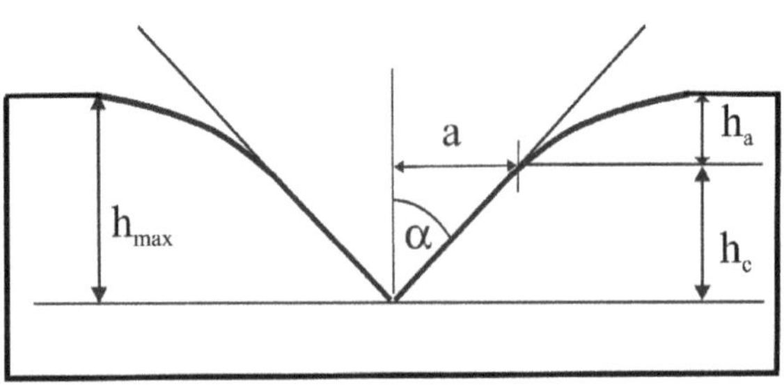

Figure 2. The contact between an elastic conical indenter and an elastic half-space under the influence of pressure P. Adapted from Ref. [3]

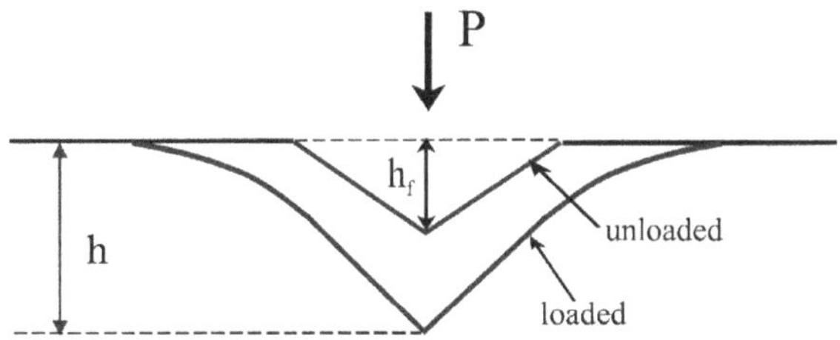

Figure 3. Schematic of the loading and unloading of a sharp indenter on an elastic–plastic half-space. Adapted from Ref. [4]

The basis of nanoindentation to extract material properties is due to the fact that by indenting an elastic–plastic material, after the indenter reached the maximum load and penetration upon unloading, only the elastic part is recovered. In other words, at the beginning of the unloading step, the load versus displacement occurs in the elastic deformation regime. Based on this fact, Oliver and Pharr introduced the method to measure the Young modulus of materials by nanoindentation.[4,5] Figure 3 shows the schematic of the loading and unloading of a sharp indenter on an elastic–plastic half-space.

By assuming that the procedure is about the unloading part, in the aforementioned equations, h is replaced by $(h - h_f)$, in which h_f is the final depth remaining due to plastic deformation. As a result, Eq. (4) becomes

$$P = \frac{4}{3} E^* \sqrt{R}(h - h_f)^{3/2}. \tag{8}$$

In hardness tests, stiffness S is defined as the derivative of the load with respect to the depth[6–8]:

$$S = \frac{dP}{dh} = 2E^* \sqrt{R}(h - h_f)^{1/2}. \tag{9}$$

By relating the depth to the contact area between the indenter and the surface, the relationship between the contact area, the stiffness, and the reduced modulus is derived, which can be used to compute the reduced modulus as shown in Eq. (10):

$$S = \frac{dP}{dh} = \frac{2}{\sqrt{\pi}} E^* \sqrt{A}. \tag{10}$$

Here, A is the projected area of an indent. The hardness H is computed simply by dividing the load by the area:

$$H = \frac{P}{A}. \tag{11}$$

Figure 4 shows the schematic of the load versus displacement of an indentation test on an elastic–plastic material, and as it is shown in the figure, stiffness is measured at the beginning of the unloading process. The load versus displacement curve is the most important data to be used for computing the material properties.

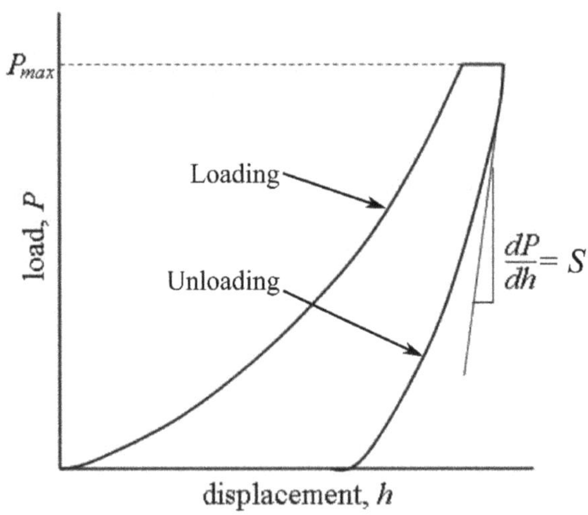

Figure 4. Schematic of the load versus displacement curve obtained from an indentation test. P_{max} is the maximum load and S is the stiffness of initial unloading

1.3. *Practical Application of Nanoindentation*

In the previous section, the underlying theory of contact mechanics and indentation was explained. In this section, the practical application of the theory is discussed based on the following assumptions:

- The tested material is half-space.
- There is no flaw, crack, or phase change in the vicinity of the indentation.
- The surface is smooth enough.
- The material behaves as elastic–plastic.
- The material is homogeneous and isotropic.

The first four assumptions are necessary to have an accurate result, for example the Young modulus, but the last assumption is required only if the obtained property is assumed to be pertaining to the whole material. For example, if the material is not homogeneous, the Young modulus obtained from indentation test is only valid for that point and if the material is anisotropic, the Young modulus obtained is only valid in a specific direction. The application of nanoindentation to test materials which violate these assumptions will be discussed later.

To apply the theory of contact mechanics to extract the material properties, additional studies are needed from experiments. It has been shown experimentally that the unloading curve obeys the following rule[5]:

$$P = \alpha (h - h_f)^m, \tag{12}$$

in which *a* and *m* are fitting constants which depend on the material. To find the relationship between depth and contact area, the sink in depth, h_s, is modeled from elastic models as in Eq. (13):

$$h_s = \frac{\epsilon P_{\max}}{S}, \tag{13}$$

where φ is a constant that depends on the geometry of the indenter. The contact area is a function of contact depth h_c, which can be deduced from Figure 3:

$$h_c = h_{\max} - \frac{\epsilon P_{\max}}{S}. \tag{14}$$

Here, it is assumed that the area is a function of contact depth, i.e. $A = F(h_c)$, and is determined from the geometry of the indenter probe as explained in the next section. By finding the contact area and substituting it in Eqs. (10) and (11), the reduced modulus and hardness can be computed. It should be noted that the reduced modulus obtained from Eq. (10) is a combination of moduli of sample and the machine, so the machine compliance should be known in order to compute the sample modulus.

1.4. *The Nanoindentation Probe and Area Function*

Depending on the types of materials being tested and the properties being explored, probes with different geometries are needed for nanoindentation. While load and penetration depth can be easily controlled and monitored during a nanoindentation test regardless of the geometry of the probe, the contact area, which is an important parameter used in Eqs. (10) and (11) to extract the nanohardness and stiffness of the material, is hard to measure directly and expected to vary significantly for probes with different geometries. An area function, which is the projected area of an indent as a polynomial function of the indenter, is thus used and should be determined carefully based on the geometry of the probe. With this area function, it is also possible to gain real-time nanohardness values from a load versus displacement curve. The most commonly used probes include Berkovich, conical, Vickers, and spherical as shown in Figure 5.

In Vickers, the half angle is $\theta = 68°$ and in Berkovich it is $\theta = 68.27°$,which has three faces. The ideal area function for different tips is summarized in Table 1. Table 1 shows the area function of different

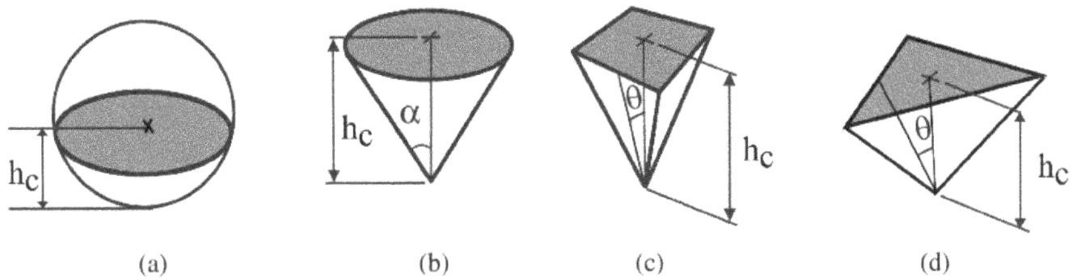

Figure 5. Indentation parameters for (a) spherical, (b) conical, (c) Vickers, and (d) Berkovich indenters. Adapted from Ref. [3]

Table 1. Area function for different probes

Tip	Area function, $A(h_c)$
Vickers	$24.504h_c^2$
Berkovich	$24.5h_c^2$
Cube corner	$2.6h_c^2$
Knoop	$108.21h_c^2$
Conical	$\pi h_c^2 \tan^2\alpha$
Spherical	$\pi(2Rh_c - h_c^2)$

probes used in nanoindentation as a function of h_c; however, these equations are for ideal probes, and for real probes they may deviate from the ideal equation. To find the real function, a number of tests at different depths is performed on a material for which Young modulus is known, then the ideal function with some constants is fitted to satisfy the testing results. In general, this procedure should be done frequently since the tip wears out and the area function can change. Generally, the actual area function is closer to the ideal one when the indentation depth is deeper.[3] Another deviation from the ideal function is the pile-up or sink-in phenomena. In pile-up, the material comes up due to indentation and causes the contact area to be bigger than a normal test, and in sink-in the material goes lower so the contact area is less than a normal test, as shown in Figure 6.

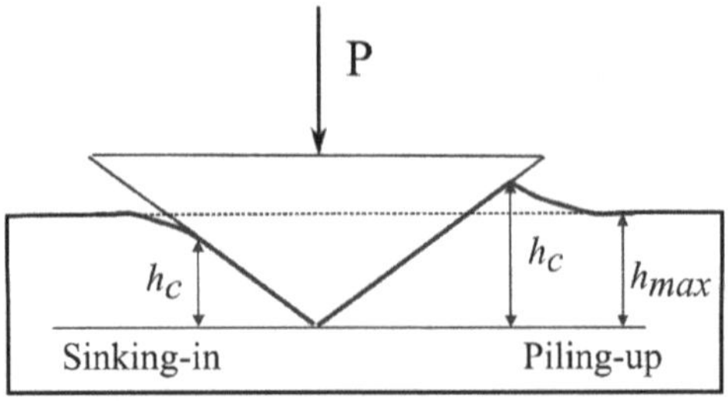

Figure 6. Schematic comparison between contact areas of sink-in and pile-up (a) cross-section view and (b) plan view. Adapted from Ref. [3]

1.5. *Operational Modes of Nanoindentation*

1.5.1. *Continuous Stiffness Measurement*

Besides vertical penetration, nanoindenters have been modified to do different tests and measure different properties. One feature that is added to a nanoindenter is called Continuous Stiffness Measurement (CSM). CSM is a mode in nanoindenation that instead of measuring only the stiffness from the unloading step of maximum load does many small loading/unloading steps during the whole loading process. It enables to have the desired quantity, for example Young modulus, at different depths from the near surface until the final depth.[9] Figure 7 shows the schematics of the load–displacement curve in the CSM mode.[9]

1.5.2. *Scanning Probe Microscopy*

Scanning Probe Microscopy (SPM) is a method of probing the surface and measuring the topography using a fine probe. SPM method can be used by the nanoindenter to give the semi *in situ* images of the tested sample surface. SPM imaging is integrated in some commercial nanoindenters, for example, the Hysitron TriboScope nanoindenters, by using the same probe for vertical penetration in a horizontal scanning mode. It can be used before and after the conventional indentation test to produce the topography of the surface and shows the impression of the indentation.

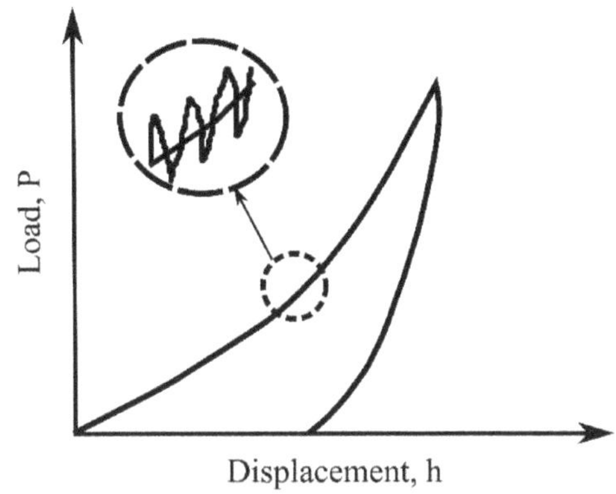

Figure 7. Load versus displacement in CSM mode

1.5.3. *Nanotribology*

Nanoindentation can also be used for scratching and wear tests as used in nanotribology.[10] In these tests, conical tips are kept in contact with the sample under specific loads and the sample is moved in this condition. Based on the testing condition, properties of wear or coefficient of friction can be obtained. Figure 8 shows the optical images of impression of a probe on the surface of ta-C coatings on Si substrate.[11]

2. Instrumentation of Nanoindentation

Testing at nanoscales has its own restrictions, and sensing and actuating up to several nanometers and micronewtons needs special instrumentation. The actuation is usually performed by inducing magnetic forces, electrostatic, spring, or piezo. Each of the above-mentioned methods have their advantages and disadvantages. For example, piezo actuators have precise accuracy at lower scales such as several nanonewtons, while magnetic inducers can exert forces up to several Newtons. Displacement measurement can be done by different methods such as optical measuring, differential capacitor, and differential transducer.

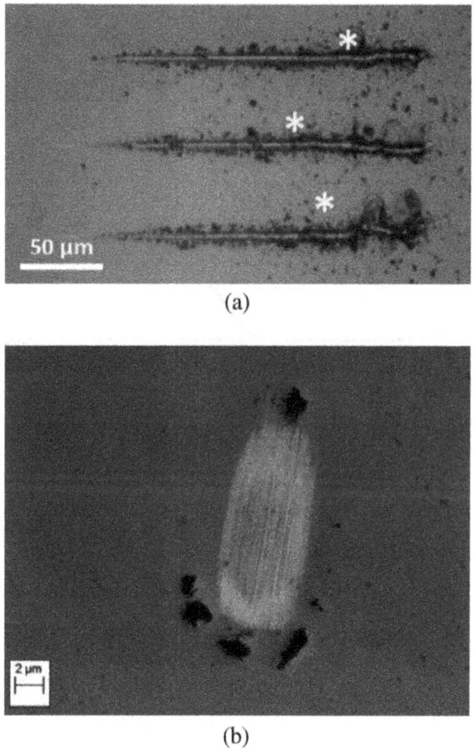

Figure 8. (a) Optical images of nanoscratch test impressions up to 300 mN on 20 nm ta-C and (b) SEM images of wear test impressions on 20 nm ta-C film at 50 mN for 3,000 cycles. Adapted from Ref. [11]

2.1. *Implementation of Major Commercial Machines*

Major producers of standalone nanoindenters are Hysitron Inc., USA, Agilent Technologies Inc., USA, and Micromaterials Ltd., UK. As one example, Figure 9 shows the Hysitron TI950 TriboIndenter. This nanoindenter has a special three-plate capacitive transducer to control the displacement of the probe.

2.2. *Atomic Force Microscope*

Atomic Force Microscope (AFM) is a device consisting of a cantilever tip which is being moved on a surface in non-contact mode and

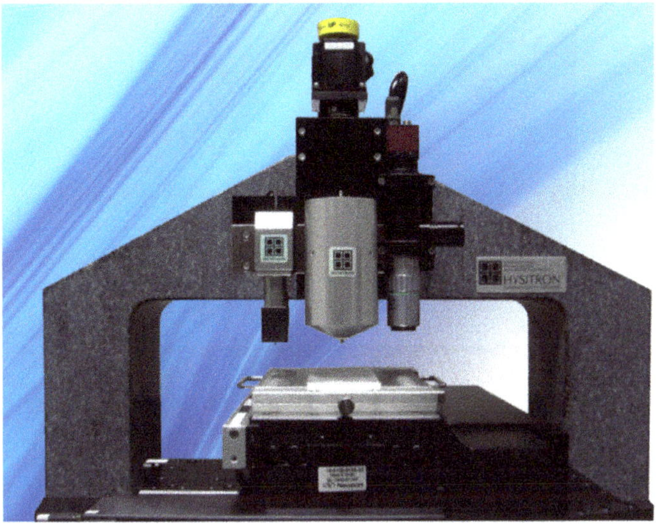

Figure 9. Hysitron TI950 TriboIndenter. Published with permission of Hysitron, INC

measures the topography of the surface by measuring the force exerted on the tip due to the interatomic forces between the tip and the surface.[12] The measurement can be done by measuring the deviation of light reflected from the cantilever or the variation in the length of a spring attached to the cantilever. AFM can also be used for nanoindentation purposes by impressing the AFM tip into the sample surface.

The advantages of using the AFM as a nanoindenter are the following: (1) the topography can be assessed prior to nanoindentation, so the indentation location can be very accurate. (2) Since AFM is very sensitive up to several nanonewtons, it can be used to indent ultrathin films up to 10 nm.[13] To use the AFM as a nanoindenter, it should comply with the assumptions in nanoindentation, i.e. tip geometry should be matched with the assumptions in nanoindentation theory.

2.3. *State of the Art: In Situ Nanoindentation*

Sometimes, it is necessary for the evolution of the tested material to be observed in real time during the nanoindentation. By placing the

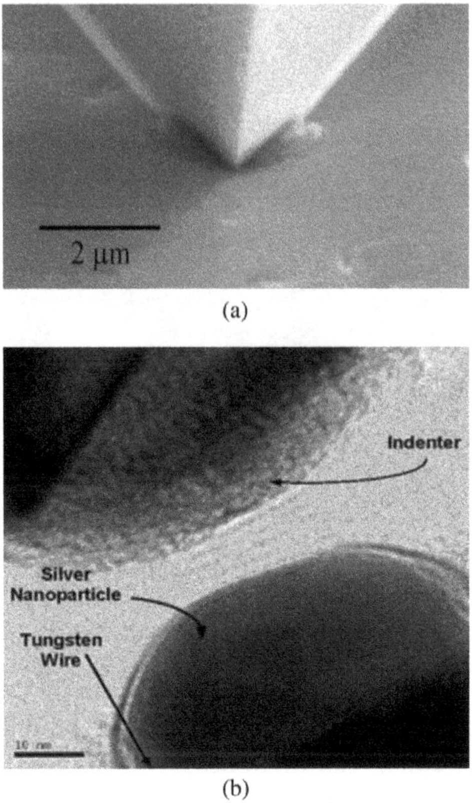

Figure 10. (a) *In situ* SEM nanoindentation of a TiN/SiN$_x$ thin film. Adapted from Ref. [16] and (b) *In situ* TEM nanoindentation of a silver nanoparticle. Adapted from Ref. [14]

nanoindenter inside a Scanning Electron Microscope (SEM) or Transmission Electron Microscope (TEM), the nanoindentation process can be viewed in great detail.[14–16] Figures 10 (a) and 10(b) shows the *in situ* SEM nanoindentation of TiN/SiN$_x$ thin coating[16] and *in situ* TEM nanoindentation of a silver nanoparticle.[14]

Nanoindentation can also be used with other instruments to perform tests in different conditions. For example, for materials that need to be in special environment, tests can be done inside a glovebox (for example, battery materials) or inside a vacuum chamber. Another adoption of nanoindentation is to have a temperature controlling stage for higher or lower temperature than ambient temperature.

3. Preliminary Considerations in Dental Materials Field

3.1. *Human Tooth*

The human tooth is made of two main components: a coronal hard upper part and a vascular pulp lower part, which is the root of the tooth. The crown consists of an outer enamel, and below it is dentin, which are hard parts of a human tooth, as shown in Figure 11. The primary application of human tooth is to cut, crush, and break the food, so it becomes easier for the digesting system.

Enamel is the hardest and stiffest tissue in body and is made of 96–98% wt. of inorganic minerals, mainly hydroxyapatite, and the rest is water and organic matrix.[18] Figure 12 shows the hierarchical structure of the enamel consisting of hydroxyapatite rods with inter-rod enamel surrounding.[19]

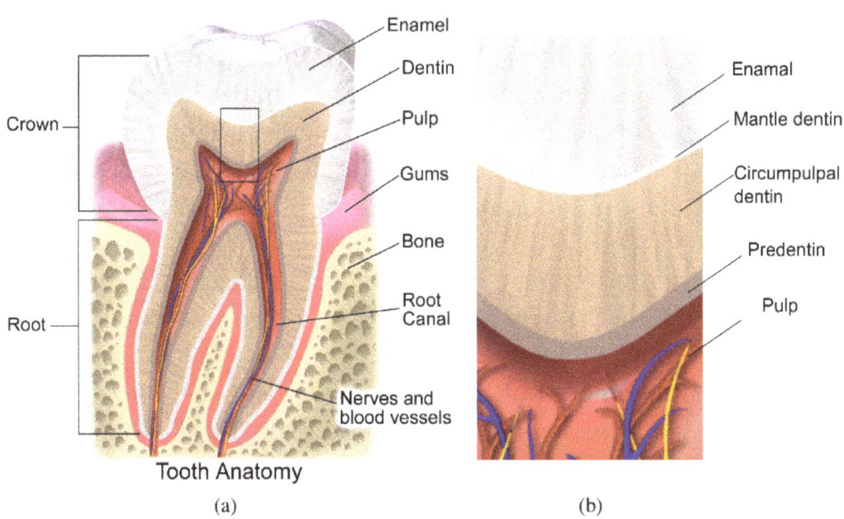

Figure 11. (a) Human tooth anatomy and (b) Zoomed view to show the different types of dentin. Adapted from Ref. [17]

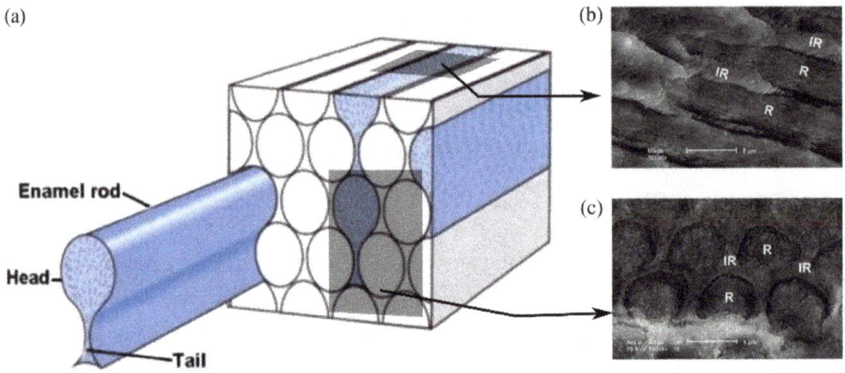

Figure 12. (a) Schematic of enamel hierarchy, (b) and (c) SEM images of different faces. Adapted from Ref. [19]

Since enamel is the outer part of the tooth which is in contact with other teeth and food and it undergoes both shear stress and normal stress up to 2.5 GPa which cannot be repaired, it has to be durable in comparison with other tissues.[20] Below the enamel sits dentin which has the same mineral as enamel but less in weight percentage (70%). Therefore, it is more elastic than enamel. Dentin contains cross-sectional tubules which extend from the interface between pulp and dentin to the interface between dentin and enamel.[18] These tubules increase the permeability of dentin. Dentin is divided into different sections from pulp to enamel: predentin, circumpulpal dentin, and mantle dentin, which are shown in Figure 11(b).

Pulp is a connective tissue which is highly vascularized and innervated and consists of the pulp chamber of the crown and root canals.[18] Pulp is made up of different cells immersed in an organic matrix, of which is 25% is composed of organic materials and the rest is water. Because of high amount of water, pulp is a soft tissue which dries when the tooth is dried and leaves a hole in the tooth. Pulp's roles are to build dentin, to supply nutrition to it, to serve as a conduit for nerves which give dentin sensitivity, and to repair dentin if needed,[21] as shown Figure 11.

3.2. *Artificial Dental Materials*

Since the emergence of dentistry in human history around 3000 B.C.,[22] a wide range of materials from gold to ivory have been used. In modern dentistry, four main categories of dental materials are being used including metals, ceramics, polymers, and their composites.[23,24] Table 2 shows the general properties of three main categories of dental materials including their mechanical properties.[25]

A good dental material should be biocompatible, form proper bonds with surroundings, be good looking, have properties close to the natural tooth material, and be capable of repairing tissues if necessary.[24] There is no permanent material to be used in dentistry; however, materials based on their application are divided into temporary and long term. On the other hand, based on the application of the materials, they can be divided into three main categories, namely, preventive, restorative, and auxiliary materials. Table 3 shows the summary of common types of preventive and restorative dental materials in terms of their applications.[24]

In this section, the mechanical properties of each group of artificial dental materials is briefly presented.

3.2.1. *Ceramics*

Ceramics are non-metallic inorganic materials which usually exhibit high hardness and brittleness. In clinical applications, aesthetics is the most important feature of ceramic materials.[27] After ceramics were first introduced in 1774, it took over 190 years until the introduction of a porcelain-fused-to-metal system which caused the demand for ceramic systems to increase significantly in the 1960s.[27] In general, porcelain-only restoratives have two major problems; one is the brittle fracture of ceramics which causes the porcelain to break suddenly, and the second is the abrasive effect of the opposing tooth, which causes the tooth moving against the porcelain to wear out. Porcelain fused to metal enables the system to have both the aesthetics of porcelain, which is the closest material to the natural tooth crown, and the strength of metal simultaneously.

Table 2. General properties of metals, ceramics, and polymers

		Metals		Ceramics		Polymers	
Properties	**Alloys**	**Intermetallic compounds**	**Inorganic salts**	**Crystalline**	**Glasses**	**Rigid**	**Rubbers**
Hardness	Medium to hard	Hard	Medium to hard	Hard	Hard	Soft	Rubbers
Strength	Medium to high	Medium	Medium	High	High	Low	Low
Toughness	High	Low	Low	Most low, some high	Low	Low	Medium
Elastic modulus	High	High	High	High	High	Low	Very Low
Electric conductivity	High	High	Low	Low	Low	Low	Low
Thermal conductivity	High	High	Low	Low	Low	Low	Low
Thermal Expansion	Low	Low	Low	Low	Low	High	High
Density	High	High	Medium	Medium	Medium	Low	Low
Translucency	None	None	Medium	High	High	High	Low
Examples	Gold-copper	Amalgam phases	Gypsum, zinc phosphate	SiO_2, Al_2O_3	Dental porcelain	Poly (methyl methacrylate)	Impression materials

Source: Adapted from Ref. [25].

Table 3. Applications and durability of preventives and restorative dental materials

Material type	Applications of products	Potential preventive benefits	Durability
Resin adhesive	A	F (certain products)	M
Resin sealant	S	S	M
Resin cement	L	F (certain products)	M
Composite	B, L, R	F	M
Hybrid ionomer	B, L, R	F	M
Glass ionomer (GI)	A, B, L, R, S	F, S	L, M
Metal-modified GI	R	F	L, M
Zinc oxide-eugenol	B, L, T	—	L,M
Zinc phosphate	B, L	—	M
Zinc polycarboxylate	B, L	—	M
Zinc silicophosphate	B, L	F	M
Resin composite	R	F (certain products)	H
Dental amalgam	R	—	H
Ceramic	R	—	H
Metal-ceramic	R	—	H
Metal-resin	R	—	M, H
Temporary acrylic resin	T	—	L
Denture acrylic	R	—	H
Cast metal	R	—	H
Wrought metal	R	—	H

Notes: A = Adhesive, B = Base, L = Luting Agent, S = Pit/Fissure Sealant, R = Restorative, T = Temporary Restorative. Potential Preventive Benefits: F = Fluoride-releasing Material, S = Sealing Agent. Durability: L = Low, M = Moderate, H = High.
Source: Adapted from Ref. [24].

3.2.2. *Composites*

Resin-based composites were first used mostly as adhesive or direct restorative in 1960s.[28] Due to aesthetic problems of amalgam and by improving the filler materials, the demand is now for resin-based composites which have good appearance and also strong bonding to tooth.[26] However, the high wear rate of composites limits their lifetime, especially in a high stress environment.

4. Nanoindentation in Dental Materials

4.1. *Adaptions of Nanoindentation for Biomaterials*

Knowing the mechanical properties of biological materials, specifically dental materials, is crucial in clinical applications.[29] Due to the hierarchical nature of biological materials and the fact that they are found in small sizes, it is hard to test them using conventional methods for testing inorganic materials. This is where alternative tools such as nanoindentation can be used. Nanoindentation, with its flexibility in testing small samples and even *in situ* testing, is an ideal tool to extract mechanical properties of tissues. Since nanoindentation can be used to measure local properties, it is useful to map the properties and examine the influence of changes in tissue on the properties.

Microindentation has been used for many years to measure mechanical properties of soft tissues such as cartilage.[30,31] For example, millimeter indentation was used to investigate the healthy and diseased cartilages.[30] One of the first applications of nanoinstruments in dentistry was to use the nanohardness test to measure mechanical properties of teeth.[32–34] Since the biological materials are usually adhesive and possess time-dependent behavior,[35] the conventional method used in nanoindentation explained in Sections I and II needs to be altered accordingly.

4.1.1. *Probe Selection*

For testing biomaterials using nanoindentation, two factors should be considered regarding the proper probe selection. The indenting probe should have a reasonable size, which means if the probe is too large compared to the testing sample, the result is under the influence of other parts, or if the sample is too big compared with the probe, the result is local and does not represent the property of the whole sample. In the same sense, sharp probes such as Berkovich and cube corner are usually used when testing small samples such as a cell and larger probes such as flat punch and spherical tips are used for tissues.

4.1.2. *Creep*

Creep is the phenomenon related to time-dependent behavior in tissues, especially soft tissues. Creep means that the material shows deformation under constant load.[36] In nanoindentation with sharp loading function, creep causes a so-called "nose" when the indenter is unloading from the maximum depth, as shown in Figure 13(a). The simplest solution to exclude the effect of creep from unloading part is to use a trapezoidal load function which causes the viscoelastic material to deform under constant load due to creep and upon unloading; only elastic deformation is involved with unloading[29,37,38] as shown in Figure 13(b). Obviously, the holding time depends on the material's characteristics and loading rate and can vary between 3 and 120 s.[29] In

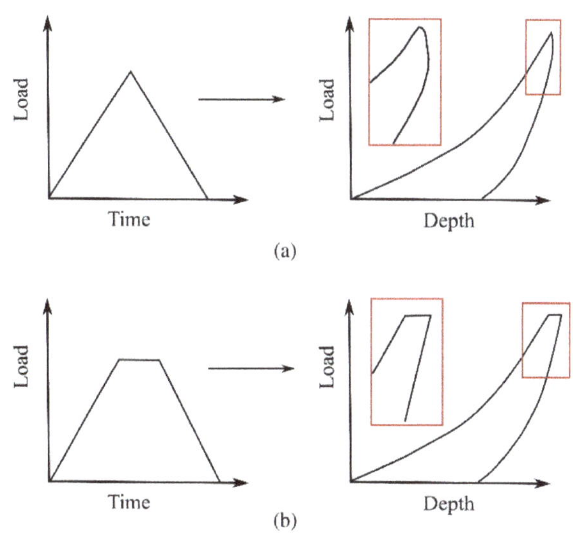

Figure 13. Schematics of (a) rectangular load function and the load–displacement curve of viscoelastic material associated with it showing nose when unloading due to creep and (b) trapezoidal load function and eliminating the creep effect in load–displacement curve. Adapted from Ref. [29]

addition to trapezoidal load function, some numerical calculations were developed to consider viscoelasticity as a more rigorous solution.[29]

4.1.3. *Viscoelasticity*

Biological tissues when exhibiting high viscoelastic behavior, especially for highly hydrated and organic tissues, cannot be fully understood with simple elastic models. A linear viscoelastic material can be modeled by

$$E = E_{str} + iE_{los}, \tag{15}$$

where E is the complex dynamic modulus, E_{str} is storage modulus, E_{los} is the loss modulus, and i is the imaginary unit. Storage modulus represents elastic behavior of the material, while loss modulus describes the viscous behavior, and in perfectly elastic material it is equal to zero. Using nanoindentation and performing dynamic test, loss and storage moduli can be determined.[37] Using Berkovich tip and assuming standard Kelvin model to describe linear viscoelastic materials, Sadr *et al.* studied four adhesive materials.[39] They reported creep compliance functions and showed that the moduli considering viscoelastic behavior is fairly less than the modulus measured and reported by the nanoindentation device.[40]

4.1.4. *Adhesion*

Adhesion is another issue related to nanoindentation of tissue materials. Adhesion means that the material sticks to the probe without using force, which causes artificial negative forces during withdrawal of the probe from the sample, as shown in Figure 14. If the adhesion force is significant, the measured E-modulus is overestimated.[35] If the indentation is performed with a spherical tip, Johnson–Kendall–Roberts method can be used to improve the accuracy.[40] In this method, the load–displacement data is acquired before the probe touches the surface, so the negative adhesion force is

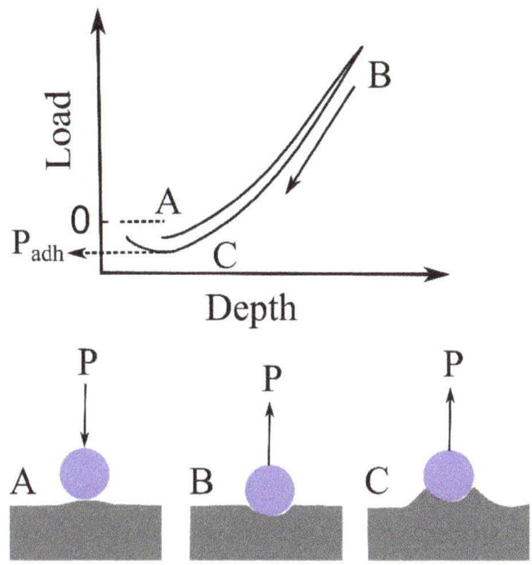

Figure 14. Force–displacement curve for indentation of a poly (dimethyl) siloxane sample. P_{adh} is the maximum adhesive force during unloading relative to reference zero before tip reaches sample. "A" shows the adhesion between sample and tip when approaching. "B" shows the unloading of tip at maximum depth. "C" shows pull-up points where, upon withdrawal of tip from sample, adhesion between tip and sample causes the nanoindenter to sense a negative force. Adapted from Ref. [29]

measured. Figure 14 shows the schematic of such a load–displacement curve.

4.1.5. *Hydration*

Hydration and dehydration also have great influence on the result of the test. Comparison between hydrated and dehydrated bone sample tests shows an increase of moduli between 11% and 28% from hydrated to dehydrated.[41,42] A demineralized dentin was tested using AFM nanoindentation and showed significant increase of one order of magnitude when desiccated. Even after rehydration, the E-modulus was still bigger than the original hydrated sample.[43] So, it should be noted that sample preparation time and condition can significantly change the properties of tissues, even hard tissues such as bone and dentin.

4.2. *Nanoindentation of Natural Dental Materials*

Knowing the mechanical properties of human teeth helps researchers to better understand the functions of different parts in teeth and to design and build proper artificial materials close to the natural materials.[44] In this section, the mechanical characterization of different parts of the human tooth by nanoindentation are briefly explained.

4.2.1. *Enamel*

Cuy *et al.* showed using nanoindentation mapping that enamel is not homogenous and its properties depend not only on chemical composition but also position and the orientation of rods.[45] They used Berkovich probe and performed tests on prepared samples of enamel, and the displacement range of the tests were typically 400 nm or 800 nm. The Poisson's ratio was selected as 0.25. They kept the samples in the ambient environment for long enough to avoid changing of material properties during tests so the results are expected to be higher than if they were conducted in wet environment. Their results are shown in Figure 15 as maps of E-modulus and hardness.[45] Based on their results, the hardest and stiffest part of the enamel is the outer part. Hardness and Young modulus decreases when moving to the inside of the tooth, and it is directly correlated to the calcium content of the enamel.[44–46]

Jeng *et al.* conducted indentation tests using AFM on enamel rods and reported that enamel head is harder and stiffer than enamel tail and the axis.[46] Furthermore, it was shown that the enamel rods are anisotropic in their axial section.[47] In this work, the effect of rotating the Berkovich probe on the sample was investigated and SEM images were taken, which found the asymmetric pile-up of indentation impressions due to anisotropic behavior of the enamel rod. Measured values of hardness and E-modulus were different based on the machine which was used, the probe, the range of load, the strain rate, and the hydration content of the sample.[44,48] For example, higher loads resulted in lower measured hardness and E-modulus.[49]

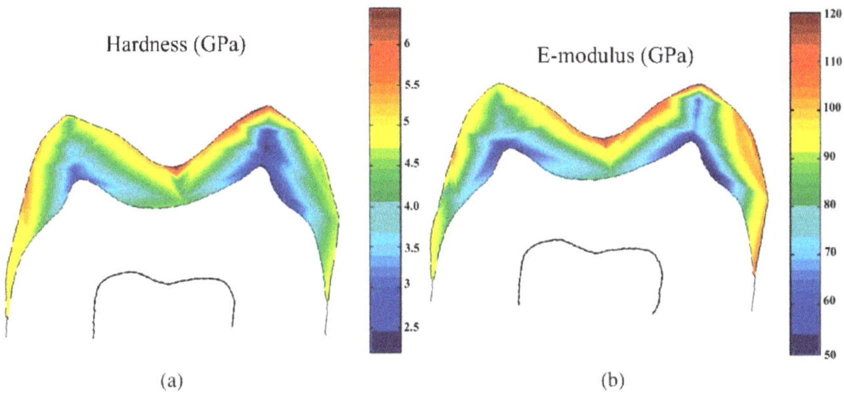

Figure 15. (a) Hardness and (b) E-modulus map of enamel. Adapted from Ref. [45]

4.2.2. *Dentin*

Dentin has a more complex structure in comparison to enamel, and it was the focus of several works to study its mechanical properties. Similar to enamel, hierarchical structure of dentin has great influence on mechanical properties. The orientation and density and mineral content of tubules and collagen fibers are parameters affecting the mechanical properties of dentin.[44,50]

Cohen *et al.* cut off the coronal dentin and embedded it in epoxy and used AFM quasi-static indentation with cube corner probe.[50] They examined a typical tubule in dentin which consists of a lumen which is a hole in the middle, PeriTubular Dentin (PTD), which is the mineralized collar around lumen and surrounding mineralized collagen-rich matrix called InterTubular Dentin (ITD). Cohen *et al.* also conducted indentations with same peak load in the radial lines from lumen outward.[50] The inset of Figure 16(b) shows the AFM image of the sample and the indentation impressions. The hardness increases from ITD with 1.2 GPa until the highest value of 4.7 GPa is seen in PTD and then decreases slightly to 4 GPa at the lumen edge, as is obvious from the size of impressions in Figure 16.[50]

Ziskind *et al.*[51] used CSM nanoindentation with Berkovich tip to extract hardness and E-modulus of the same sample as Cohen *et al.*[50]

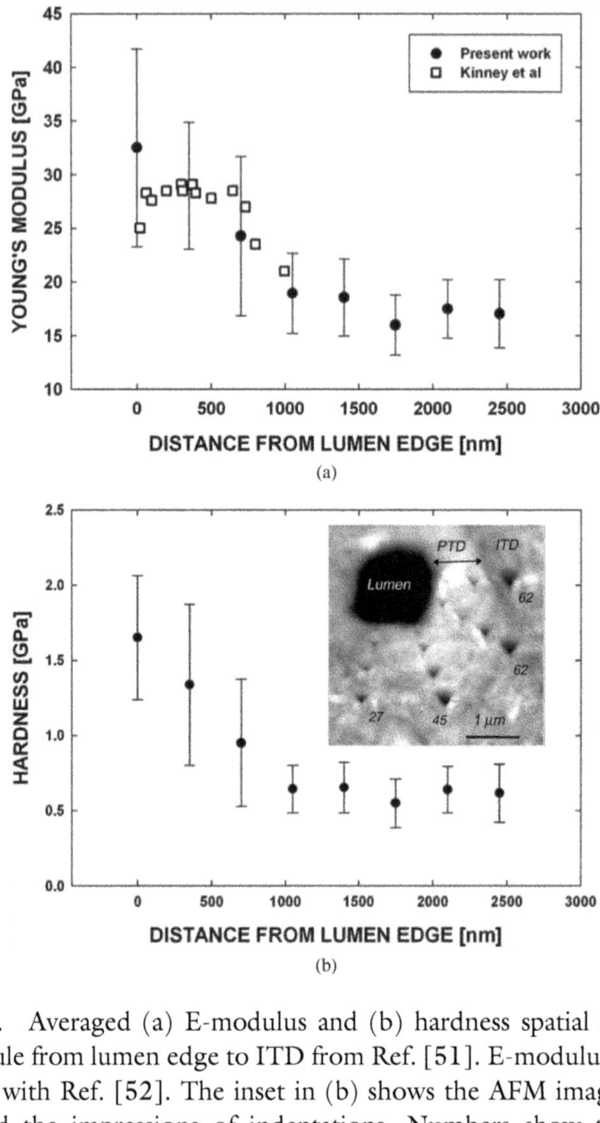

Figure 16. Averaged (a) E-modulus and (b) hardness spatial results of a single tubule from lumen edge to ITD from Ref. [51]. E-modulus results are compared with Ref. [52]. The inset in (b) shows the AFM image of single tubule and the impressions of indentations. Numbers show the load in micronewton. Adapted from Ref. [50]

mentioned above. The E-modulus and hardness values decreased gradually when traveling from lumen edge to ITD, as shown in Figure 16. As expected, although the trend of results is the same as mentioned in Ref. [50], due to the change in testing situation, the measured E-modulus and hardness from a Berkovich probe are lower than the results obtained by using a cube corner probe.

The decay in hardness and stiffness of dentin was also shown to be exponentially correlated to the mineral content of the tissue.[53] In addition, environmental parameters such as hydration level and temperature significantly influence dentin mechanical properties. For example, by testing different samples that were dehydrated and wet and previously frozen and not frozen, it was shown that dehydrated samples have higher hardness and E-modulus. For previously frozen hydrated samples, the E-modulus and hardness decreased significantly in comparison with not-frozen wet samples, which is attributed to the damage caused by water inside the tissue during freezing. However, since dry samples have less water content, freezing did not change the properties significantly.[54] Using nanoindentation and measuring the energy dissipation, it was shown that dry dentin exhibits stronger elastic–inelastic behavior than wet dentin.[55] In a comparative work by using the Berkovich probe, the conventional method of nanoindentation was compared with the CSM method. It was shown that the CSM method measures higher values than the conventional method for both enamel and dentin at different peak loads.[56]

4.3. *Nanoindentation of Artificial Dental Materials*

The best materials to be used in clinical dentistry are the ones that are closer to the characteristics of real tooth materials. This is the motivation to test the dental materials and to evaluate their performance. Basically, tests to be done on artificial and natural dental materials are the same; so in this section, some of the methods used in characterizing artificial dental materials are only highlighted briefly.

A wide range of nanoindentation tests have been done on restorative materials to extract their mechanical properties.[57,58] For example, nanoindentation with conical probe has been used to extract stress–strain curve from load–displacement response of some dental restoratives based on approximations that relate the maximum displacement and load to strain and stress, respectively.[57] Based on the stress–strain curves, it was found that Wiron alloy has the closest stress–strain behavior to enamel, while Mark II and VM9 ceramics have higher strength. Ilie and Hickel also used nanoindentation to investigate the nanomechanical properties of different composite materials.[59] They measured the hardness, elastic modulus, and dynamical properties such as storage and loss moduli of materials in two different conditions. They concluded that silorane-based composites exhibit good properties which make them suitable for clinical applications.[59]

4.4. *Other Types of Tests on Dental Materials Enabled by Nanoindentation*

Nanoindentation can be used to extract other properties of tooth tissues such as the tribological[26,60–62] and dynamic[37,63–65] properties. For example, using AFM with cube corner tip, Balooch *et al.*[64] measured the maximum width of the DEJ to be 2–3 μm, which is much less than the previous reported data, and the storage modulus of enamel close to the DEJ to be in the range of 51–74 GPa (average 63 GPa). Other types of mechanical tests on dental materials enabled by nanoindentation are explained in the following paragraphs.

4.4.1. *Viscoelastic Properties*

Balooch *et al.*[43] measured the viscoelastic constants of demineralized dentin under three conditions using a flat punch probe for AFM and assuming the standard linear solid model. In particular, the relaxed elastic modulus and relaxation time constants under constant strain and constant stress have been measured.

4.4.2. *Creep Behavior*

Creep behavior in enamel has been studied by He and Swain using nanoindentation with Berkovich probe.[66] They applied trapezoidal load function, held the maximum force for 900 s, and recorded the displacement at this step as creep. And for back creep, they held the probe on the sample at the minimum load for 900 s. Figure 17 shows the creep and back creep when this method is used to investigate the influence of ambient conditions on creep behavior of

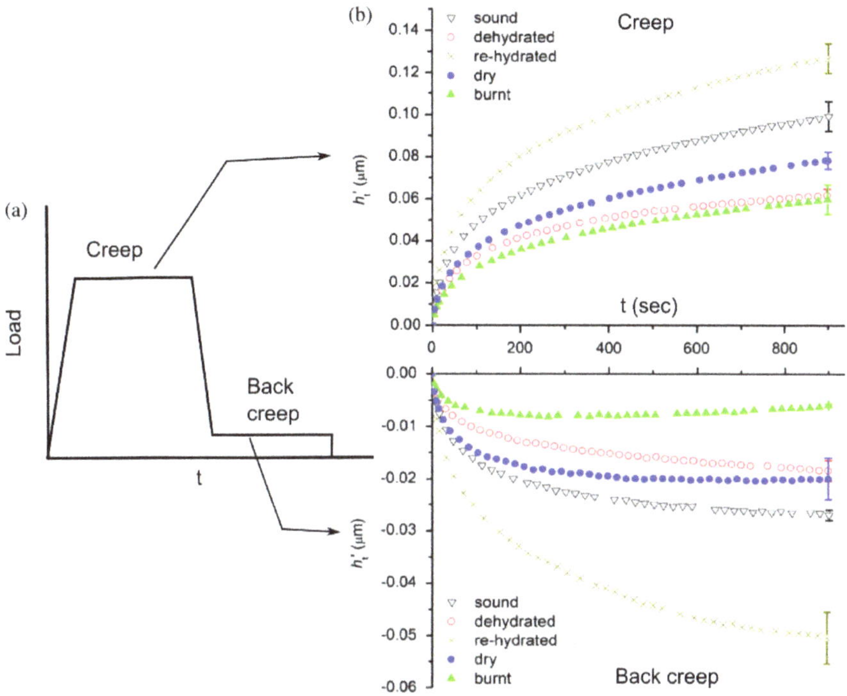

Figure 17. (a) Trapezoidal load function in nanoindentation for creep and back creep test. (b) Displacement versus time for holding time at maximum load (creep) and minimum load (back creep). Adapted from Ref. [66]

enamel.[66] The results implied that different environmental mediums may influence both the creep and the back creep behavior of enamel regardless of the load.

4.4.3. *Fracture Toughness*

Originally developed for Vickers hardness, fracture toughness from nanoindentation is estimated based on the following equation[50,68]:

$$K_c = \alpha \sqrt{\frac{E}{H}} \frac{P}{c^{3/2}}, \quad (16)$$

in which K_c is fracture toughness, P is applied load, H is hardness, E is E-modulus, c is the length of the crack from the center of the indentation on surface, and α is an empirical calibration constant. This procedure has significant uncertainty, and on top of that it only works for brittle materials. The most brittle part of tooth is enamel, which has been studied using this method using a cube corner tip.[67] The advantage of using a sharp indenter is to initiate the crack with lower applied load. As an example, Marshall *et al.* reported fracture roughness of 0.6–0.9 $\text{MPa}\cdot\text{m}^{1/2}$ for DEJ using a cube corner,[68] and Ayatollahi and Karimzadeh reported the maximum value of 1.06 $\text{MPa}\cdot\text{m}^{1/2}$ for intact enamel.[69]

4.4.4. *Nanotribology*

The nanotribological properties of tooth is another interesting topic to study using nanoindentation including both scratch and wear tests. Guidoni *et al.* used a conical probe and an increasing load function to perform single scratch tests on dry and wet enamel samples.[70] By comparing results of wet and dry enamels, it is shown that plastic deformation plays an important role on the abrasive behavior of enamels. They also performed a wear test by scanning an area with the probe at certain loads and concluded that the plastic deformation occurred in the first scan. After that, the probe slid much smoother over the deformed surface and caused fatigue deformation.[70] Rod and interrod sections in enamel have also been studied under nanoscratch tests by using a conical probe.[62] It was shown that interrod enamel is less resistant to wear. Furthermore, the wear and scratch tests have been performed on tooth enamel to investigate the effect of bleaching on enamel.[61] The wear rate, which is the rate of volume of surface removed during the test, and friction coefficient have been measured[61] from this work by using a Berkovich probe.

5. Concluding Remarks and Outlook

In biology and specifically dentistry, understanding the properties of tissues is crucial for clinical purposes. Since dental materials are usually small and heterogeneous at micrometer or even nanometer scales, conventional methods for testing bulk materials are generally not applicable. In this respect, nanoindentation as a powerful non-destructive tool to extract mechanical properties at small scales has been widely used in recent years to test dental materials. With proper adaptations, various nanoindentation techniques have been used to extract the mechanical properties of both natural and artificial dental materials, including the elastic modulus, hardness, viscoelastic properties, and nanotribological properties. It is expected that in the near future, with the increasing popularity of state-of-the-art nanoindentation techniques such as *in situ* nanoindentation, the mechanical properties of dental materials can be mapped more accurately with their hierarchical microstructures than currently available, which will have a profound impact on revealing the wear and decay mechanisms of dental materials during clinical use.

Acknowledgment

This work was supported by NSERC Discovery Grant under RGPIN 430800-2013, Canada.

References

1. Hertz, H. *J. Reine. Angew. Math.* **1881**, *92*, 156–171.
2. Hertz, H. *Verh. Ver. Beförd. Gewerbe Fleisses* **1882**, *61*, 410.
3. Fischer-Cripps, A. C. *Nanoindentation*, Springer, New York: **2011**. doi:10.1007/978-1-4419-9872-9.
4. Oliver, W. C.; Pharr, G. M. *J. Mater. Res.* **2004**, *19*, 3–20.
5. Oliver, W. C.; Pharr, G. M. *J. Mater. Res.* **1992**, *7*, 1564–1583.
6. Bulychev, S. I.; Alekhin, V. P.; Shorshorov, M. K.; Ternovskii, A. P.; Shnyrev, G. D. *Zavod. Lab.* **1975**, *41*, 1137–1140.
7. Ternovskij, A. P.; Alekhin, V. P.; Shorshorov, M. K.; Khrushchov, M. M.; Skvortsov, V. N. *Zavod. Lab.* **1973**, *39*, 1242–1247.
8. Bulychev, S. I.; Alekhin, V. P.; Shorshorov, M. K.; Ternovskii, A. P. *Strength Mater.* **1976**, *8*, 1084–1089.
9. Li, X.; Bhushan, B. *Mater. Charact.* **2002**, *48*, 11–36.

10. Beake, B. D.; Harris, A. J.; Liskiewicz, T. W. Review of recent progress in nanoscratch testing. Available at: http://dx.doi.org/10.1179/1751584X13Y.0000000037 (**2013**).
11. Beake, B. D.; Davies, M. I.; Liskiewicz, T. W.; Vishnyakov, V. M.; Goodes, S. R. *Wear* **2013**, *301*, 575–582.
12. Binnig, G.; Quate, C. F.; Gerber, C. *Phys. Rev. Lett.* **1986**, *56*, 930–933.
13. Bhushan, B.; Koinkar, V. N. *Appl. Phys. Lett.* **1994**, *64*, 1653.
14. Carlton, C. E.; Ferreira, P. J. *Micron* **2012**, *43*, 1134–1139.
15. Chen, L. J.; Wu, W. W. *Mater. Sci. Eng. R Rep.* **2010**, *70*, 303–319.
16. Rabe, R. *et al. Thin Solid Films* **2004**, *469*, 206–213.
17. Blausen.com staff. *Wikiversity J. Med.* **2014,** *1.*
18. Kaitsas, V.; Olivi, G. *Lasers in Restorative Dentistry* 3–22, Springer, Berlin, Heidelberg: **2015**.
19. Schneider, G. A.; He, L. H.; Swain, M. V. *J. Appl. Phys.* **2008**, *103*, 14701.
20. He, L. H.; Swain, M. V. *J. Mech. Behav. Biomed. Mater.* **2008**, *1*, 18–29.
21. Nanci, A. *Ten Cate's Oral Histology: Development, Structure, and Function*, Elsevier, Amsterdam: **2013**.
22. Hoffmann-Axthelm, W. *History of Dentistry*, Quintessence Publishing Company, Incorporated, Hanover Park: **1981**.
23. Rudolf, R.; Anžel, I.; Stamenković, D. *Metalurgija* **2008**, *14*, 135–142.
24. Anusavice, K. J.; Shen, C.; Rawls, H. R. *Phillips' Science of Dental Materials*, Elsevier Health Sciences, Amsterdam: **2013**.
25. O'Brien, W. J. *Dental Materials and Their Selection*, Quintessence Publishing Company, Hanover Park: **2008**.
26. Zhou, Z. R. *et al. J. Phys. Appl. Phys.* **2008**, *41*, 113001.
27. Rosenblum, M. A.; Schulman, A. *J. Am. Dent. Assoc.* **1997**, *128*, 297–307.
28. Nicholson, J. W. *Int. J. Adhes. Adhes.* **2000**, *20*, 11–16.
29. Ebenstein, D. M.; Pruitt, L. A. *Nano Today* **2006**, *1*, 26–33.
30. Mow, V. C.; Gibbs, M. C.; Lai, W. M.; Zhu, W. B.; Athanasiou, K. A. *J. Biomech.* **1989**, *22*, 853–861.
31. Kempson, G. E.; Freeman, M. A. R.; Swanson, S. A. V. *J. Biomech.* **1971**, *4*, 239–250.
32. Waters, N. E. *Symp. Soc. Exp. Biol.* **1980**, *34*, 99–135.
33. Wang, R.; Weiner, S. *Connect. Tissue Res.* **1998**, *39*, 269–279.
34. Weaver, J. K. *J. Bone Joint Surg. Am.* **1966**, *48*, 273–88.

35. Carrillo, F. *et al. J. Mater. Res.* **2005**, *20*, 2820–2830.
36. Gittus, J. Creep, viscoelasticity, and creep fracture in solids. **1975**.
37. Lewis, G.; Nyman, J. S. *J. Biomed. Mater. Res. B Appl. Biomater.* **2008**, *87B*, 286–301.
38. Fischer-Cripps, A. C. *Surf. Coat. Technol.* **2006**, *200*, 4153–4165.
39. Sadr, A.; Shimada, Y.; Lu, H.; Tagami, J. *Dent. Mater.* **2009**, *25*, 13–19.
40. Johnson, K. L.; Kendall, K.; Roberts, A. D. *Proc. R. Soc. Math. Phys. Eng. Sci.* **1971**, *324*, 301–313.
41. Hengsberger, S.; Kulik, A.; Zysset, P. *Bone* **2002**, *30*, 178–184.
42. Rho, J.-Y.; Pharr, G. M. *J. Mater. Sci. Mater. Med.* **1999**, *10*, 485–488.
43. Balooch, M. *et al. J. Biomed. Mater. Res.* **1998**, *40*, 539–544.
44. Zhang, Y.-R.; Du, W.; Zhou, X.-D.; Yu, H.-Y. *Int. J. Oral Sci.* **2014**, *6*, 61–69.
45. Cuy, J. L. *et al. Arch. Oral Biol.* **2002**, *47*, 281–91.
46. Jeng, Y.-R.; Lin, T.-T.; Hsu, H.-M.; Chang, H.-J.; Shieh, D.-B. *J. Mech. Behav. Biomed. Mater.* **2011**, *4*, 515–522.
47. Cheng, Z. *et al. J. Mater. Sci. Mater. Med.* **2010**, *21*, 1811–1816.
48. He, L. H.; Fujisawa, N.; Swain, M. V. *Biomaterials* **2006**, *27*, 4388–4398.
49. Park, S. *et al. Dent. Mater.* **2008**, *24*, 1477–1485.
50. Cohen, S. R. *et al. J. Chem.* **2008**, *48*, 65–72.
51. Ziskind, D.; Hasday, M.; Cohen, S. R.; Wagner, H. D. *J. Struct. Biol.* **2011**, *174*, 23–30.
52. Kinney, J.; Balooch, M.; Marshall, G.; Marshall, S. *Arch. Oral Biol.* **1999**, *44*, 813–822.
53. Angker, L. *et al. Arch. Oral Biol.* 2004, *49*, 369–378.
54. Guidoni, G.; Denkmayr, J.; Schöberl, T.; Jäger, I. *Philos. Mag.* **2006**, *86*, 5705–5714.
55. Bertassoni, L. E.; Swain, M. V. *J. Biomech.* **2012**, *45*, 1679–1683.
56. de Luis, I. G.; Garrido, M. A.; del Rio, T. G.; Ceballos, L.; Rodriguez, J. *Boletin Soc. Esp. Cerámica Vidr.* **2010**, *49*, 177–182.
57. He, L. H.; Swain, M. V. *Dent. Mater.* **2007**, *23*, 814–821.
58. Al-Haik, M. S. *et al. Int. J. Theor. Appl. Multiscale Mech.* **2009**, *1*, 1–15.
59. Ilie, N.; Hickel, R. *Dent. Mater.* **2009**, *25*, 810–819.
60. Zheng, J. *et al. Wear* **2013**, *301*, 316–323.
61. Garrido, M. A.; Giráldez, I.; Ceballos, L.; Río, M. T. G. Del; Rodríguez, J. *Wear* **2011**, *271*, 2334–2339.

62. Zheng, S. Y. *et al. Wear* **2011**, *271*, 2290–2296.
63. Ryou, H.; Romberg, E.; Pashley, D. H.; Tay, F. R.; Arola, D. *J. Mech. Behav. Biomed. Mater.* **2012**, *7*, 3–16.
64. Balooch, G. *et al. J. Biomech.* **2004**, *37*, 1223–1232.
65. He, L. H.; Swain, M. V. *J. Biomed. Mater. Res. A* **2007**, *81A*, 484–492.
66. He, L. H.; Swain, M. V. *Biomaterials* **2007**, *28*, 4512–4520.
67. Kruzic, J. J.; Kim, D. K.; Koester, K. J.; Ritchie, R. O. *J. Mech. Behav. Biomed. Mater.* **2009**, *2*, 384–395.
68. Marshall, G. W.; Balooch, M.; Gallagher, R. R.; Gansky, S. A.; Marshall, S. J. *J. Biomed. Mater. Res.* **2001**, *54*, 87–95.
69. Ayatollahi, M. R.; Karimzadeh, A. *Int. J. Fract.* **2013**, *183*, 113–118.
70. Guidoni, G.; Swain, M.; Jäger, I. *J. Mater. Sci. Mater. Med.* **2010**, *21*, 1195–1203.

Chapter 3

Finite Element Analysis in Dentistry

Josete B. C. Meira*,§, Alice N. Jikihara*,
Pavel Capetillo*, Marina G. Roscoe†,
Paolo M. Cattaneo‡, and Rafael Y. Ballester*

**Department of Biomaterials and Oral Biology, University of São Paulo São Paulo, SP, Brazil*
†Department of Orthodontics and Restorative Dentistry, University of Guarulhos São Paulo, SP, Brazil
‡Section of Orthodontics, Department of Dentistry, Faculty of Health Science, Aarhus University, Aarhus, Denmark

§jo@usp.br

Finite element analysis (FEA) presents a wide range of application in dentistry. FEA models can precisely calculate the material stress in conditions of geometry and boundaries that can properly represent the clinical reality. However, like any research model, the FEA requires some simplifications to be feasible. The researcher's challenge is to distinguish between the necessary simplifications and the misrepresentative ones. This chapter presents some information to help FEA users to improve their FEA result interpretation. In addition, it will help readers who are not familiar with this technique to understand the power of this tool and enable them to critically analyze the published FEA studies.

1. Introduction

The experimental tests explored in the previous chapter enable the mechanical characterization of dental materials and the comparison between analogous materials in standard conditions. Once the mechanical characteristics are set, it is possible to go forward in predicting the material behavior a "quasi-real" scenario by using finite element analysis (FEA). The real shape of the test object and actual loading application can be represented in the FEA model.[1,2] FEA has been used to provide a better understanding of experimental tests,[3] so, this chapter will focus on the "clinical scenario" studies.

In the last decade, there was a large increase in the number of FEA papers in dentistry. It is expected that in this large pool of articles, we can find studies with important errors in model generation and/or with fundamental flaws in result interpretation. The great challenge for the readers is to recognize the studies with major faults and critically evaluate the limitations of the generated conclusions. Still, it is important to remember that finite element models are always simplified representations of the reality. Experimental models are also simplifications of reality. It is possible to say that all models present some limitations. Therefore, the researcher's challenge is to distinguish between the necessary or required simplifications from the misrepresentative ones, for either the experimental models or the FEA ones.

2. How the Model Geometry is Defined and Obtained?

2.1. *Two- or Three-Dimensional Models?*

A consistent FEA can be developed either with a simple two-dimensional (2D) geometry or with a more complex 3D patient-based model. Between these two extremes, there is a wide range of geometric complexity that can be used for modeling. Frequently, models of teeth with 2D geometry are criticized due to errors generated by limitations inherent to 2D models (see Section 2.2). However, planar representations are still well accepted in studies involving the simulation of complex phenomena, such as crack propagation[4] and fatigue.[5] 2D models are also recommended in the early stages of a simulation. The strategy is to start the investigation with simple models and then gradually increase the degree of complexity throughout the study.

The construction of a 2D geometry can be easily performed with the computer-aided design (CAD) features of the finite element software. In patient-based models, the geometry is obtained using modern methods of image acquisition (see Section 2.3). These models have become increasingly common, due to technological advances in medical imaging technology and computation fields. Equipment and technology, previously restricted to selected research groups, have become more widespread in the dental clinics and in dental academia. However, it is important to notice that the results obtained in a model based on precise measurements of a single patient might be more limited with respect to the generalization of their findings than those obtained in anatomically simplified models with average measurements of a population. In addition, an excess of anatomical details can create "noise" that may compromise or conceal the relevant results.

2.2. *Limitations of 2D Models*

In 2D FEA models, the geometry is drawn in two dimensions, but the software considers that the real object is in fact a 3D entity. The plane models (plane stress and plane strain) assume that the object has the same geometry along the non-represented axis (z-axis), while the axisymmetric models assume a 360° revolution around the symmetric axis (Figure 1). Furthermore, the plane stress model considers that the thickness in z direction is very small when compared to x and y dimensions, which makes the stress in z insignificant. It justifies the simplification of $\sigma_z = 0$ used for these models. On the other hand, the plane strain models consider that the thickness in z is very large, which makes the strain in z insignificant. Therefore, $\varepsilon_z = 0$.

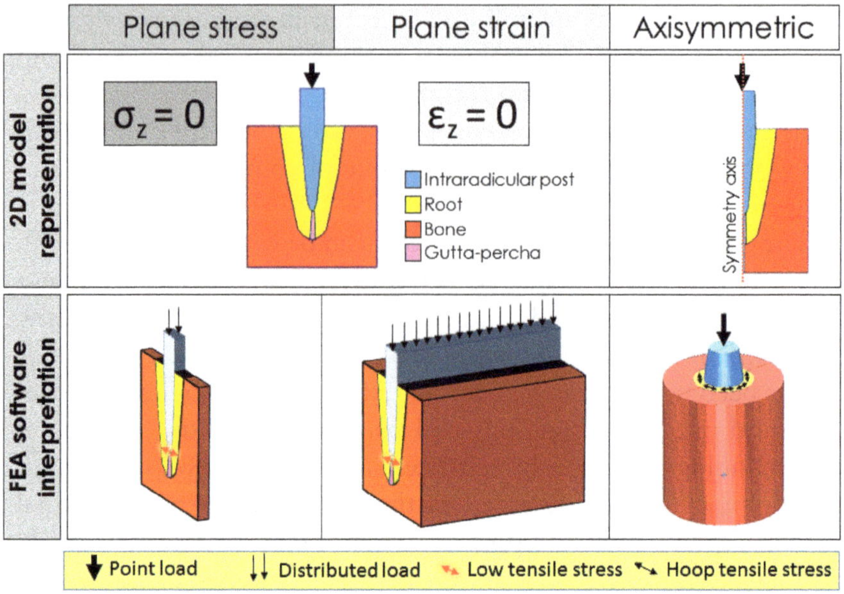

Figure 1. 2D models of a root with an intraradicular post. In plane stress and plane strain models, no hoop tensile stress is generated due to the interpretation of the software regarding the real object geometry. In axisymmetric model, the hoop tensile stress is present

Because of these geometric assumptions, both plane models are not able to represent the tensile hoop stresses generated in the real root due to the intrusion of an intraradicular post, for example Ref. [6]. However, axisymmetric models can satisfactorily represent this wedge effect, since they reproduce the real structural stiffness of the root. The main limitation of this model is its inability to simulate clinically relevant oblique loading conditions.

2.3. *Strategies for Geometry Acquirement*

The anatomic geometry can be obtained by different approaches. In this chapter, we focus in three geometry sources: literature data, 3D scanners, and computer tomography (CT). Regardless of the image data source, the anatomic model is converted into a

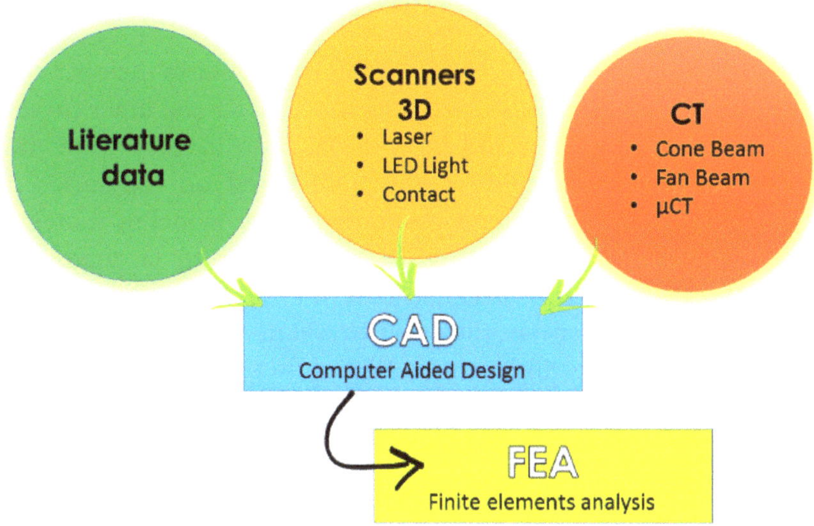

Figure 2. Overview of different approaches used for FEA models construction

parameterized model by the CAD software and, finally, to a discretized model by the FEA software (Figure 2).

2.3.1. *Geometry Based on Literature Data*

The geometric shape and measurement data of the anatomic structure are collected from the literature. A well-known source for dental anatomy parameters is available in Wheeler's *Dental Anatomy, Physiology, and Occlusion.*[7] The book presents, in a grid of 1 mm^2, accurate figures of tooth external contours from five standard aspects: labial, lingual (or palatal), mesial, distal, and occlusal (or incisal). Tables with average values of key measurements of each type of tooth are also offered: length of crown, length of root, mesiodistal diameter of crown, mesiodistal diameter of crown at cervix, buccolingual diameter of crown, buccolingual diameter of crown at the cervix, curvature of cementoenamel junction, and curvature of cementoenamel junction on distal. The authors also dedicate a chapter to pulp chambers and root canal in which the internal anatomy of the tooth is explained in detail.

Drawing the anatomic model from this data requires the operator to be highly skilled in CAD software. First, the outer and inner curves are drawn, then the outer and inner surfaces are created from the curves, and finally the solids are created, based on the surfaces. During this process, it is interesting to divide the model in strategic planes (for example, buccolingual or mesiodistal) to facilitate the viewing of the details. It is also important to avoid gaps and interpenetration of solids. Otherwise, the operator will have problems to mesh the model after transferring it to the FEA software.

2.3.2. *Geometry Based on 3D Scanning*

In the last decade, the CAD/CAM technology has become more and more widespread in dentistry; thus, dentists and prosthetic technicians had the possibility to familiarize themselves with 3D scanners. There are three types of 3D scanners: laser, LED light, and contact. In general, resolution (number of dots per unit area measured by the device), trueness (degree of closeness to the true value), precision (deviation of measurements from the mean value), and accuracy (sum of trueness and precision) do not depend directly on the type of scanner. Thus, different types may have the same resolution and accuracy, depending on specific technical characteristics of the appliance.

The accuracy of contact scanners is dependent on the capacity of the scanning tip to reach the desired surface. Therefore, it can present limitations in copying some of the details. Moreover, the object must necessarily be coupled to a support, so it is restricted to extraoral scanning. A recent study[8] evaluated some parameters of different types of extraoral 3D scanners and found values between 34.3 points/mm^2 and 299.8 points/mm^2 for the resolution, and 29–46 μm for trueness.

The data are typically recorded in an STL file,[a] a format taken from the 3D-printing technology, in which only the 3D-surface

[a]The STL has several after-the-fact backronyms such as "Standard Triangle Language" and "Standard Tessellation Language".

geometry is described in a triangular mesh. Generally, the STL mesh guides the construction of the geometric model, but not the FEA mesh, since it does not have sufficient quality, and/or is characterized by triangles with compromised edges.

The acquisition of geometry by 3D scanning is limited to the external surfaces of the object. In order to obtain the internal geometry of interest for FEA models, it is necessary to use other methods of image acquisition, such as drawing from literature data, as described in Section 2.3.1, or in combination with CT data.[9]

2.3.3. *Geometry Based on Computed Tomography*

Two types of CT are used for clinical application in dentistry: cone-beam-CT (CBCT) and fan-beam-CT (FBCT). CBCT is used more as a complementary diagnostic test for guiding dental treatment, especially in implantology. It allows a considerable decrease of the radiation dose when compared to FBCT, reducing patient exposure to ionizing radiation. When details of tooth geometry are important for the FEA model, the anatomical volume view has to be limited to the region corresponding to few teeth. FBCT is usually indicated as a medical complementary test, and it can offer high resolution for a whole skull model, due to its higher radiation power.

The resolution of CTs is low when compared to that from micro-CTs (μCT). While the voxel from CT is around $0.3 \times 0.3 \times 0.3$ mm^3, that from μCT is in the range of 1–50 μm. Therefore, μ-tomography is preferred for low scale-models (see Section 2.4). However, μ-CT is not feasible for large size models due to dimensional limitation of the equipment, in which only small objects can be scanned, and by the fact that the radiation level is much higher, when compared to clinical tomography. Therefore, these features limit the use of μCT as an "*in vivo*" investigation tool, at least for humans. Only geometries of extracted teeth models or those from human autopsy, excised bone samples, or small animal models can be scanned with this strategy.

An important feature of CTs is that they can provide not only the external contours but also the internal geometry of the anatomical structures in a non-destructive and non-invasive way. The method applies a segmentation process, based on differences in pixel gray-level values in the image, which is dependent on the radiopacity of the tissue.

Recently, some specific software have been created and improved to convert medical images of DICOM[b] files into 3D FEA models.[10–12] They offer intuitive tools to provide fast and consistent image segmentation. Furthermore, its finite element mesh preparation workflow allows the user to obtain high-quality volumetric meshes that can easily be converted into finite element mesh by the FEA software.

2.4. *Represented Structures and Model Scale*

The decision about the structures that should be represented depends on the purpose of the study. Generally, all essential structures should be represented and well discretized (see Section 3). However, sometimes it is not so easy to define which structures are essential for a specific study. If non-essential structures are represented (or if the mesh density is exaggerated in regions of less interest — see Section 3), there will be no gains, but an unnecessary computational cost.

Let us give an example: for studying the stress polymerization of a class II composite restoration, it is not useful to represent the whole root. Representing just the cervical portion of the root ensures that the boundary restriction remains sufficiently far away from the region of interest.[13,14]

If the researcher is unsure about the extension of the root that should be represented, some preliminary exploratory analysis is recommended. The strategy to be used in this process is similar to that used for obtaining the convergence curve (see Section 3): run a series of models with different root length representation, and then analyze the selected result parameter at the region of interest as a function of

---

[b]DICOM is the abbreviation for Digital Imaging and Communications in Medicine and corresponds to a series of standardization of medical images in order to create a common language between professionals and between medical imaging devices.

root extension. The ideal model will be the one in which a minimal root length is represented for independent results.

Another important aspect related to the discretization process is that the model must represent only compatible size structure. When representing a thin structure, the suitable element will be very small, because the structure should have at least three layers of elements. Therefore, if a complete large structure is represented in the same model, the number of elements would be excessively high, which may make it unfeasible. What is the solution? Avoid representing structures of very different order of magnitude in a single model.

For didactic and practical purposes, this chapter divided FEA models for dentistry into three scale levels, according to the size of the represented structures (Figure 3). Still, sometimes, it is impossible or unproductive to represent all the structures of interest in a single

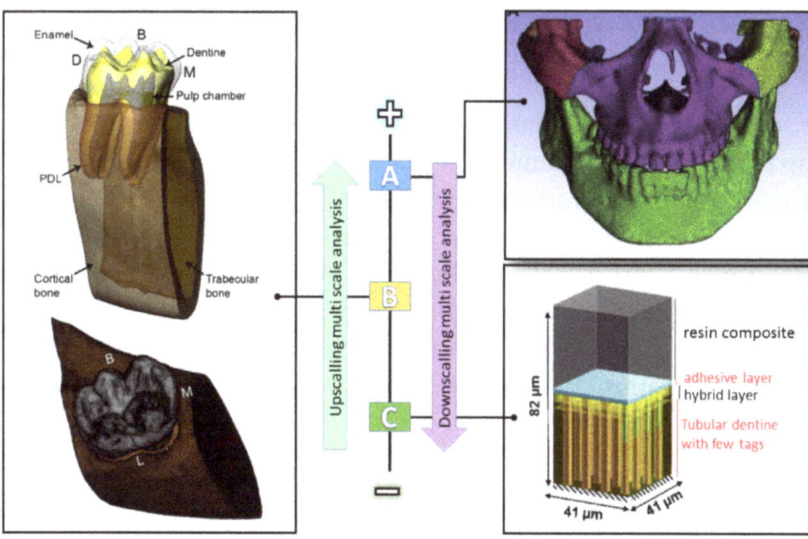

Figure 3. Didactic classification of FEA model scales: Level A — simulation of a whole maxilla, jaw, or skull represented (example from Ref. [12]); Level B — simulation of a tooth or few teeth (example from Ref. [15]); Level C — simulation of micro- or nanostructure of a material. Adapted from Ref. [16]

model due to the computational cost. Multiscale modeling represents a solution for those cases.

2.4.1. *Level A*

This scale refers to FEA models in which the whole maxilla, jaw, or skull are represented. This type of model is becoming more frequent due to the facilities in acquisition of anatomic geometry from DICOM tomography files (see Section 2.3.3) and increased advances in computer science. In this scale, the tooth is usually represented as a single body, as if it was composed of a single material.[10,11,17,18] In some cases, the distinction between cortical and trabecular bone is not represented.[12,19,20] In general, only thick structures like tooth, bone, and implants are represented in these models. Yet, in some studies the periodontal ligament (of 0.2–0.3 mm thickness) is also simulated.[10,11,19,20]

2.4.2. *Level B*

This scale refers to FEA models in which a tooth (or part of it) or a group of teeth are represented. In this scale, the tooth is represented with more details, including enamel, dentin, and pulp. Depending on the study focus, restorations,[21,22] cavities,[23,24] and intraradicular posts[25] are also represented. The bone is sometimes represented distinguishing cortical from trabecular,[26] and sometimes only the cortical layer is considered. Contrary to level A models, structures as thin as 0.3 mm, such as periodontal ligament, are generally represented.[26]

2.4.3. *Level C*

This scale refers to FEA models in which the micro- or nanostructure of a material or a multilayer adhesion is represented. The large increase of articles using this scale in the last decade can be attributed to the possibility of obtaining experimentally the mechanical properties of the materials in micro- or nanoscales from tests like nanoindentation, atomic force microscopy, or micropillar compression experiments.

This scale has been well explored in studies of adhesive interfaces in which microscopic structures, such as intertubular dentin, hybrid layer, adhesive layer, adhesive tags, and smear plugs are represented.[16,27] Parameters such as thickness of the layer of dentin infiltrated by adhesive, thickness of the adhesive layer, etc., are based on images achieved from scanning electron microscopy. Yet, the structures have been represented by primitive geometries (such as rectangles, triangles, parallelepipeds, cylinders cones, spheres), ignoring the precise irregular shapes disclosed by microscopy.

2.4.4. *Multiscale*

In a multiscale analysis, two or more models, with different scale levels, are related. The results of the first one are used as an input for the next scale level in two ways: upscaling or downscaling. The upscaling approach has been used in studies of mechanical characterization of enamel[28–31] and bone,[32] while the downscaling approach has been used in studies of adhesion and dental trauma.[33]

3. Mesh Quality and Mesh Convergence

It is well known that a finer mesh results in a more accurate solution. However, using the finest mesh in the whole model is usually a bad strategy because unnecessary calculation will be performed, producing a useless computational cost. The mesh convergence study enables the acquisition of a mesh that satisfactorily balances accuracy and rationalization of computing resources.

3.1. *Reducing the Element Size*

Generally, the mesh is refined by reducing the element size. A good approach in FEA simulation is to start the study with a coarse mesh.

Although this mesh gives an inaccurate solution, it is very useful in the early stages of the analysis, when some model verifications are required (e.g. check of the applied loads and constraints). After these verifications, the mesh is systematically refined and the convergence curve is created.

In order to obtain the convergence curve, a selected result parameter at the region of interest is plotted as a function of a measure of "mesh density" (Figure 4), such as the number of elements in the whole model or in the region of interest. Although the decrease of element size is somehow an indicator of increase in mesh density, the element size should not be used in the *x*-axis of the convergence curve. The convergence is achieved at the ideal mesh density point, in which the result does not change significantly with the increase of the refinement. This is also a guarantee that unnecessary calculation will not be performed.

In some cases, each increase of mesh density in the convergence curve is achieved by splitting all the elements in the model. However, the local mesh refinement is preferable instead of refining the whole mesh model (Figure 5). In that case, it is important to create transition regions to gradate the element size from coarse to fine meshes. The elements away from regions of interest can be considerably larger than those in regions of interest, without jeopardizing the analysis accuracy.

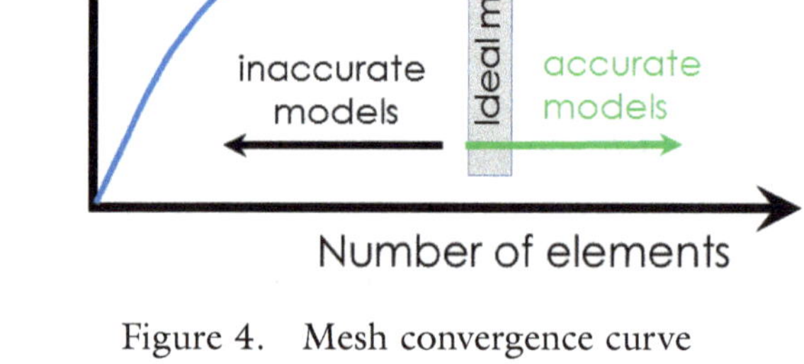

Figure 4. Mesh convergence curve

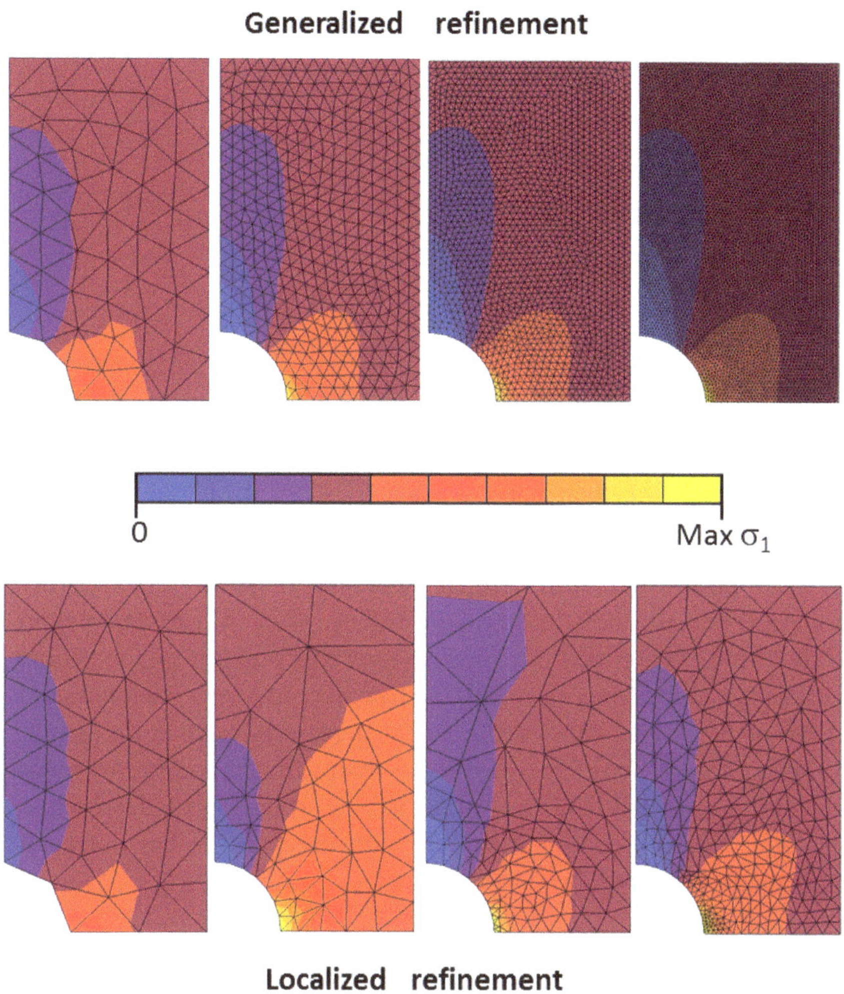

Figure 5. Mesh convergence by reducing element size: generalized and localized refinement

3.2. *Increasing Element Order*

The mesh can also be refined by increasing the element order. In this case, the geometry and the number of elements in the mesh are not modified. It continues the same, but with a higher-order element. For example, if a first-order element (like a linear triangular one, which

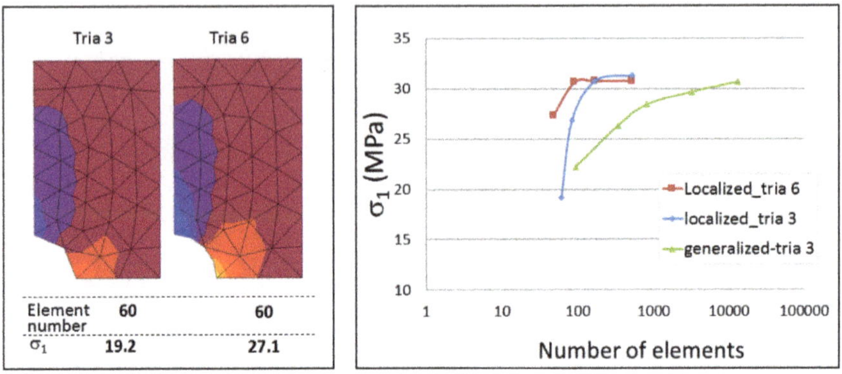

Figure. 6. (a) Comparison between the results of first-order element (tria 3) with a second-order element (tria 6). (b) Mesh convergence curve of different refinement technique

has three nodes) has been used in the coarse model, a second-order element (like a parabolic triangular element, which has six nodes) can be chosen for the refined model. This is an easy and fast way to refine, because no remeshing is needed. However, as every element and region of the model receives the same increase in calculating power, the computational costs increase faster than with the local refinement previously presented. This technique is interesting for a quick evaluation of a "final model" in which the convergence test has not been performed (Figure 6).

4. Issues Related to Properties of Biological Materials

Usually, the material properties data used in FEA models are obtained from published experimental studies. Researchers are faced with the problem of a large dispersion of data recorded for the biological structures. There are two main reasons for this dispersion: (1) biological materials are not homogeneous and standardized, since they vary as a function of individual aspects (genetic, age, gender, etc.); and (2) the methods used to obtain the mechanical properties of biological materials are not as standardized as those of materials for engineering analysis.

Dispersion motivates some researchers to perform their own experimental tests in order to obtain the required material properties inputs for FEA models.[34] This approach does not solve the dispersion problem, as the new result will be one more in the spectrum of the available data. Nevertheless, it is interesting because the authors are not limited to published data and more specific and accurate input for the particular conditions of the study can be obtained. On the other hand, an approach that is usually not encouraged by journal reviewers is to use properties from other FEA studies. Although that would be not critical for some cases, it can propagate inaccuracies.

Many FEA studies represent biological materials as isotropic, linear, and elastic. In these cases, only two parameters are necessary: the modulus of elasticity and the Poisson's ratio. However, biological materials are usually more complex, and do not behave as an isotropic, linear and elastic material.[35] On the other hand, the more complex the material properties to be modeled, the higher the risk for inaccuracy or misinterpretation of the results.

Nonlinear elastic and viscoelastic models are frequently used for periodontal ligament. This thin soft connective tissue that links tooth to bone is composed of two basic components: the collagen fibers (which are arranged in different directions along the root contour) and the fluid interstitial matrix. This histologic arrangement allows the PDL to perform as both a shock absorber and a load transmitter from tooth to bone.

Experimental studies have shown that periodontal ligament acts as a viscoelastic, anisotropic, and heterogeneous material.[36] Therefore, the way it behaves during loading and unloading conditions varies depending both on the velocity of force application as well as from its duration. In FEA studies, the PDL has been simulated using distinct constitutive models, which have been organized into two groups: (1) models for instantaneous or short-term loading cases; and (2) models for delayed or long-term loading cases. The first group contains different elastic constitutive laws, like linear-elastic, hiperelastic, or nonlinear.[37] The second group includes viscoelastic, poroelastic,[38] and multiphase models.

5. Boundary Conditions and Loading

The boundary conditions define the loading and the constraints applied to the model (usually to the nodes), and therefore determine the FEA output. In general, in a 2D model, each free node has 4 degrees of freedom (2 translations and 2 rotations), while in a 3D model each free node has 6 degrees of freedom (3 translations and 3 rotations).

Constraints represent imposition of displacements on a finite element model, which might be null to enable the software to reach a numerical solution in the analysis. These restrictions of displacements concern rotations and translations around *X*, *Y*, and, for the 3D models, *Z*-axes.

Loadings can be applied using different methods, such as point loads, pressure, distributed loads across a specific area, as well as loads simulated by the contact of the antagonist tooth. Regardless of the loading method, high magnitude of stresses is always expected around the loaded nodes. Still, these are not realistic stress concentrations, thus in all finite element models, loading and constraints should remain sufficiently far from the region of interest to ensure accuracy of the results.

6. Interpretation of FEA Output

Interpretation of the results is a very critical stage of biomechanics FEA simulation. It requires a thorough knowledge of the FEA methodology, of the related mechanical concepts, and of the biological phenomenon under study. Integrating all these forms of knowledge is not an easy task. It usually requires time, practice, reflection, and patience. Therefore, the learning curve in this step is usually more prolonged than that of the previous steps. It takes longer for the beginner to acquire autonomy to choose the sound failure criterion and to describe the generated data.

An additional difficulty appears because the failure, while usually evident in experimental tests, in FEA is mostly not directly discernable. For example, in an FEA simulation of a tooth restored with a post and a metal-ceramic crown, the stress distribution map obtained by the FEA is not enough for determining the risk of root fracture. It is necessary to compare the stress values generated in each structure with the correspondent strength of its material.

6.1. *The Failure Criteria*

In a simplified approach, we can say that the fracture of brittle materials is governed by the magnitude of tensile stresses. Therefore, the maximum principal stress (σ_1) is frequently used as the failure criteria for these materials, since it represents the maximum tensile stress. In addition, one important measure that needs be taken care of when analyzing these cases is checking the compressive stresses, especially the maximum compressive stresses, given by the minimum principal stress criteria (σ_3). The compressive stress promotes a protective effect in the brittle material because it hinders the propagation of cracks that grow in the perpendicular direction to the compression. With regard to ductile materials, they usually fail before the fracture, because the plastic deformation that appears beyond the yield strength tends to jeopardize the object function. As the plastic deformation is mainly governed by the shear stress, Tresca or Von Mises criterion is generally used to assess the risk of failure of ductile materials.

In biomechanical simulations, the choice of the failure criterion is based not only on the nature of the material under study (brittle or ductile), but also on the biological mechanisms involved in the failure process. Furthermore, the chosen failure criteria result must be consistent with clinical outcome of published randomized controlled trials (RCT). Therefore, specified failure criteria have been created in the FEA studies in Dentistry and Medicine, such as algorithms for bone remodeling.[39,40]

6.2. *The Biological Mechanism*

The orthodontically induced inflammatory root resorption (OIIRR) treatment is a very didactic example to demonstrate the importance of integrating the theoretical concepts of failure criteria with the

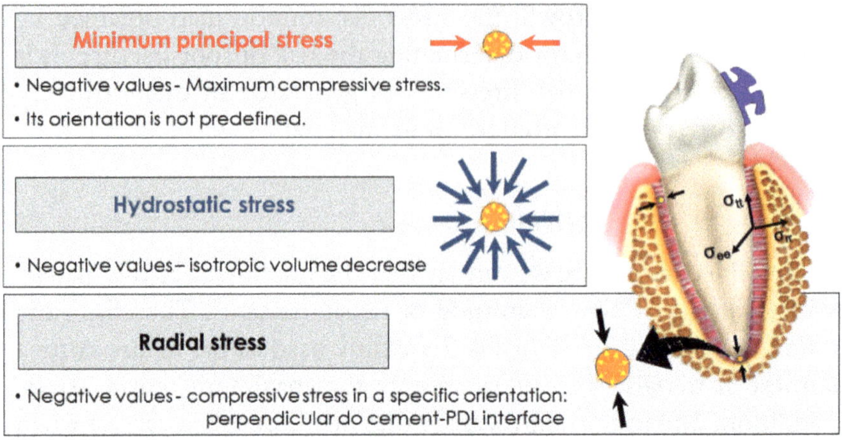

Figure 7. Compressive stresses that have been used to predict the obstruction of PDL vessels: minimum principal stress, hydrostatic stress, and radial stress. The coordinate system in the radial stress image exhibits the orientation of radial (rr), tangential (tt), and hoop (qq) stresses

biological mechanisms involved in the phenomenon under study. Although the resorption occurs in the root, it is not linked with the stress supported by dentin or cement, as suggested in some studies.[41–43] It is well described in the literature that the biological mechanisms associated with OIIRR is the obstruction of PDL vessels in overcompressed areas,[44–49] Therefore, the failure criteria need to take into account what happens in PDL that favors the blood stasis. The minimal principal stress or the compressive values of hydrostatic or radial stresses have been used to predict OIIRR by FEA[50–53] (Figure 7). It seems coherent that if these compressive stresses exceed the capillary hydrostatic pressure (4.7 kPa), the risk of obstruction and resorption is high.[50–52]

6.3. *Importance of Results Presentation*

FEA software usually present results as a map of the distribution of the response of interest (pressure, strain, displacement, etc.), in which each color represents a range of values. Although the programs automatically set the scale, it is interesting to the user to make some manual adjustments to improve the viewing and interpretation of the outcomes. For example, when displaying the map of the maximum principal stress (σ_1), it is interesting to set the minimum value to zero, to easily differentiate the regions with positive σ_1 values from those with negative values. Likewise, for the minimum principal stress (σ_3) the maximum value should be set in zero (Figure 8). While positive values of σ_1 refer to the maximum tensile stress, negative values indicate tension-free region. While negative values of σ_3 refer to the maximum compressive stress, positive values indicate compression-free region. The simple adjustment on the scale already helps to visualize these different areas. In addition, the distribution map of the figure can be complemented with a figure of the orientation of σ_1 or σ_3.[54]

In many cases, the presentation in maps may not be enlightening to the phenomenon under study. The researcher can then use other reports provided by the software to build, in an intelligent but laborious way, other modes of most enlightening presentation. For instance, results on interfaces are better represented using graphs instead of the

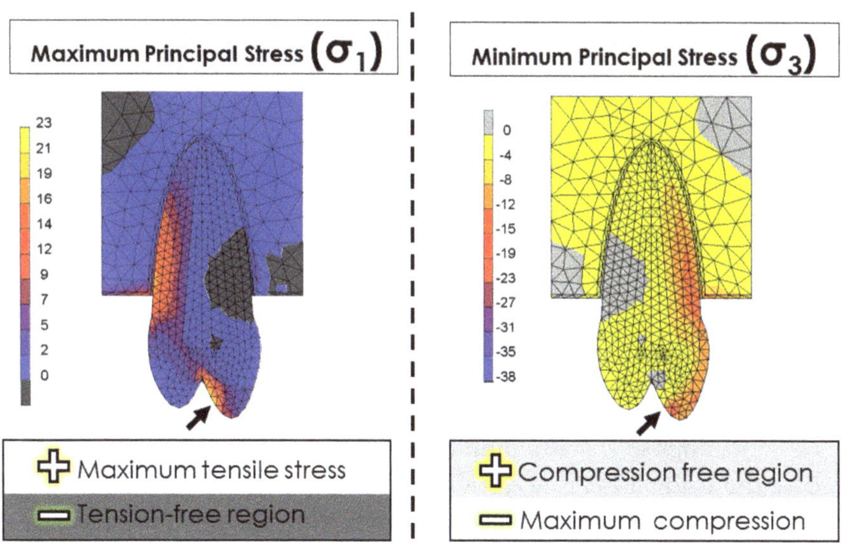

Figure 8. Map distribution of maximum principal stress

habitual map-distributed figure. The response is usually plotted as a function of cumulative selected nodes distance.[55] It is important to define which side of the interface will be explored. For example, in a cement–post interface, the user can chose to plot the stress in the cement or the stress in the post. The two curves should also be plotted, but the presentation of average stress (of cement and post) is not recommended because it lacks a physical sense.

Another important issue is that the statistical analysis is usually dispensable in FEA studies for comparing results among different models. It is not well acknowledged among researchers habituated with clinical or experimental study design, in which the variability is inherent. Therefore, it is a common (but unsuitable) criticism from some journals reviewers. The absence of statistic is explained due to absence of experimental error. It is useless to run a certain FEA model more than once, waiting for random variation in the response. The response will be exactly the same in different runs (if the model is the same regarding input data and mesh). The judgment as to whether the differences are significant or not will be aided only by the good sense of the researcher in recognizing that the discrepancy significantly interferes in practice. For instance, a stress difference about only 1% should be considered irrelevant for studies on specimen shape subjected to resistance test if the real tests vary by more than 10%. In some specific FEA study designs, the statistical analysis is used, but it is the exception, not the rule.

7. Final Remarks

- FEA presents a wide range of application in dentistry. Some stress studies can only be performed using this methodology, since stresses are not visible experimentally.
- Simplifications are inherent to any model (even experimental models) and impose specific limitations that do not necessarily invalidate the study. FEA is no different. The researcher's challenge is to distinguish the necessary simplifications from the misrepresentative ones.

- Meticulousness and thoroughness in organizing and displaying the FEA results facilitate the interpretation of the authors and the understanding of the reader.

Acknowledgments

We would like to thank CNPq for Alice Jikihara's PhD scholarship of Capes and also for Pavel Capetillo's PhD scholarship, which were essential for the writing of this chapter. We would also want to thank FAPESP for the constant financial support in our FEA studies.

References

1. Ichim, I.; Swain, M. V.; Kieser, J. A. *J. Biomech.* **2006**, *39* (10), 1903–1913.
2. Liao, Z. *et al. J. Biomech.* **2015**, *48* (16), 4214–4220.
3. Meira, J. B. *et al. J. Dent. Res.* **2011**, *90*, 365–370.
4. Barani, A. *et al. Acta Biomater.* **2015**, *15*, 237–243.
5. Li, H. *et al. Dent. Mater.* **2011**, *27* (7), e125–e133.
6. Meira, J. B. *et al. J. Biomed. Mater. Res. A* **2008**, *84* (2), 442–426.
7. Ash, N. *Wheeler's Dental Anatomy, Physiology, and Occlusion*, 9th edn. (Amsterdam: Elsevier, **2010**), p. 401.
8. Gonzalez de Villaumbrosia, P.; Martinez-Rus, F.; Garcia-Orejas, A.; Salido, M. P.; Pradies, G. *J. Prosthet. Dent.* **2016**, *116*, 543–550.e1.
9. Dejak, B.; Mlotkowski, A. *Dent. Mater.* **2013**, *29* (9), e227–e237.
10. Ammar, H. H. *et al. Am. J. Orthod. Dentofacial Orthop.* **2011**, *139* (1), e59–e571.
11. Kim, K.Y. *et al. Eur. J. Orthod.* **2015**, *37* (3), 275–283.
12. Liu; C., Zhu; X.; Zhang, X. *Am. J. Orthod. Dentofacial Orthop.* **2015**, *148* (3), 466–478.
13. Ausiello, P. *et al. Dent. Mater.* **2011**, *27* (5), 423–430.
14. Meriwether, L. A. *et al. Dent. Mater.* **2013**, *29* (5), 573–579.
15. Benazzi, S. *et al. PLoS One* **2013**, *8* (7), e69990.
16. Junior, M. M. *et al. Int. J. Adhes. Adhes.* **2012**, *35*, 114–119.

17. Ludwig, B. *et al. Am. J. Orthod. Dentofacial Orthop.* **2013**, *143* (3), 426–435.
18. Lee, N. K.; Baek, S. H. *Am. J. Orthod. Dentofacial Orthop.* **2012**, *141* (3), 345–351.
19. Tominaga, J. Y. *et al. Am. J. Orthod. Dentofacial Orthop.* **2014**, *146* (2), 166–174.
20. Yu, I. J. *et al. Eur. J. Orthod.* **2014**, *36* (4), 394–402.
21. Dejak, B.; Mlotkowski, A. *Dent. Mater.* **2013**, *29* (12), e309–e317.
22. Ichim, I. P. *et al. Dent. Mater.* **2007**, *23* (12), 1562–1569.
23. Rodrigues, F. P. *et al. Dent. Mater.* **2012**, *28* (2), 123–132.
24. Cuddihy, M. *et al. Dent. Mater.* **2013**, *29* (6), 626–634.
25. Ausiello, P. *et al. Dent. Mater.* **2011**, *27* (12), 1285–1294.
26. Mattos, C. M. *et al. J. Dent.* **2012**, *40* (5), 423–432.
27. Anchieta, R. B. *et al. Dent. Mater.* **2015**, *31* (2), 141–153.
28. An, B.; Wang, R.; Zhang, D. *Acta Biomater.* **2012**, *8* (10), 3784–3793.
29. Scheider, I. *et al. Acta Biomater.* **2015**, *15*, 244–253.
30. Ma, S; Scheider, I.; Bargmann, S. *J. Mech. Behav. Biomed. Mater.* **2016**, *62*, 515–533.
31. An, B. *et al. J. Mech. Behav. Biomed. Mater.* **2015**, *42*, 1–9.
32. Podshivalov, L.; Fischer, A.; Bar-Yoseph, P. Z. *J. Mech. Behav. Biomed. Mater.* **2011**, *4* (6), 888–899.
33. Miura, J. *et al. Dent. Mater.* **2009**, *25* (1), 67–73.
34. van Driel, W. D. *et al. Proc. Inst. Mech. Eng. H* **2000**, *214* (5), 497–504.
35. Huo, B. *J. Biomech.* **2005**, *38* (3), 587–594.
36. Fill, T. S. *et al. J. Biomech.* **2012**, *45* (1), 9–16.
37. Toms, S. R.; Eberhardt, A. W. *Am. J. Orthod. Dentofacial Orthop.* **2003**, *123* (6), 657–665.
38. Bergomi, M. *et al. J. Biomech.* **2011**, *44* (1), 34–38.
39. Chen, J. *et al. J. Biomech.* **2014**, *47* (7), 1689–1695.
40. Eser, A. *et al. J. Biomech.* **2013**, *46* (13), 2250–2257.
41. Oyama, K. *et al. Eur. J. Orthod.* **2007**, *29* (2), 113–117.
42. Rudolph, D. J.; Willes, P. M. G.; Sameshima, G. T. *Angle Orthod.* **2001**, *71* (2), 127–131.
43. Kamble, R.H. *et al. Angle Orthod.* **2012**, 82 (5), 799–805.
44. Roscoe, M. G.; Meira, J. B.; Cattaneo, P. M. *Am. J. Orthod. Dentofacial Orthop.* **2015**, *147* (5), 610–626.

45. Schwarz, A. M. *Int. J. Orhodontia.* **1932**, 18, 331–352.
46. Chan, E.; Darendeliler, M. A. *Am. J. Orthod. Dentofacial Orthop.* **2005**, *127* (2), 186–195.
47. Chan, E.; Darendeliler, M. A. *Am. J. Orthod. Dentofacial Orthop.* **2006**, *129* (4), 504–510.
48. Barbagallo, L. J. *et al. Am. J. Orthod. Dentofacial Orthop.* **2008**, *133* (2) 218–227.
49. Paetyangkul, A. *et al. Am. J. Orthod. Dentofacial Orthop.* **2009**, *136* (4) 492 e1–e9; discussion 492–493.
50. Hohmann, A. *et al. Angle Orthod.* **2007**, *77* (4), 653–659.
51. Hohmann, A. *et al. Comput. Methods Programs Biomed.* **2009**, *93* (2), 155–161.
52. Field, C. *et al. Am. J. Orthod. Dentofacial Orthop.* **2009**, *135* (2), 174–181.
53. Viecilli, R. F. *et al. Am. J. Orthod. Dentofacial Orthop.* **2008**, *133* (6), 791 e11–e26.
54. Meira, J. B. *et al. Dent. Mater.* **2013**, *29* (5), 594–601.
55. Santos, A. F. V. *et al. J. Dent. Res.* **2010**, *89* (6), 587–591.

Chapter 4

Preventive Dental Material

Larissa Bubnowicz and Rodrigo França*

Department of Restorative Dentistry University of Manitoba, 780 Bannatyne Ave., Winnipeg, Canada

**Rodrigo.franca@umanitoba.ca*

Fluoride is routinely used within the preventive clinical practice of the oral healthcare profession, as it is the only therapeutic agent to effectively control dental caries. It is therefore expected that dental materials with the ability to release fluoride may control the recurrence of caries to the surrounding dental surfaces and reduce caries incidence in the entire dentition. This chapter begins with an overview of dental caries as a multifactorial disease; its causes and determinant factors, the limitations of the anti-caries effect of fluoride, and how former theoretical concepts are no longer deemed acceptable are subsequently discussed. The preventive effect of fluoride on dentition details the processes of undersaturation versus supersaturation, the fluoride physicochemical reaction mechanism theories, and the newly proposed structure model of enamel fluoridation. Overall, this provides a comprehensive understanding of the mode of action of topical fluorides and aids in the development of new caries treatment strategies. As an oral healthcare practitioner, it can be challenging to decide which combinations of methods of fluoride delivery should be recommended, and the treatment decisions for disease management vary among practicing professionals. In spite of considerable evidence that supports modern management of caries and a minimally invasive treatment approach, "traditional dentistry" is still widely practiced. In conclusion, for caries prevention and therapeutic fluoride regimens, the movement of evidence-based research to the practicing oral healthcare team is crucially important.

1. Introduction

It is firmly established that fluoride is the only therapeutic agent known for effective caries control[1] and has been attributed to the decline of the prevalence, and severity, of dental caries in most developed countries.[2–5] The routine application of topical fluoride, a well-known preventive clinical practice within the oral healthcare profession, reduces demineralization of tooth enamel from acid production, a main contributing factor to tooth decay and dental caries.[6] It is expected that dental materials with the ability to release fluoride may control the recurrence of caries to the surrounding dental surfaces, even contributing to the reduction of caries incidence in the entire dentition.[1]

2. Preventive Effect of Fluoride on Dentition

Dental caries is a multifactorial disease, caused by a complex and dynamic interplay among bacterial pathogenic activity, nutritional diet, and the host itself.[8] More simply stated, caries is a biofilm-sugar-dependent disease, each of which is a negative determinant factor in caries progression in any dental surface, be it intact, sealed, or restored.[1,6]

The presence of fermentable sugar carbohydrates[1,7] with that of biofilm adhesion and accumulation on the tooth surface results in the production of acid.[8] Specifically, the presence of dietary sugars aids in this, specially sucrose which is the most cariogenic. Besides being easily fermented into acids, sucrose is the only carbohydrate that changes the biofilm matrix, enabling the bacteria to synthesize extracellular polysaccharides that enhances the overall cariogenicity of the biofilm.[1,8–11]

At the molecular level, this induces mineral loss from the underlying tooth structure and eventually the dissolution of the enamels' mineral hydroxyapatite (HAp, $Ca_{10}(PO_4)_6(OH)_2$).[12]

Saliva and fluoride are two other determinant factors in the development of the disease. Both function to have substantial, positive effects on the reduction of enamel mineral loss.

Saliva acts to clear the fermentable substrates and/or buffer the acids produced, and fluoride acts to enhance mineral precipitation back on the teeth. Fluoride frequently available to the aqueous oral environment (fluid phase of biofilm or saliva) as a free soluble is ideal; it interferes with the caries process by effectively reducing demineralization and enhancing remineralization of tooth enamel and dentin.

The limitations of the anti-caries effect of fluoride need to be acknowledged. It is important to clarify that neither are able to prevent the development of carious lesions, as they do not impede the formation of biofilm on any dental surface, inhibit acid production from sugars, or affect bacterial metabolism.[8,13]

Therefore, concepts that were once deemed to be theoretically reasonable, such as "fluoride strengthens teeth", "increases the resistance of teeth to acids", and "reduces the acid produced by bacteria", are no longer deemed acceptable theories with regard to caries reduction associated with fluoride use.[8,13,14] The effect of fluoride in the oral cavity is its presence in a soluble, ionic form to reduce mineral loss, through the precipitation of fluorapatite on the tooth structure.[8,15,16]

2.1. *Undersaturation versus Supersaturation*

In its stable state, at a neutral pH of 7, dental enamel hard tissue has sufficient calcium (Ca^{2+}), phosphate ($(PO_4)_{3-}$), hydroxyl (OH^-), and fluoride (F^-) ions in the immediate vicinity of its crystal lattice to maintain equilibrium with the surrounding oral fluid. When not in equilibrium, one of two results: undersaturation, where hydroxyapatite dissolves, or supersaturation, where minerals from the oral environment are deposited in the enamel, occurs (Figure 1).

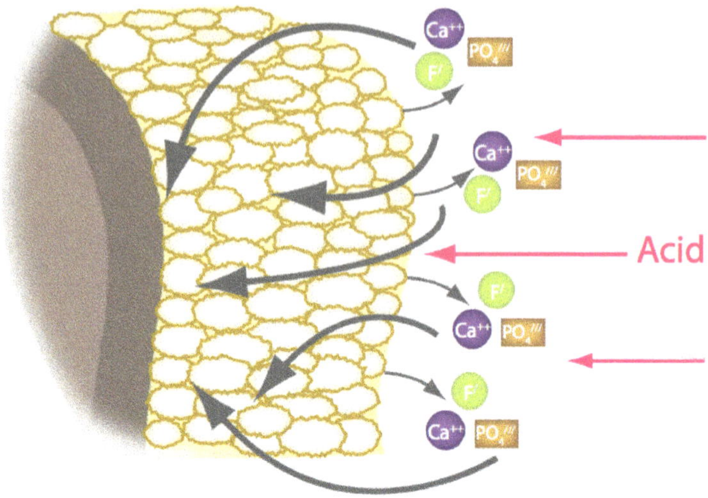

Figure 1. Ions of a cariogenic acid attack. Adapted from Ref. [17]

During a cariogenic acid attack, pathogenic bacteria *Streptococcus mutans* existing in the plaque biofilm form organic acids from any available carbohydrates.[1,8] This production of acid lowers the pH value of the oral environment, and thus the process of undersaturation begins.

As the acids dissociate, proton ions (H^+) are released, increasing the H^+ concentration in the plaque surrounding the tooth. As a result, the concentration of hydroxyl ions decreases, protonating phosphate ions. In order to maintain equilibrium between the oral environmental fluid and the vicinity of the tooth surface, both phosphate and hydroxyl ions dissolve out of the tooth. This process eventually leads to the dissolution of calcium from hard tooth structure, causing tooth demineralization (Figure 2(a)).

When the ingestion of sugar ceases and as the pH increases, the process of supersaturation commences, initiated with the precipitation of minerals back into the tooth structure. Remineralization (Figure 2(b)) begins specifically when calcium and phosphate ions

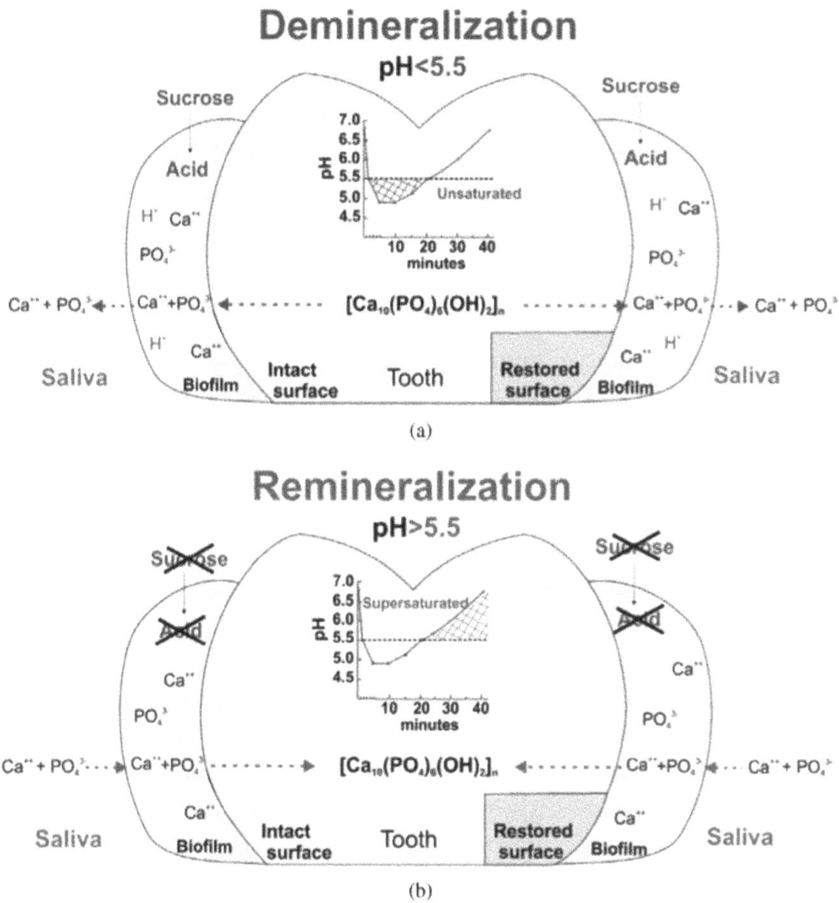

Figure 2. The processes of enamel demineralization and remineralization. (a) During a cariogenic attack, acid production lowers the pH value of the oral environment, initiating undersaturation. This process leads to the dissolution and demineralization of tooth mineral (hydroxyapatite) from an intact surface, or adjacent to a dental restoration. (b) As saliva clears out sugar and buffers the produced acid, the pH increases and the process of supersaturation commences. Remineralization occurs in the surfaces previously demineralized. Adapted from Ref. [1]

are redeposited into the crystal voids of demineralized enamel, re-forming the hydroxyapatite crystalline enamel structure.

The natural phenomenon of remineralization is enhanced if fluoride is present in the oral environment, as the mineral ion accelerates and promotes the overall process, even at very low concentrations (Figure 3).[8] As long as fluoride is present in the oral cavity at this time, fluorapatite will form first and more rapidly, over that of hydroxyapatite.[1]

In contrast, fluorapatite has a lower solubility product, which means it remains stable even at low pH values and is more acid-resistant than the original hydroxyapatite (demineralization starts as pH~5.5 for HAp and ~4.6 for FAp).[19] Therefore, fewer minerals are lost, and at a slower rate, to dissolution during cariogenic acid attacks, ultimately slowing the progression of caries development[1] and clinical observation.[3]

But even in its presence, if there is significant mineral loss, fluoride is unable to replenish the porous area inside the enamel and the clinical signs become visible in the form of a white spot lesion. However, fluoride will help to impair this process by arresting the caries lesion progression. Remineralization in the presence of fluoride results in the white spot eventually having a shiny surface, but its white aspect, from the porous areas underneath, will always partially remain.[8,14]

These processes, as described above, occur every single time sugar is ingested, resulting in an acidogenic challenge. Their complexity depends on a multitude of dynamic and influential factors, all of which play an important role in caries activity and vary from individual to individual based on enamel composition, pathogenic bacteria present in the plaque biofilm surrounding the tooth, saliva mineral content, frequency of sugar consumption, daily oral hygiene habits, and access to routine oral healthcare.

2.2. *Fluoride Physicochemical Reaction Mechanism Theories*

Even though fluoride has been known as a caries preventive agent for decades,[20] controversy nevertheless remains on the exact

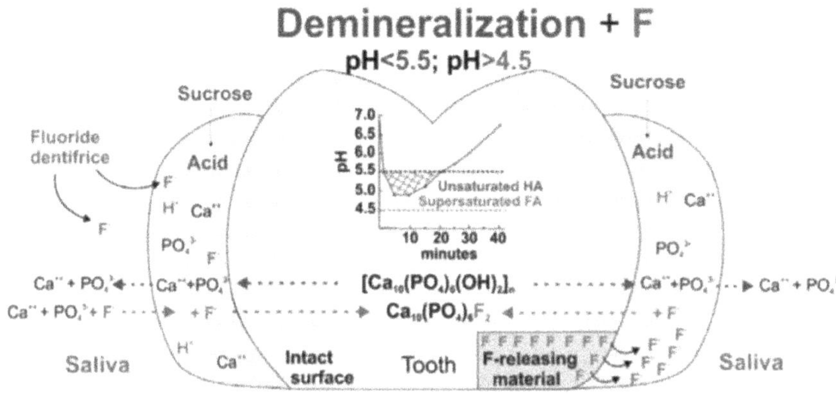

(a)

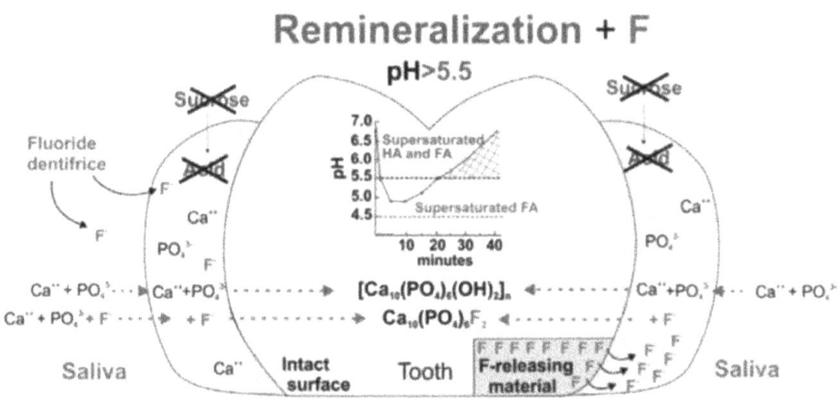

(b)

Figure 3. The mode of action of fluoride on the enamel tooth structure. (a) The mechanism of fluoride on the inhibition of enamel demineralization. If fluoride is delivered to the biofilm or saliva from a fluoride reservoir, the event described in Figure 2(a) is lessened; fewer minerals are lost as a slower rate to dissolution. Fluoride reservoirs, as depicted, are fluoridated dentifrice (left) or fluoride-releasing restorative dental materials (right). (b) The effect of fluoride on the process of enamel remineralization, described in Figure 2(b), is enhanced by fluoride sources made available to the plaque biofilm and saliva, precipitating the formation of the more stable and acid-resistant fluorapatite mineral. Adapted from Ref. [1]

physicochemical reaction mechanism and products after teeth fluoridation. Pure, direct substitution to form fluorapatite (FAp), or incomplete substituted products creating calcium fluoride (CaF_2), are discussed as two of the major fluoride reactivity theories.

One of the two major fluoride reactivity theories describes how elemental fluoride reacts with hydroxyapatite crystals, ($Ca5(PO_4)_3OH$), of dental enamel to become isostructural fluorapatite, ($Ca5(PO_4)_3F$), thus creating firmly bound fluoride within the enamel crystal rod structure. It is the lower solubility of fluorapatite, (FAp), which more strongly resists demineralization, and therefore carious lesion formation, in an acidic oral environment.[21]

The second theory suggests that free fluoride ions chemically react with calcium, released from hydroxyapatite dissolution, to create calcium fluoride, (CaF_2), an alternative loosely bound form of fluoride on the enamel crystallite surface.

Forms of fluoride reactivity can be described in the following equations[22]:

Iso-ionic exchange of F^- for OH^- in apatite:

$$Ca_{10}(PO_4)_6OH_2 + 2\ F^- \rightarrow Ca_{10}(PO_4)_6F_2 + 2\ OH^- \qquad (1)$$

Apatite dissolution with CaF_2 formation:

$$Ca_{10}(PO_4)_6OH_2 + 20\ F^- \rightarrow 10\ CaF_2 + 6\ PO_4^{3-} + 2\ OH^- \qquad (2)$$

Equations (1) and (2) describe the current theorized forms of fluoride reactivity mechanisms Eq. (1) demonstrates the pure substitution of the hydroxyl groups, OH^-, with that of free solution fluoride ions to form FAp. Equation (2) shows how the free solution fluoride ions chemically react with released calcium from demineralized hydroxyapatite to create CaF_2.

Currently, it remains rather inconclusive which reaction mechanism theory is responsible for the caries-preventive effect of fluoride.[6] Regardless, in healthy human enamel, it is apparent that fluorapatite is indeed present in addition to hydroxyapatite, ultimately resulting in increased stabilization of the overall apatite structure.[23]

2.3. *Molecular-Based Structural Model of Enamel After Fluoridation*

After fluoridation by an acidic agent, the surface of enamel can be described by a three-layer model, containing calcium fluoride (CaF_2), calcium hydroxide ($Ca(OH)_2$), fluorapatite (FAp, $Ca_5(PO_4)_3F$), and hydroxyapatite (HAp, $Ca_5(PO_4)_3OH$).[18,24] This newly proposed structure model of fluoridated enamel helps with the comprehension of the influence of topical fluoride application in the pathogenic mechanism of dental caries and tooth decay.

Topical fluoridation of enamel results in changes in the surface structure of HAp by the formation of other compounds. Many studies[18,24] have shown that FAp is found in highest concentration within a thin layer next to the original bulk enamel, which agrees with previously published results.[21] It is well known that its acid-resistant properties protect the enamels' HAp from dissolution and demineralization, as previously discussed.

Previously published research[18,25,26] has consistently found that an atomic layer of CaF_2 exists on the enamel surface. It is theorized that when fluoride is present in greater quantities than is necessary for the crystallization of FAp, precipitation of CaF_2 occurs.[27] That this superficial layer is both acid soluble and accumulates on the surface enamel suggests that it acts as a fluoride reservoir, releasing fluoride ions for further FAp formation or enzyme induction.

$$Ca^{2+} + 2F^{-} \rightarrow CaF_2. \tag{3}$$

Equation (3) describes large, residual quantities of free soluble fluoride ions (F^-) precipitate CaF_2. As adapted from Gerth *et al.*, 2007.[18]

Between the layer of FAp and CaF_2, a layer of antimicrobial effective calcium hydroxide, $Ca(OH)_2$, has been identified and is thought to be the product of the reaction of immediately formed CaF_2 and unreacted HAp.[18] The efficiency of calcium hydroxide is based on its antimicrobial effect and potential for inducing mineralization.[28,29] Because of its basic pH value, it acts as a neutralizing agent and stops the dissolution of teeth by the acidic milieu of bacteria causing caries.[30]

Even though calcium hydroxide has various practices in dentistry, such as its use as medication during root canal treatment, until recently, it has not been described as a product of enamel fluoridation. Based on the current findings of recent evidence and research studies, there is strong support to identify this compound as part of the suggested structure model (Figure 4).[18]

Therefore, this discovery and more detailed understanding may provide deeper insight into the mode of action of topical fluorides and for the development of new caries treatment strategies.

$$2\ HAp + CaF_2 \rightarrow 2\ FAp + Ca(OH)_2. \qquad (4)$$

Equation (4) describes Calcium hydroxide ($Ca(OH)_2$) as the product of the reaction mechanism between immediately formed calcium fluoride (CaF_2) and unreacted hydroxyapatite (HAp). As adapted from Gerth *et al.*, 2007.[18]

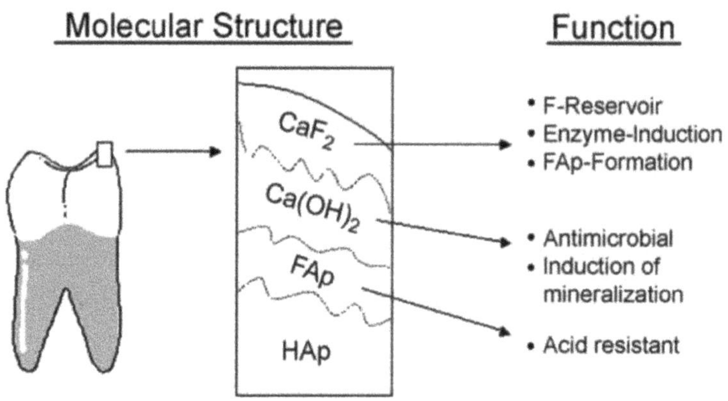

Figure 4. Three-layer molecular-based structural model of fluoridated enamel and its relationship to the pathogenic mechanisms of caries. Adapted from Ref. [18]

3. Methods of Fluoridation

Fluoride is known to elicit an anti-cariogenic effect when available continuously at very low concentrations in the oral cavity, by the same mode of action irrespective of the means of fluoride delivery. The methods of fluoride delivery that will be discussed here are meant to continuously supply the oral cavity and environment with this ion, thus reducing the development and progression of caries lesions.[8]

3.1. *Community-Based Methods of Fluoride Use*

3.1.1. *Water Fluoridation*

Almost all water contains some low levels of naturally occurring fluoride. Many communities adjust the fluoride level of the water supply to an optimal concentration known to reduce tooth decay and promote good oral health. This practice is known as community water fluoridation. Because of the drastic decline in tooth decay since its initiation, the Centers for Disease Control and Prevention (CDC) named "fluoridation of drinking water to prevent dental caries as one of 10 great public health interventions of the 20th century".[3] Years of research attest to its effectiveness and safety,[31] and support community water fluoridation as the most successful and cost-effective mode of delivering fluoride on a population basis to all people.

In the 1930s, scientists studied the epidemiology of fluorine and dental caries, and found that children who drank water with naturally high levels of fluoride had less tooth decay.[32] After much research, in 1945, the city of Grand Rapids, Michigan, was the first to add fluoride to its city water system in order to provide residents with its benefits.

When fluoride is systemically ingested, it returns to the oral cavity through salivary secretions. For this mechanism of action to be effective, fluoridated water must be ingested continuously. There is a measurable effect of having the dentition continuously bathed by fluoride-enriched saliva; a previous study[33] has demonstrated that even a micromolar increase, from 0.01 to 0.02 ppm, in fluoride concentration in saliva has a tremendous and significant effect to caries control.

When fluoridated water is used for food preparation and/or for cooking meals, fluoride is made available to the oral environment upon consumption. The benefits of cooking with fluoridated water are discussed in a recent paper[34]; while foods cooked with fluoridated water are being chewed, an increase in fluoride concentration in saliva is observed prior to swallowing. This supports the concept that a prolonged fluoride effect is accomplished by low concentrations returning to the oral cavity via saliva.

In 2001, the CDC[3] published recommendations on the use of fluoride to prevent and control dental caries.[35] Based on the evidence that frequent exposure to low concentrations of fluoride daily will effectively reduce dental caries risk in all age groups, the CDC recommends all dentate individuals drink water with an optimal level of fluoride.

3.1.2. *Professionally Applied Methods of Topical Fluoride Use*

It was the acknowledgment of the role of fluoridated water in caries reduction that initiated the development of other modes of fluoride delivery, specifically professional topical fluoride application of high-concentration gels (from 9,000 to 12,300 ppm F) and varnishes (22,500 ppm F).[17]

The main mechanism is a reaction between the soluble fluoride, of the manufactured topical product, and the enamel tooth mineral, precipitating calcium fluoride-like deposits (CaF_2). These deposits act as a fluoride reservoir, slowly dissolving and releasing fluoride into the oral environment.[36] These fluoridated products must be reapplied to maintain their caries-preventive effect.[17]

There is a clear evidence[37–39] of the anti-caries effect of professional applications of topical fluoride.[40] The evidence supports that individuals with moderate and high risk of dental caries may benefit most from professionally applied fluoride adjuncts[41]; however, they are also used in those with additional needs.[17] The level of evidence-based documentation differs by method of topical fluoride use and among age groups.[17]

Table 1. The American Dental Association's Council on scientific affairs published recommendations on the use of professionally applied topical fluorides for individuals of moderate and high caries risk for all age groups

	Moderate risk	High risk
Under age 6	Fluoride varnish at 6-month intervals	Fluoride varnish; 2–4 times per year (6- or 3 month intervals)
6–18 years of age	Fluoride varnish or gel at 6 month intervals	Fluoride varnish or gel; 2–4 times per year (6 or 3 month intervals)
Over 18 years of age	Fluoride varnish or gel at 6 month intervals	Fluoride varnish or gel; 2–4 times per year (6 or 3 month intervals)

Note: Low-risk patients may not benefit from professional topical fluoride applications.
Source: Adapted from Refs. [17, 42].

Based on clinical trials and evidence-based studies, the American Dental Association's Council of Scientific Affairs recently published recommendations on the use of fluoride gel and varnish for professional topical fluoride treatments, with the choice dependent on age and risk category (Table 1).[42] Evidence-based clinical practice requires that the oral healthcare practitioner assess caries risk level prior to recommendation and implementation of treatment.[17,42]

3.1.3. *Topical Fluoride Gels*

Traditionally, the administration of high-concentration topical fluoride gel in trays was the standard of professionally applied fluoride treatments. Common fluoride gel products include acidulated phosphate fluoride (APF) and sodium fluoride (NaF).[41] It is still the method most frequently used clinically by oral healthcare practitioners as specific caries-preventive agents in adult clients.[2]

Miller and Vann[43] expanded on the above recommendations of the ADA Council of Scientific Affairs (Table 1), addressing topical fluoride use in children under the age of 6, with special healthcare needs, and attention span or cooperation concerns.[17]

3.1.4. *Topical Fluoride Foam and Rinses*

Topical fluoride foam was introduced into dental practices in the 1990s and since has been commonly used. However, topical foam is not clinically recommended,[17] as evidence shows that its clinical efficacy is not as strong as that for fluoride gel and varnish.[17,41] There is no evidence to support rinses.[17]

3.1.5. *Topical Fluoride Varnish*

Topical fluoride varnish is a resin-based, 5% sodium fluoride treatment material for the prevention of enamel and root surface caries. This dental material facilitates prolonged adherence to the tooth surface structures, is able to deposit large amounts of fluoride on enamel, and acts as a sustained fluoride source.[17,44–47]

Additional attractions are that administration takes less time, creates less discomfort, and is widely accepted amongst patients. Sodium fluoride varnish was first introduced as a desensitizing agent, for dentinal hypersensitivity associated with exposed root surfaces and as a cavity liner.[17]

Prior to fluoride varnish, there was no safe way to administer topical fluoride to children under the age of 3. Their limited ability to control swallowing and spit effectively eliminates gels, foams, and rinses as viable treatment options.

For children 6 years or younger, there is strong evidence from systematic reviews of randomized controlled trials[48,49] to support fluoride varnish applications at 6-month intervals, for moderate- and high-risk patients, and every 3 months in high-risk patients.[50,17]

For children between the ages of 6 and 18 years, with moderate and high risk of caries, systematic reviews support fluoride varnish application every 6 months, and every 3 months in high-risk children. Marinho *et al.*[50] conducted an evidence-based review of randomized, and quasi-randomized, controlled trials with blind outcome assessment in children up to 16 years for the duration of at least 1 year.[35] This review indicates a substantial caries-inhibiting effect of fluoride varnish in both deciduous and permanent dentition.

This age range is when orthodontic treatment typically commences, and the appliances involved increase the risk for enamel demineralization. Investigations[51–53] have demonstrated that fluoride varnish has the capability to reduce or minimize enamel demineralization adjacent to orthodontic brackets.[17]

The main uses of fluoride varnish in adults are for remineralization and control of root caries, caries prevention for those at high risk, and treatment of dentinal sensitivity. For individuals over 18 years of age, there is some evidence to support administration at 6-month intervals for those at moderate and high risk, and every 3 months for patients at high risk.[50] However, this level of evidence is low as it is centered on expert committee reports and opinions, rather than prospective, randomized clinical trials.[17]

Petersson *et al.*[54] conducted a systematic search of the literature published between 1966 and August 2003 to evaluate the caries-preventive effect of professional fluoride varnish treatments.[35] Of the 24 reports included from randomized and controlled clinical trials, the results suggest limited evidence for permanent dentition.

3.2. *Individual Methods of Fluoride Use*

3.2.1. *Fluoridated Dentifrices*

Among individual methods of fluoride delivery, the use of fluoridated dentifrices is by far the most important and shall be the basis of our discussion.

Daily use of fluoride dentifrices forms the foundation of caries prophylaxis in all age groups,[55] as it combines the caries-protective processes of fluoride with the mechanical removal of plaque biofilm. Its practice is strongly supported by unequivocal evidence-based research[37,56] and has been a main contributing factor in the caries decline observed in both developed[57] and developing countries.[58,59]

Fluoride dentifrices can control caries incidence in originally intact dental surfaces, interfere with caries lesion progression adjacent to dental restorations, and can be spread throughout the mouth enriching the oral environment, saliva,[60,61] and even biofilm not perfectly removed.[55,62,63] The effectiveness and efficacy of this mode of fluoride delivery is based largely on client compliance; the effect increases with frequent toothbrushing.[23,55]

Many high-quality, randomized, and controlled studies conducted in the previous decade have proven conventional fluoride toothpastes, those containing 1,000–1,500 ppm F, as highly effective for caries control.[55]

Marinho *et al.*[64] conducted a search of the Cochrane Oral Health Group's Trial Register and supplementary databases on randomized, or quasi-randomized, controlled trials with blind outcomes assessment for analysis of comparative caries-prevention data for fluoridated dentifrice.[35] The search firmly established the benefits of fluoride toothpaste.

Twetman *et al.*[65] systematically reviewed and evaluated the scientific literature between 1966 and 2003 on the caries-preventive effect of fluoride toothpastes in various age groups.[35] The results suggest that toothpastes containing 1,500 ppm F have a superior caries-preventive effect, than those of 1,000 ppm F, and that there is a strong evidence for the daily use of fluoride toothpaste to prevent carious lesions.

Based on the evidence that frequent exposure to low concentrations of fluoride daily will effectively reduce dental caries risk in all age groups, in 2001, the CDC[3] recommended that all dentate individuals should brush their teeth twice a day with fluoride toothpaste.[35]

Toothpastes of increased fluoride concentration of 5,000 ppm F have been recently introduced with the purpose of controlling root caries. There is some evidence[66] on the effectiveness of these toothpastes, when compared to the conventional, but a literature review is still non-existent.

Recently in the last few years, a quantity of clinical studies[67] and systematic reviews[68,69] of the literature have been published on low fluoride concentration dentifrices, 250–500 ppm F.

In summary, low-concentration fluoridated toothpastes are not able to control caries under a high cariogenic challenge,[67] are not as effective as the conventional fluoridated pastes,[68] and are effective to control caries only in caries-inactive, but not caries-active, children.[70]

The following studies and reviews also validated the effectiveness of fluoride in conventional strength dentifrice formulations,[69] its ability to manage caries in caries inactive children,[70] and control the appearance of new lesions.[70]

3.3. *Fluoride-Releasing Dental Materials*

Increasing evidence suggest that decay around dental restorations is due to the occurrence of a new carious lesion adjacent to pre-existing one.[71] It is expected that dental materials with the ability to release fluoride may control this recurrence of caries to surrounding dental surfaces, even contributing to the reduction of caries incidence in the entire dentition.[1]

Fluoride-releasing dental materials may be considered the ideal as they supply the oral cavity with a constant source of slow-release fluoride and the effects are not dependent on client compliance.[1] At this time, these materials still lack clinical basis to confirm an anti-caries effect.[1]

3.3.1. *Pit and Fissure Dental Sealants*

In the late 1960s, sealing anatomical pit and fissures of occlusal surfaces with a thin layer of resin dental material was introduced as a caries-preventive method,[2,72] and this has now evolved to incorporate fluoride into the newest materials.[73] Guidelines recently developed by the American Dental Association Council on Scientific Affairs[74] recommend dental sealants for all age groups.[2]

When compared to no sealants, the evidence suggests sealing the occlusal surfaces of permanent molars with resin-based sealants to prevent caries,[1] even over existing bacteria.[2,75] The conclusion of a Cochrane Review, by Ahovuo-Saloranta *et al.*[76] of sealants in the permanent dentition of 5–10-year-old children, supports this recommendation.[35]

The potential of glass ionomer cements (GIC) to release fluoride is a strong incentive for their use as pit and fissure sealing materials, especially in deciduous and partially erupted posterior permanent dentition.[77] However, the evidence presently available remains inconclusive as to the effectiveness of materials, other than resin-based ones.[78,79]

Mejare *et al.*[66,73] performed a systematic review and concluded there is limited evidence to substantiate that fissure sealing with resin-based materials has a caries-preventive effect and that evidence is incomplete for glass ionomers used as pit and fissure dental sealants.

Current findings suggest, among oral healthcare practitioners, that dental sealants are an infrequent caries-prevention choice for adults, and therefore potential candidates may not be receiving treatment.[2] Studies[80,81] found that sealants are placed more frequently by dentists with knowledge of the benefits and cost-effectiveness, those who recently attended continuing education about prevention for children, by recent graduates, and independent of the insurance variable.[2]

3.3.2. *Glass Ionomer Cements (GIC)*

As non-metallic restorative dental materials, with ease of use, good retention, reduced post-operative sensitivity, and anti-cariogenic properties, GIC are an excellent therapeutic alternative.

Along with the ability to release fluoride, these cements can be recharged with the ion from an alternative source, such as fluoridated dentifrices. In fact, Benelli *et al.*[82] established that plaque biofilms which adhesively form on glass ionomer restorations become enriched with GIC-released fluoride, leading to confirmed inhibition of demineralization around these restorations.

This anti-cariogenic ability is just one motivation for their current use for restorations, common use as an orthodontic bracket adhesive, and potential future use as pit and fissure sealing materials.

At this time, systematic literature reviews fail to confirm the greater benefit of glass ionomers to reduce caries around restorations,[83] when compared to composite resin, and the available scientific evidence is unconfirmed as to whether glass ionomer or resin-modified glass ionomer are equally effective to those of resin-based dental sealants.[1]

These indeterminate outcomes were also observed[8,63,84] when restorations of glass ionomer and composite resin were tested against the use of fluoridated and non-fluoridated dentifrice. The concomitant use of fluoride toothpaste may explain why studies fail to demonstrate clinical effectiveness,[8,83] as the caries-preventive effect can be substituted by fluoride delivered from dentifrice.

3.3.3. *Orthodontic Bonding Agents*

During the stages of orthodontic treatment, the presence of orthodontic appliances increases retentive sites in the dentition and may cause pain and discomfort.[85] As a result, there is often increased biofilm accumulation and risk of carious lesion development, as it more difficult for individuals to properly perform daily oral hygiene routines.

Initial enamel lesions have the potential to develop as early as 6 months after the bonding of orthodontic appliances.[86,87] Enhancing fluoride bioavailability during the course of the duration of orthodontic treatment compensates for this increased caries risk and is achieved by using fluoride-releasing orthodontic bonding, adhesives and/or cements. These materials act as fluoride reservoirs reducing the incidence of white spot lesions.[1]

Because of the absence of studies meeting inclusion criteria, a Cochrane systematic review[85] could not reach a conclusion of whether the usage of these bonding materials, during orthodontic treatment, decreases the occurrence and severity of white spot lesions. Additional systematic reviews[85,88–91] were unable to deduce evidence-based recommendations for their effectiveness to adhere orthodontic appliances on these developing lesions.

3.3.4. *Restorative Dental Material*

Fluoride-releasing restorative dental materials are highly favored by the clinician as multipurposed; besides restoring the dentition, they help to prevent the development of new decay and carious lesions.[1]

Very few clinical trials and systematic reviews have been conducted that consider anti-caries effect as the outcome measure. Therefore, it remains unknown whether fluoride-releasing restoratives significantly reduce caries risk in comparison to non-fluoride-releasing restoratives.

Based on *in vitro* and *in situ* experimental studies, fluoride-releasing dental materials present the necessary properties to be clinically effective on caries control; however, this effectiveness is not still proven.[1] In summary (Table 2),[1] there is a clear need for further investigation of well-designed, randomized controlled clinical trials to investigate the anti-caries benefit of fluoride-releasing dental materials.

3.4. *Combination of Methods of Fluoridation*

As an oral healthcare practitioner, it can be challenging to decide which combinations of methods of fluoride delivery should be recommended. Most doubt stems from the clinician's difficulty in comprehending the mechanism of action of each method of fluoride and how fluoride is supplied to the oral cavity, as previously discussed in the preceding sections.

Universal consideration is that both drinking water with an optimal fluoride concentration and fluoridated dentifrice be recommended for all individuals.[8] Data and evidence-based studies[91,92] support their effectiveness to control caries and that the current low caries prevalence is as a result of their continuous use by many populations.[8]

Additional fluoride sources and measures might require recommendation for individuals at moderate and high risk for dental caries (Table 3).[8,46,92,93] These may include professional topical fluoride application and the use of fluoride-releasing dental materials. The study of Splieth *et al.*[94] found that, over the past two decades, fluoride application routinely administered in a dental office plus the use of fluoride toothpaste achieved significant caries reductions (Figure 5).[35] The investigators suggest that in high caries risk groups, topical fluoride applications six or more times per year in combination with effective plaque removal can successfully prevent caries. And

Table 2. Summary of the conclusions of presently available evidence-based research on fluoride-releasing dental materials

Type of dental material	Systematic reviews	RCT	Conclusions
Pit and fissure sealants	Ref. [73] Ref. [79] Ref. [78] Ref. [73]		Fissure sealing with resin-based materials has a caries preventive effect. It is still not known whether F-releasing resin-based sealants provide any additional benefit. There is still uncertainty concerning the effectiveness of fissure sealing with other materials
Bonding orthodontic materials	Ref. [90] Ref. [88] Ref. [91] Ref. [89] Ref. [85]	None	The evidence on the effectiveness of using F-releasing material to bond or cement orthodontic appliances on white lesion spots development is still inconclusive
Restorative materials	Ref. [90]		It is still not known whether F-releasing restoratives reduce caries risk in comparison to non F-releasing restoratives, There is weak evidence that GIC confers greater caries protection than amalgam in single-surface restoration in permanent teeth

Source: Adapted from Ref. [1].

Table 3. Recommendations on methods of fluoride delivery at a community-based, individual, and professionally applied level of approach

Method of delivery	Community-based	Individual	Professionally applied	Recommendations
Fluoridated water	X			Recommended to all individuals; no restrictions
Fluoridated dentifrice (1,000–1,500 ppm F)		X		Daily use recommended to all individuals; young children should use a small amount
Topical fluoride application (gel, varnish)			X	According to caries risk or activity, at the community or individual levels
Combinations of methods	According to caries risk or activity, at the community or individual levels			

Source: Adapted from Refs. [8, 91–92].

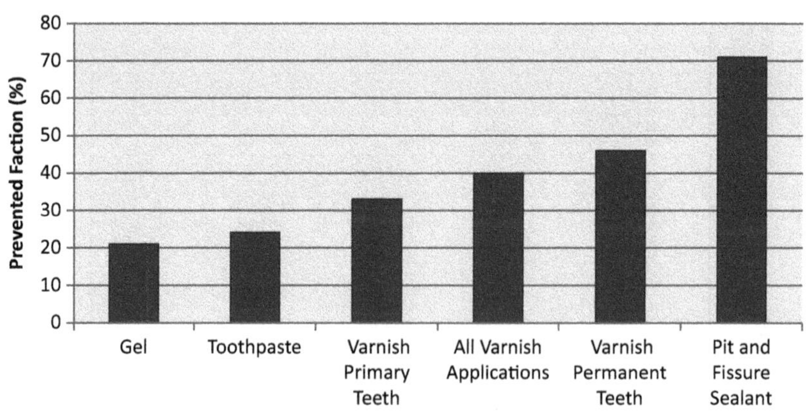

Figure 5. Prevented fraction (%) of decayed, missing, and filled tooth surfaces (ΔDMFS) for various fluoride prevention methods. Adapted from Ref. [35]

Table 4. Different levels of approach for fluoride use and mode for its delivery in the oral environment

Approach for fluoride use	Mode (examples)
Community level	Water fluoridation
Individual level	Fluoridated dentifrice
Professionally applied	Fluoride-releasing dental materials, topical fluoride application (gel, varnish)
Combinations	Fluoridated dentifrice + fluoride-releasing dental materials

Source: Adapted from Ref. [1].

Marinho *et al.*[95] concluded that topical fluorides used in addition to fluoridated toothpaste achieved a modest caries reduction compared to toothpaste alone.[35]

However, there also is evidence[55] that regular use, 3 times per day, of fluoridated toothpaste is able to achieve a level of enamel demineralization inhibition that cannot be improved with the association of a professional fluoride application; no significant improvement of the combined effect is observed.[8] This is confirmed by a literature review by Marinho *et al.*[96] on the combination of methods of fluoride versus fluoride toothpaste alone.[8] The same was observed[63] when restorations of glass ionomer and composite resin were tested.

Ultimately when considering the evidence, though contradictory, when fluoridated dentifrice is used on a regular basis and caries activity is under control, no additional method of fluoride use is recommended. For persons at moderate to high risk of caries, professional topical fluoride application and fluoride-releasing dental materials may be considered complementary methods of fluoride delivery.[8]

4. Clinical Applications and Recommendations of Preventive Fluoride

Although it has been known for many years that dental caries is an infectious disease, the management of the disease and treatment decisions for caries management vary considerably among practicing oral healthcare professionals.[35,97–105] Current surveys indicate that "traditional drill, fill and bill dentistry" is still widely practiced in spite of considerable evidence that supports modern management of caries and a minimally invasive treatment approach.[35]

Certain clinicians lack confidence in their ability to detect early lesions,[35] to arrest the disease, and to remineralize enamel[106]; therefore, restorations are often placed early and unwarrantedly. Others practice minimally invasive dentistry, monitoring early lesions and providing preventive therapeutic treatment aimed to arrest caries and remineralize enamel.[35,99,107–115] Thus, there is extensive variability in caries risk assessment, caries lesion detection, decisions on when and how to treat carious lesions, the best treatment options for high-risk patients, and the best method for monitoring disease.

There is some evidence[2] to support this variability and the notion that dentists use prevention based on caries treatment philosophy learned in dental training,[35] uncertainty of overall caries activity,[35] payment method and insurance coverage,[35] patient understanding of caries as a disease,[35] patient recall interval,[35] economic status,[116] and/or community expectations for standards of care.[35]

A profound demonstration of this is that Riley *et al.*[2] confirms patients with dental insurance were significantly associated with greater use of in-office preventive modalities (Figure 6).

Minimally invasive dentistry is based on the principles of modern caries management. Its focus is to that of traditional prevention, prophylaxis and fluoride, and minimal intervention of caries risk and prevention assessment, carious lesion monitoring and delayed intervention.[35] More specifically, these include accurate lesion detection, classification of lesion severity, assessment of caries risk, matching of treatment to the risk level, monitoring of non-cavitated carious tooth surfaces, remineralization therapies, and appropriate recall intervals according to treatment outcomes and current risk levels.

From a survey of Yorty and Brown,[117] and among Dental Practice-Based Research Networks (DPBRN) practices,[2,118–119] it is clear that concepts of minimal intervention dentistry are becoming more widely

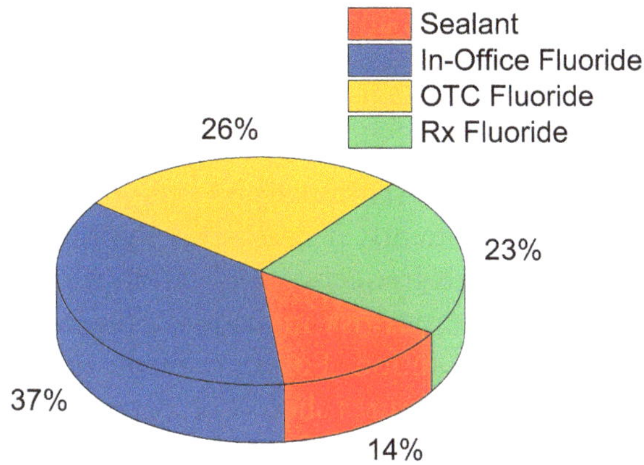

Figure 6. Frequency of use of preventive fluoride methods by dentists among Dental Practice-Based Research Networks. OTC, over-the-counter; Rx, prescription. Adapted from Ref. [2]

accepted, as emphasized by an obvious shift in dental schools toward modern management of the disease, assessment of caries risk, and delayed cavitation restoration.[35]

Evidence[2,120] show that dentists who report more conservative decisions in clinical treatment scenarios were more likely to use caries preventive agents, and oral healthcare practitioners who most frequently use caries prevention were also those who regularly perform caries risk assessment and individualized caries prevention. These findings are validated by the case scenarios of Riley *et al.*[2]; dentists who delay restoration until a more-advanced lesion depth use prevention with a higher frequency in their practices, and frequency of fluoride and sealant use are highly associated with the conservative–aggressive caries management continuum.

It is encouraged that oral healthcare professionals clinically practice caries risk assessment strategies on a routine basis. It is only after the identification of caries risk status that appropriate preventive regimens and treatment may be determined, recommended, and implemented. Risk of developing dental caries exists on a continuum and changes over time as the risk factors change. Therefore, it is imperative that for modern management of caries to be successful, lesion severity be monitored during any active treatment method[105,121] and caries risk status be re-evaluated on a continual, recurrent basis (Figure 7).[35,50]

Conscientious use of conventional prevention methods is sufficient for most low-risk patients; if additional fluoride treatment is indicated, a low-dose/high-frequency application is recommended. For moderate- and high caries risk individuals, fluoride prevention therapy alone is not the solution. For each client, the health intervention of caries control measures should be determined by a combination of considerations and risk factors: practical, based on individual client-centered needs and patient preference; scientific, that which demonstrates the greatest effect in preventing caries based on evidence-based research, daily oral hygiene habits, nutrition and diet, high levels of *S. mutans* in saliva (>10^6 CFU/mL saliva), access to routine oral healthcare and fluoride exposure, existence of exposed root surfaces, and multisurface restorations; and other socio-economic factors.[8,17]

It is suggested that some oral healthcare practitioners currently lack what is considered to be the best evidence-based clinical practice. Cooperation and communicating recent research findings between Practice-Based Research Networks, organized oral healthcare, and educational institutes is important in advancing scientific evidence

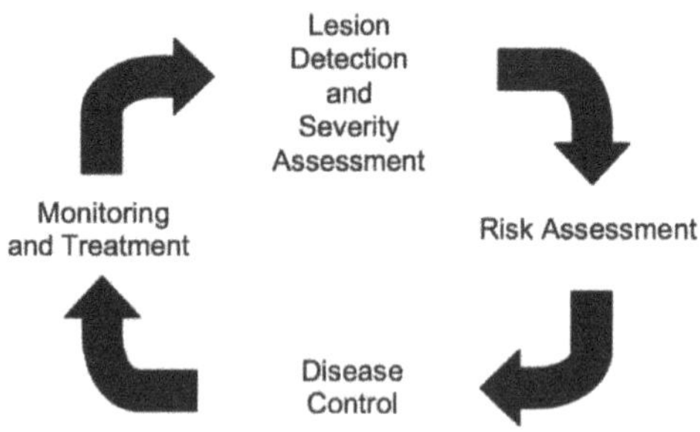

Figure 7. Minimally invasive dentistry treatment approach and modern caries management plan of dental caries as an infectious disease. Adapted from Ref. [35]

into the daily clinical practice of all oral healthcare providers. For caries prevention and therapeutic fluoride regimens in particular, this movement of evidence-based research to the practicing oral healthcare team is crucially important.

References

1. Cury, J. A.; de Oliveira, B. H. ; dos Santos, A. P. P.; Tenuta, L. M. A. *Dent. Mater.* **2016**, *32*, 323–333.
2. Riley, J. L. III; Gordan, V. V.; Rindal, D. B.; Fellows, J. L.; Ajmo, C. T.; Amundson, C.; Anderson, G. A. *Community Dent. Oral. Epidemiol.* **2010**, *38*, 360–370.
3. Centers for Disease Control and Prevention. Recommendations for using fluoride to prevent and control dental caries in the United States, MMWR, **2001**, *50*, 1–42.
4. Burt, B. A. *Acta Odontol. Scand.* **1998**, *56*, 3.
5. Featherstone, J. D. *J. Am. Dent. Assoc.* **2000**, *131*, 887–899.
6. Arends. J.; Christoffersen, J. *J. Dent. Res.* **1990**, *69* (Special Issue), 601–605.
7. Sheiham, A.; James, W. P. *J. Dent. Res.* **2015**, *94*, 1341–1347.
8. Tenuta, L. M. A.; Cury, J. A. *Braz. Oral. Res.* **2010**, *24* (Special Issue 1), 9–17.
9. Dibdin, G. H.; Shellis, R. P. *J. Dent. Res.* **1988**, *67* (6), 890–895.
10. van Houte, J.; Russo, J.; Prostak, K. S. *J. Dent. Res.* **1989**, *68* (3), 451–459.
11. Paes Leme, A. K.; Koo, H.; Bellato, C. M.; Bedi, G.; Cury, J. A. *J. Dent. Res.* **2006**, *85*, 878–887.
12. Loesche, W. J. *Microbiol. Rev.* **1986**, *50*, 353–380.
13. Emilson, C. G. *J. Dent. Res.* **1994**, *73*, 682–691.
14. Proceedings of a Joint IADR/ORCA International Symposium on Fluorides: Mechanisms of an action and recommendations for use, March 21–24, **1989**. Callaway Gardens Conference Center, Pine Mountain, Georgia. *J. Dent. Res.* **1990**, *69* (Special Issue).
15. Cury, J. A.; Tenuta, L. M. A. *Braz. Oral Res.* **2009**, *23* (Suppl 1), 23–30.
16. Cury, J. A.; Tenuta, L. M. *Adv. Dent. Res.* **2008**, *20* (1), 13–16.

17. Seale, N. S.; Daubert, D. M. The use and efficacy of professional topical fluorides, **2010**. Available at: https://www.dentalacademyofce.com/courses/2081/pdf/1103ceivarnish_web.pdf (Consulted July 2016).
18. Gerth, H. U. V.; Dammaschke, T.; Schafer, E.; Zuchner, H. *Dent. Mater.* **2007**, *23*, 1521–1528.
19. Featherstone, J. D. B.; Ten Cate, J. M. In: *Fluroide in Dentistry.* Ekstrand, J.; Fejerskov, O.; Silverstone, L. M., eds. (Copenhagen: Munskgaard International Publishers, **1988**), pp. 125–149.
20. Dean, H. T. *Publ. Health Rep.* **1938**, *53*, 1443–1452.
21. Chow, L. C. *J. Dent. Res.* **1990**, *69* (Special Issue), 595–600.
22. White, D. J.; Nancollas, G. H. *J. Dent. Res.* **1990**, *69* (Special Issue), 587–594.
23. Lussi, A.; Hellwig, E.; Klimek, J. *Schweiz Monatsschr Zahnmed,* **2012**, *122*, 1030–1036.
24. Muller, F.; Zeitz, C.; Ehses, K.; H.; Soldera, F.; Schmauch, J.; Hannig, M.; Hufner, S.; Jacobs, K. *Langmuir* **2010**, *26* (24), 18750–18759.
25. Gerould, C. H. *J. Dent. Res.* **1945**, *24*, 223–233.
26. Larson, M. J.; Richard, A. *Caries Res.* **2001**, *35*, 57–60.
27. Van den Hoek, W. G. M.; Feenstra, T. P.; De Bruyn, P. L. *J. Phys. Chem.* **1980**, *84*, 3312–3317.
28. Carrotte, P. *Br. Dent. J.* **2004**,*25*,735–743.
29. Schäfer, E.; Bössmann, K. *J. Endod.* **2005**, *31*, 53–56.
30. Dammaschke, T.; Eickmeier, M.; Schäfer, E.; Danesh, G.; Ott, K. H. R. *Acta Odontol. Scand.* **2005**, *63*, 110–114.
31. McDonagh, M. S.; Whiting, P. F.; Wilson, P. M.; Sutton, A. J.; Chestnutt, I.; Cooper, J.; Misso, K.; Bradley, M.; Treasure, E. *BMJ.* **2000**, 7, *321* (7265), 855–859.
32. Dean H. T. On the epidemiology of fluorine and dental caries. In: Gies W. J., ed. *Fluorine in Dental Public Health* (New York, NY: New York Institute of Clinical Oral Pathology, **1945**), pp. 19–30.
33. Oliveby, A.; Twetman, S.; Ekstrand, J. *Caries Res.* **1990**, *24* (1), 44–47.
34. Casarin, R. C.; Fernandes, D. R.; Lima-Arsati, Y. B.; Cury, J. A. *Rev Saude Publica.* **2007**, *41* (4), 549–556.
35. Anusavice, K. J. *J. Dent. Educ.* **2005**, *69*, 538–554.

36. Tenuta, L. M.; Cerezetti, R. V.; Del Bel Cury, A. A.; Tabchoury, C. P.; Cury, J. A. *J. Dent. Res.* **2008**, *87* (11), 1032–1036.
37. Marinho, V. C.; Higgins, J. P.; Sheiham, A.; Logan, S. *Cochrane Database Syst. Rev.* **2004**, (1), CD002781.
38. Marinho, V. C. *Adv. Dent. Res.* **2008**, *20*, 3–7.
39. Marinho, V. C.; Higgins, J. P.; Logan, S.; Sheiham, A. *J. Dent. Edu.* **2003**, *67*, 448–458.
40. Calvo, A. F. B.; Tabchoury, C. P. M.; Del Bel Cury, A. A.; Tenuta, L. M. A.; da Silva, W. J.; Cury, J. A. *Caries Res.* **2012**, *46*, 31–37.
41. American Dental Association. *JADA* **2006**, *137*, 1151–1158.
42. ADA. *JADA* **2006**, *137* (8), 1151–1159.
43. Miller, E. K.; Vann, W. F. *J. Clin. Pediatri. Dent.* **2008**, *32* (4), 259–264.
44. Fejerskov, O.; Thylstrup, A.; Larsen, M. J. *Acta Odontol Scand.* **1981**, *39*, 241–249.
45. Ogaard, D.; Seppa, L.; Rolla, G. *Adv. Dent. Res.* **1994**, *8*, 190–201.
46. Ten Cate, J. M. *Eur. J. Oral. Sci.* **1997**, *222*, 219–227.
47. Beltran-Aguilar, E. D.; Goldstein, J. W.; Lockwood, S. A. *J. Am. Dent. Assoc.* **2000**, *131*, 589–596.
48. Weintraub, J. A.; Ramos-Gomez, F.; Jue, B.; Shain, S.; Hoover, C.; Featherstone, J.; Gansky, S. *J. Dent. Res.* **2006**, *85*, 172–176.
49. Stearns, S. C.; Rozier, R. G.; Pahel, B. T.; Park, J. Y.; Quinonez, R. B. (ppt presentation). https://studylib.net/doc/11616531/effects-of-expanding-preventive-dental-care-in-medical-of (Accessed in July 2016).
50. Marinho, V. C. C.; Higgins, J. P. T.; Logan, S.; Sheiham, A., *Cochrane Database Syst. Rev.* **2003**, (1), D002278.
51. Farhadian, N.; Miresmaeili, A.; Eslami, B.; Mehrabi, S. *Am. J. Ortho Dentofacial Orthop.* **2008**, *133* (Suppl 4), S95–S98.
52. Vivaldi-Rodrigues, G.; Demito, C. F.; Bowman, S. J.; Ramos, A. L. *World J. Orthod.* **2006**, *7* (2), 138–144.
53. Gontijo, L.; de Almedia Cruz, R.; Brandao, P. R. *Braz. Dent. J.* **2007**, *18* (1), 49–53.
54. Petersson, L.; Twetman, S.; Dahlgren, H.; Norlund, A.; Holm, A-K.; Nordenram, G. *et al. Ata Odontol. Scand.* **2004**, *62* (3), 170–176.
55. Paes Leme, A. F.; Dalcico, R.; Tabchoury, C. P.; Del Bel Curry, A. A.; Rosalen, P. L.; Cury, J. A. *J. Dent. Res.* **2004**, *83* (1), 71–75.

56. Marinho, V. C. C.; Higgins, J. P. T.; Logan, S.; Sheiham, A. *Cochrane Database Syst. Rev.* **2003**, (1), CD002278.
57. Bratthall, D.; Hansel-Petersson, G.; Sundberg, H. *Eur. J. Oral. Sci.* **1996**, *104*, 416–422.
58. Cury, J. A.; Tenuta, L. M.; Ribeiro, C. C.; Paes Leme, A. F. *Braz. Dent. J.* **2004**, *15* (3), 167–174.
59. World Heath Organization. *The World Oral Health Report 2003* (Geneva: WHO, **2003**), pp. 4–19.
60. Serra, M. C.; Cury, J. A. *Rev. Assoc. Paul. Cir. Dent.* **1992**, *46* (5), 875–878 (in Portuguese).
61. Zamataro, C. B.; Tenuta, L. M.; Cury, J. A. *Eur. Arch. Paediatr. Dent.*. **2008**, *9* (2), 90–93.
62. Tenuta, L. M.; Zamataro, C. B.; Del Bel Cury, A. A.; Tabchoury, C. P.; Cury, J. A. *Caries Res.* **2009**, 43(4), 278–285.
63. Cenci, M. S.; Tenuta, L. M.; Pereira-Cenci, T.; Del Bel Cury, A. A.; ten Cate, J. M.; Cury, J. A. *Caries Res.* **2008**, *42* (5), 369–379.
64. Marinho, V. C.; Higgins, J. P.; Logan, S.; Sheiham, A., *Cochrane Database Syst. Rev.* **2003**, (4), CD002782.
65. Twetman, S.; Axelsson, S.; Dahlgren, H.; Holm, A. K.; Kallestal, C.; Lagerlof, F. *et al. Acta Odontol. Scand.* **2003**, *61* (6), 247–255.
66. Baysan, A.; Lynch, E.; Ellwood, R.; Davies, R.; Petersson, L.; Borsboom, P. *Caries Res.* **2001**, *35* (1), 41–46.
67. Cury, J. A.; do Amaral, R. C.; Tenuta, L. M. A.; Del Bel Cury, A. A.; Tabchoury, C. P. M., *Eur. J. Oral. Sci.* **2010**, *118* (4), 370–375.
68. Ammari, A. B.; Bloch-Zupan, A.; Ashley, P. F. *Caries Res.* **2003**, *37* (2), 85–92.
69. Walsh, T.; Worthington, H. V.; Glenny, A. M.; Appelbe, P.; Marinho, V. C.; Shi, X. *Cochrane Database Syst. Rev.* **2010**, *20* (1), CD007868.
70. Lima, T. J.; Ribeiro, C. C. C.; Tenuta, L. M. A.; Cury, J. A., *Caries Res.* **2008**, 42(1), 46–50.
71. Kidd, E. A. M.; Fejerskov, O. *J. Dent. Res.* **2004**, *83* (Special N° C), C35–C38.
72. Griffin, S. O.; Regnier, E.; Griffin, P. M.; Huntley V. *J. Dent. Res.* **2007**, *86*, 410–415.
73. Mejare, I.; Lingstrom, P.; Petersson, L. G.; Holm, A. K.; Twetman, S.; Kallestal, C. *et al. Acta Odontol. Scand.* **2003**, *61* (6), 321–330.

74. Beauchamp, J.; Caufield, P. W.; Crall, J. J.; Donyl. K.; Feigal, R.; Gooch, B. *et al. J. Am. Dent. Assoc.* **2008**, *139*, 257–268.
75. Oong, E. M.; Griffin, S. O.; Kohn, W. G.; Gooch, B. F.; Caufield, P. W. *J. Am. Dent. Assoc.* **2008**, *139*, 271–278.
76. Ahovuo-Saloranta, A.; Hiiri, A.; Nordblad, A.; Worthington, H.; Mäkelä, M. *Cochrane Database Syst Rev.* **2008**, *8*(4), CD001830.
77. Uribe, S. *Evid. Based Dent.* **2005**, *6*, 35.
78. Ahovuo-Saloranta, A.; Forss, H.; Walsh, T.; Hiiri, A.; Nordblad, A.; Makela, M. *et al. Cochrane Database Syst. Rev.* **2013**, *3*, CD001830.
79. Chadwick, B. L.; Treasure, E. T.; Playle, R. A. *Caries Res.* **2005**, *39*, 34–40.
80. Main, P. A.; Lewis, D. W.; Hawkins, R. J. *J. Can. Dent. Assoc.* **1997**, *63*, 542.
81. Clarkson, J.E.; Turner, S.; Grimshaw, J. M.; Ramsay, C. R.; Johnston, M.; Scott, A. *et al. J. Dent. Res.* **2008**, *87*, 640–644.
82. Benelli, E. M.; Serra, M. C.; Rodrigues Jr, A. L.; Cury, J. A. *Caries Res.* **1993**, *27* (4), 280–284.
83. Randall, R. C.; Wilson, N. H. *J. Dent. Res.* **1999**, *78* (2), 628–637.
84. Hara, A. T.; Turssi, C. P.; Ando, M.; González-Cabezas, C.; Zero, D. T.; Rodrigues, A. L. Jr; Serra, M. C.; Cury, J. A. *Caries Res.* **2006**, *40* (5), 435–439.
85. Benson, P. E.; Parkin, N.; Dyer, F.; Millett, D. T.; Furness, S.; Germain, P. *Cochrane Database Syst. Rev.* **2013**, *12*, CD003809.
86. Tufekci, E.; Dixon, J. S.; Gunsolley, J. C.; Lindauer, S. J. *Angle Orthod.* **2011**, *81*, 206–210.
87. Lucchese, A.; Gherlone, E. *Eur. J. Orthod.* **2013**, *35*, 664–648.
88. Millett, D. T.; Glenny, A. M.; Mattick, C. R.; Hickman, J.; Mandall, N. A. *Cochrane Database Syst. Rev.* **2007**, CD004485.
89. Millet, D. T.; Mandall, N. A.; Mattick, R. C.; Hickman, J.; Glenny, A. M. *Cochrane Database Syst. Rev.* **2011**, CD008236.
90. Derks, A.; Katsaros, C.; Frencken, J. E.; van't Hof, M. A.; Kuijpers-Jagtman, A. M. *Caries Res.* **2004**, *38*, 413–420.
91. Rogers, S.; Chadwick, B.; Treasure, E., *AMJ Orthod. Dentofac. Orthop.* **2010**, *138*, 390. e1-e8, discussion-1.
92. Tenuta, L. M. A.; Cury, J. A. *Fluoreto na práctica de promoção de saúde individual e coletiva* (Rio de Janeiro: ABOPREV, **2005**). Cadernos da ABOPREV IV, in Portuguese.

93. Brasil. Ministério da Saúde. *Guia de recomendações para o uso de fluoretos no Brasil* (Brasília: Ministério da Saúde, **2009**), p. 53, in Portuguese.
94. Splieth, C. H.; Nourallah, A. W.; Konig, K. G. *Clin. Oral. Investig.* **2004**, *8* (1), 6–10.
95. Marinho, V. C.; Higgins, J. P.; Sheiham, A.; Logan, S. *Fluoride Toothpastes for Preventing Dental Caries in Children and Adolescents* (Chichester, UK: John Wiley & Sons, **2004**).
96. Marinho, V. C.; Higgins, J. P.; Sheiham, A.; Logan, S. *Cochrane Database Syst. Rev.* **2007**, (1), CD002781.
97. Anusavice, K. J.; Denn, D. K. *Crit. Rev. Oral Biol. Med.* **2001**, *12* (5), 368–372.
98. Bader, J. D.; Shugars, D. A. *J. Dent. Res.* **1993**, *72* (5), 891–896.
99. Bader, J. D.; Shugars, D. A. *J. Dent. Educ.* **1995**, *59* (1), 61–95.
100. Bader, J. D.; Shugars, D. A. *J. Public Health Dent.* **1995**, *55* (3), 181–188.
101. Lewis, D. W.; Kay, E. J.; Main, P. A.; Pharoah, M. G.; Csima, A. *J. Public Health Dent.* **1996**, *56* (4), 176–181.
102. Söderholm, K-J; Antonsson, D. E; Fischlschweiger, W. In: *Quality Evaluation of Dental Restorations: Criteria for Placement and Replacement*, Anusavice, K. J., ed. (Chicago: Quintessence Publishing Co. 1989), pp. 95–108.
103. Jensen, O. E.; Handelman, S. L.; Iker, H. P. *Oral Surg. Oral Med. Oral Pathol.* **1987**, *63*(3), 254–257.
104. Ekstrand, K. R.; Ricketts, D. N.; Kidd, E. A.; Qvist, V.; Schou, S. *Caries Res.* **1998**, *32* (4), 247–254.
105. Anderson, M. H.; Bales, D. J.; Omnell, K-A. *J. Am. Dent. Assoc.* **1993**, *124*, 37–44.
106. Bader, J. D.; Shugars, D. A. *J. Evid. Based Dent. Pract.* **2006**, *6*, 91–100.
107. Hudson, P. *J. Am. Dent. Assoc.* **2004**, *135* (6), 760–764.
108. Nicholson, J. W. *Tex. Dent. J.* **2003**, *120* (10), 960–969.
109. Murdoch-Kinch, C. A.; McLean, M. E. *J. Am. Dent. Assoc.* **2003**, 134(1), 87–95.
110. Peters, M. C.; McLean, M. E. *J. Adhes. Dent.* **2001**, *3* (1), 7–16.
111. Peters, M. C.; McLean, M. E. *J. Adhes. Dent.* **2001**, *3* (1), 17–31.

112. Tyas, M. J.; Anusavice, K. J.; Frencken, J. E.; Mount, G. J. *Int. Dent. J.* **2000**, *50* (1), 1–12.
113. Leben, J. R. *J. Am. Dent. Assoc.* **1997**, *128* (10), 1356.
114. McIntyre, J. *Ann. R. Australas Coll. Dent. Surg.* **1994**, *12*, 72–79.
115. Simonsen, R. J. *Compendium* **1987**, *8* (6), 428–430, 432.
116. Brennan, D. S.; Spencer, A. J. *J. Dent.* **2007**, *35*, 570–577.
117. Yorty, J. S.; Brown, K. B. *J. Dent. Educ.* **1999**, *63* (10), 745–747.
118. Brennan, D. S.; Spencer, A. J. *Community Dent. Oral Epidemiol.* **2005**, *33*, 181–195.
119. Thomas, R. K. *Mkt. Hlth. Svcs.* **2000**, *20*, 13–18.
120. de la Cruz, G. G.; Rozier, R. G.; Slade, G. *Pediatrics* **2004**, *114*, 642–652.
121. Anusavice, K. J. *J. Dent. Educ.* **1997**, *61* (11), 895–905.
122. Scheie, A. A. In: *Clinical and Biological Aspects of Dentifrices*, Embery, G.; Rölla G., eds. (Oxford: Oxford University Press, **1992**), Chapter 5; pp. 29–39.
123. Kay, E.; Locker, D. *Community Dent. Health.* **1998**, *15* (3), 132–144.
124. Bertassoni, L.E.; Habelitz, S.; Mashall, S. J.; Marshall, G. W. *J Biomech* **2011**, *44* (1), 176–181.
125. Chan, J. T.; Warren, D. P.; Henson, H. A. *J. Gt. Houst. Dent. Soc.* **1996**, *68*, 22–24.
126. Hebling, J.; Santos-Pinto, L. M.; Cury, J. A. *Rev. Bras. Odontol.* **1995**, *52*, 30–35.
127. Marsh, P. D. *Int. J. Dent. Hyg.* **2006**, *4* (Suppl 1), 3–10, discussion 50–52.
128. Mendes, S.; Souza, I. P.; Cury, J. A. *Rev. Odontol. Univ. São Paulo* **1996**, *10*, 281–285 (in Portuguese).
129. Piexoto, E. M. C.; Silva, M. F. A. *Rev. Bras. Odontol.* **1992**, *4*, 1–4 (in Portuguese).
130. Ripa, L.W. *J. Dent. Res.* **1990**, *69* (Special Issue), 786–796.
131. Rolla, G.; Saxegaard, E. *J. Dent. Res.* **1990**, *69* (Special Issue), 780–785.
132. Tanka, M.; Moreno, E. C.; Margolis, H. C. *Archs. Oral Biol.* **1993**, *38* (10), 863–869.
133. ten Cate, J. M.; Simons, Y. M.; van-Strijp, A. J. *J. Dent. Res.* **1988**, *67*, 114.

134. Tsuda, H.; Arends, J. *Caries Res.* **1993**, *27*, 249–257.
135. Villena, R.S.; Tenuta, L. M. A.; Cury, J. A. *Braz. Dent. J.* **2009**, *20* (1), 37–41.
136. Wefel, J. S.; Wei, S. H. Y. *Pediatr. Dent.* **1979**, *1*, 97–99.
137. Wei, S. H. Y.; Hattab, F. M. *J. Dent. Res.* **1987**, *66*, 242, Abst. No. 1086.
138. Wei, S. H. Y.; Lau, E. W. S.; Hattab, F. N. *J. Dent. Res.* **1988**, *67*, 114, Abst. No. 13.

Chapter 5

Mercury Toxicity

Gelson Luis Adabo

Department of Dental Materials and Prosthodontics, Faculty of Dentistry of Araraquara, UNESP. R. Humaitá, 1680, Araraquara — SP, 14801-385, Brazil

Mercury is a highly toxic heavy metal that is in liquid state at ambient temperature. It exists naturally, and is released from the earth's crust, by rock outgassing, or volcanic activity. Mercury residues are also produced by anthropogenic activities, such as mercury extraction, petroleum industry, coal-burning power stations, residential heating systems, waste incinerators, and gold mining. Mercury vapor remains in the atmosphere for months and can be found in the metallic or elemental form (Hg^0), inorganic form (Hg^{1+} and Hg^{2+}), and organic form (carbon-containing compounds). Mercury is hazardous to human health. It may affect mainly the respiratory, nervous, renal, and immune system, and is considered by the World Health Organization (WHO) as one of the 10 chemicals that are a major public health concern.[1] It spreads globally by atmospheric transport and can impair human health directly or by bioaccumulation via ecosystems.

1. Introduction

Dental amalgam is the most popular material for direct restoration in posterior teeth. Silver–tin–copper–zinc alloy particles are mixed together with elemental mercury (typically 1:1 by weight) producing an amalgam that is inserted into a tooth cavity, and carved into the tooth's form. The crystallized amalgam acquires mechanical properties to resist the chewing force, and it may last in the mouth for more than 20 years. It was introduced in 1830, and at the beginning of the 1900s, the first approved formulation was developed. Since its introduction, it has been used because of its suitable physical properties, high longevity, low cost, low technical sensitivity, and efficient sealing at the interface to dental tissues. These characteristics make dental amalgam highly relevant to use in large dental care programs for poor populations. Regardless of the efficacy of this biomaterial, the lack of esthetics and concerns about the effect of the mercury on the health of patients and professionals, as well as environmental issues, place dental amalgam at the center of a great debate.

2. Historical

The controversy is as old as dental amalgam. In 1848, the American Society of Dental Surgeons stated that using mercury-based restorations constituted malpractice.[2] The toxicity of mercury is fairly known, but some dentists and dental professional organizations, such as the Fédération Dentaire Internationale (FDI),[3] the European Union agency "Scientific Committee on Emerging and Newly Identified Health Risks (SCENIHR),[4] and the American Dental Association (ADA),[5] have considered amalgam safe for patients because they believe that amalgam has a minimal amount of unreacted mercury after setting. On the other hand, these agencies recognize the risks for dental staff because of mercury vapor produced during manipulation to insert a new restoration or for removal of an old one. In addition, mercury vapor can be released into the dental office from spread mercury and solid fresh amalgam residue. However, those agencies have considered that the occupational risks can be managed if simple hygiene precautions and technical procedures to minimize the exposition to mercury are followed.

The Minamata Bay disaster, in Japan, highlighted how hazardous mercury can be. In 1956, an unknown disease affected about 3,000 people, characterized by severe neurologic signs and symptoms. Minamata was a poor fishing village, where in the 1930s a plant was built for manufacturing acetaldehyde and polyvinyl chloride using mercury. The company began to discharge mercury residues into the bay, and after decades, the ecosystem reached a critical pollution level. The metallic mercury was converted into methylmercury by water organisms, and this lead to the contamination of the entire food chain — especially shellfish and predator fish — which is a typical food for that population. Eventually, "Minamata Disease", as it was known at that time, was diagnosed as result of poisoning by methylmercury. Approximately 700 people who developed the disease, died. In 1971, another famous mercury poisoning occurred in Iraq, known as the "Basra poison grain disaster", when the population made flour to cook bread using grain for planting that had been treated with a methylmercury fungicide. This caused mercury poisoning in more than 6,000 people and lead to 500 deaths. These tragedies brought into question the safety of mercury for all applications, including dentistry.

Beginning in the 1990s, several non-expert newspaper and magazines published news articles, and there were television programs showing the dangers of amalgam restoration. It spread the controversy to the public, and patients became anxious about the effects of mercury from amalgam restorations on their general health, asking for amalgam fillings in tooth-colored restorations to be replaced. One of the most striking pieces of news was presented on the "60 Minutes" news program (CBS television). An interview with Dr. Murray Vimy (University of Calgary) who performed an experiment adding radioactive marker in amalgam fillings in sheep's teeth showed how quickly mercury could be identified in the organs, especially in the kidney. Since then, replacement of amalgam restorations with mercury-free materials has been indicated by some orthomolecular medicine practitioners, claiming that the mercury is responsible for several systemic diseases or chronic illness.[6]

3. Toxicology

Mercury toxicity depends on its form (elemental, mercury salts, organic), time of exposure, and dose, which may have different target organs. Organomercury, as ethylmercury that was widely used as a preservative in some vaccines and especially methylmercury (MeHg) found in seafood, is the most hazardous for human health. Elemental mercury (Hg^0) from the atmosphere or wastewater accumulates in water and is converted into organic mercury by microorganisms, which contaminate the food chain of aquatic organisms, particularly fish. Even though acute poisoning is rare, chronic consumption of contaminated fish remains relevant, especially for pregnant women and infants. MeHg from mercury-rich food enters the human body via intestinal absorption, and when it reaches the bloodstream, it adheres mainly to cysteine that is delivered to the whole body. The maximum level in the blood occurs at about 2 days after exposure. After 4 days, MeHg is distributed throughout the body and can be found in the brain, peripheral nerves, bone marrow, liver, and kidneys.[7] MeHg can cross the placenta and the blood–brain barrier (BBB), and depending on the intensity and individual susceptibility, it may impair the growth and migration of neurons in fetal brain.[8]

Mercury salts may be found in cosmetics and can be absorbed through the skin. Chronic poisoning is difficult to diagnose because the symptoms may be confused with other diseases. In addition, acute poisoning does not impair the neural system, but a high dose affects the gastrointestinal tract, causing severe symptoms such as vomiting, hematemesis, intestinal perforation, proctitis, and may evolve to cardiovascular collapse and renal failure.[9]

Chronic poisoning by mercuric mercury may occur associated with mercury vapor poisoning in workers who are occupationally exposed. The target organs are the kidneys, which lead to renal tubular necrosis and/or autoimmune glomerulonephritis. However, mercurous mercury is less dangerous. It was used as a laxative and is poorly absorbed by the intestine, but a part of it is transformed into mercuric mercury that can be absorbed and cause some toxicity. Acute poisoning with mercury salts can also lead to death.[9]

Elemental mercury (Hg^0) is a liquid and vaporizes at room temperature, but the vapor will not be perceived because it does not have an odor or a color. Hg^0 is highly lipid soluble — 80% of the inhaled mercury vapor is retained in the body. It is absorbed by the lungs and enters in the alveolar membranes, where it is quickly distributed to the whole body. When it reaches the bloodstream, part of the H^0, which is a significant neural toxin, will remain in plasma and part will be rapidly converted into its inorganic form (Hg^{2+}) by the red blood cells, but this reaction is not quick enough to prevent a small portion from crossing the BBB. In the central nervous system (CNS), the oxidized form is unable to cross the BBB because of its low lipophilicity; the inorganic mercury will be attached to the sulfidryl groups in proteins to be immobilized in brain for years to decades as mercuric selenide, especially in the cerebellum. The half-life of the oxidized mercury in blood is quite short (1–4 days), and it is slowly excreted in urine, feces, and breast milk for up to 90 days. However, part of the mercury remains mainly in the kidney, brain, and in lower amounts in the lung, breast, thyroid, adrenals, pancreas, liver, gastrointestinal tract, testes, prostate, muscles, exocrine glands, and immune system cells.

Chronic poisoning produces mainly neurological dysfunction, which varies according to the severity. Acute elemental mercury poisoning is rare, and signs and symptoms include weakness, myalgia, chills, fever, nausea, vomiting, diarrhea, dyspnea, cough, and chest pain. Lungs are more severely affected, and the pulmonary toxicity may lead to necrotizing bronchitis and pneumonitis, compromising respiratory function. There is risk of death, but recovery may be complete or partial with subsequent residual interstitial fibrosis.[10] Symptoms of chronic poisoning resulting from a low dose include subtle neurological effects impairing psychomotor and cognitive functions. People poisoned with a low dose describe fatigue, weakness, anorexia, and gastrointestinal disturbance, which are non-specific, and low-dose poisoning is difficult to diagnose. However, high levels of chronic poisoning produce tremor, depression, loss of memory, severe behavior and personality changes, emotional excitability, fatigue, psychotic reactions (delirium, hallucinations, and suicidal tendency) and gingivitis, which characterize the erethism syndromes. In the kidneys, mercury produces reactive oxygen species, which have nephrotoxic effect even in subcytotoxic doses.

The kidney is composed of tubular segments with different functions, and is an excretion route for waste products from metabolic process, drugs, and xenobiotics, which can potentially lead to kidney injury. Because of injury to tubular cells, cytoplasmic proteins are released into the urine, which can indicate renal tubular damage, and which might indicate a potential toxicant based on the eliminated protein. Theoretically, mercury accumulates in the proximal tubules, and the presence of glutathione-S-transferases-α in urine suggests proximal tubule damage and possible kidney injury. Albumin is another biomarker of interest, if this protein is almost totally filtered by the proximal tubules. When the albumin concentration is high, it can indicate a reduction in glomerular filtration and tubular absorptive capacity. It may predict a renal disease or nephrotoxicant exposure.[11]

Mercury concentration in blood and urine are commonly used to measure the risk of poisoning, but these tests are not able to indicate the mercury load in the organs. Considering that the half-life of mercury in bloodstream is short (up to 4 days), it is not feasible to quantify the amount of mercury accumulated in the body once the blood exam reports a picture of that short period. The mercury concentration in urine represents a better measure because it shows an estimative of mercury intake, but it does not indicate mercury in the target tissues.[12] Moreover, interpersonal variations should be considered.

Taking into account that CNS is one of mercury's main target organs, neurological tests are proposed to aid in diagnosing mercury poisoning. Neuropsychologic and neurophysiologic status may include tests of attention, short-term memory, verbal memory, visual memory, manual dexterity, verbal fluency, visuomotor ability, depression and anxiety inventories, and electromyography and nerve conduction testing. The objective of the neurological tests is to correlate their results with a high concentration of mercury in the air, blood, and urine, as well as examinations to measure biomarkers of renal damage.

4. Mercury in Dentistry

Since the 1990s, the concerns about the effects of mercury from dental amalgam have started a major debate that pitted the US Food and Drug Administration (FDA),[13] FDI[3] and ADA,[1] which have defended the continued use of dental amalgam, against the recommendation of the WHO,[1] US Environmental Protection Agency (EPA), and other organizations, which propose banning amalgam. Eventually, in 2013, the Minamata Convention on Mercury, an international treaty signed by 140 countries, agreed to phase out production and trade of products containing mercury until 2020. However, even after the use of amalgam is phased out, it is not known how many teeth have been restored with amalgam. Therefore, the concern will remain for decades, because existing amalgam restorations may be negatively affecting patients' health, and removal of old amalgam restorations will produce mercury vapor and amalgam particles, putting dentists at an occupational risk and also having a negative effect on the environment.

4.1. *Amalgam Safety for Patients*

According to the WHO, dental amalgam is the primary intake source of mercury for the general population, which is higher than that found in food, water, and air.[1] Patients are exposed to some amalgam vapor for up to 2 weeks when the restorations are placed or removed for replacement. After placement, small quantities of mercury vapor leach continuously from the restoration, which is absorbed by inhalation (80%), for the lifetime of the restoration.

The actual mercury level in the body tissues may be directly verified only via autopsy. Guzzi *et al.*[14] reported on amalgam restorations and their relationship to mercury retained in brain, thyroid, and kidney in 18 cadavers. Cadavers with 12 or more restored teeth showed more mercury accumulated in the tissues than cadavers that had three or less restored teeth. Brain tissues (frontal lobe cortex and pituitary glands) showed significantly higher mercury level compared to thyroid and kidney tissues. Bjorkman *et al.*[15] found a strong correlation between the number of amalgam restorations and mercury in the occipital cortex and pituitary and thyroid glands. Additionally, the kidneys are recognized as an important target organ, but autopsies have not found a large amount of mercury in these organs. Alcohol abuse may reduce the mercury load, but it is unclear how alcohol interferes with the metabolism of mercury.[16]

The maximum value of urinary mercury concentration (HgU) that is considered safe for most people in the general population is less than 10 μg Hg/L. There is a positive correlation between HgU and the number of amalgam surfaces. Each amalgam restoration surface will add approximately 0.1 μg Hg/L to the HgU.[16] However, mercury concentration in blood and urine seems not to be correlated with disease symptoms that are associated with amalgam restorations.

Based on the number of restorations, the patient's eating habits, and chewing gum and bruxism, daily mercury uptake may reach 22 μg/d, but for most people the dose is below to 5 μg/d.[18] If the limit exposure to mercury vapor (0.3 mg/m^3) is taken, then the exposure is estimated to be equivalent to 4.9 μg/d intake.[19] In other words, people who have large amount of amalgam restorations would have exposure to mercury as if they were in an environment with the maximum of mercury vapor acceptable as safe. In 2011, Richardson *et al.*[16] estimated that 67.2 million Americans exceeded those conditions. However, while most people are resistant to long-term, low-level mercury exposure, part of the population is sensitive to its toxic effects, even those who have normal blood and urine mercury levels.[10]

"Amalgam-disease", which has symptoms that include buccal discomfort, diffuse body pain, weakness, fatigue, and dizziness, and some diseases such as thyroid dysfunction, anemia, cardiopathy, and renal disease, has been self-reported by patients who suspect being chronically poisoned by amalgam restorations. However, this "disease" might be related to psychological factors, and it has been found in patients who have a tendency toward somatization.[20] Björkman *et al.*[21] studied the concentrations of immune mediators (cytokines, chemokines, and growth factors) in serum in patients with health complaints attributed to amalgam after removal of all dental amalgam restorations and compared with a healthy group. At baseline, patients with health complaints had slightly higher value in immune mediators in serum, but 12 months after amalgam removal, the concentrations of Th1-type proinflammatory marker decreased to the same extent as what was reported for the reference group. Gottwald *et al.*[22] studied the relationship between toxicological, allergological, and psychological aspects in patients with amalgam-associated complaints with a group with similar numbers of amalgam fillings. There was higher atopic predisposition, psychic strain, and depression scores in the group of patients with complaints, but toxic exposure to mercury was not different from the control group.[22] Sjursen *et al.*[23] compared a group of patients who attributed health complaints to amalgam filling to a control group with no intervention. Amalgam restorations were replaced with mercury-free material, and the subjective health complaints were measured after 3 months, and at 1 and 3 years after intervention. The results showed a reduction in the symptoms, but it was not possible to conclude if the subjective improvement in health was a result of a psychological effect of the elimination of the "amalgam anxiety".[23] Melchart *et al.*[24] treated patients with subjective complaints, which could not be explained by a medical or psychological disorder, using three different strategies, removal of dental amalgam, removal in combination with high-dose vitamin, and trace element therapy, with a non-removal group whose patients participated in a health promotion program only. The authors observed similar reduction in the subjective complaints, for both the group with amalgam removal and the non-removal group that was treated by therapy of health promotion program.[24] In a complementary study, Weidenhammer *et al.*[25] investigated the effect of amalgam removal on women using a questionnaire comprising affective symptoms, neuropsychological symptoms, general somatic complaints, and some intraoral symptoms at baseline and after 12 months. There was no statistical difference between the group that had an amalgam restoration removed and the control group that was treated based on a psychological model as a strategy to enhance general health. Irrespective of amalgam removal, patients' symptoms decreased.[25]

However, the psychological role in "amalgam disease" may not completely explain the symptoms. Sensitive people who have certain genetic polymorphisms may exhibit different effects of mercury cytotoxicity. Thus, amalgam filling removal can effectively induce health improvement.[26]

The major concern is to estimate the actual risk for pregnant women and children. Considering that children are more susceptible to poisoning, the association of exposure from amalgam fillings in pregnant women or lactating mothers with neurodevelopmental disabilities in children has been investigated. There is evidence that elemental mercury can be found in amniotic fluid, placenta, and umbilical cord blood, as well as in fetal liver, kidney, and brain. Inhaled mercury vapor enters into the placenta and can cross the fetal BBB, leading to a concern about potential neurological damage. Moreover, lactating women may excrete mercury in colostrum and breast milk.[9,27–30] Regardless of the knowledge that breast milk can contain mercury, the WHO[1] recognizes the minimal risks of breastfeeding.

The impact of amalgam restorations on children has been studied by several authors. Bellinger *et al.*[31] is one of the most-cited studies. The authors compared the neuropsychological outcome of full-scale IQ scores, tests of memory and visuomotor ability, and renal glomerular function in 534 children who had teeth restored using amalgam (n = 267) or mercury-free materials (n = 267) during a 5-year follow-up period. No statistically significant differences were found between children in the two groups, either with regard to neuropsychological aspects or renal integrity; there was, however, a higher mean urinary mercury level in children with amalgam fillings.[31] DeRouen *et al.*[32] reported the results of a 7-year follow-up study after restorative procedures in children with amalgam restorations or composite restorations. Urinary mercury concentrations increased in children after placement of amalgam restorations, but there were no statistically significant differences in neurobehavioral and neurological tests between the groups.[32] A similar conclusion was drawn by Ye *et al.*[33] who measured the effect of mercury from amalgam fillings in children, aged 7–11 years, on renal function and neurobehavioral and neuropsychological performance, and concluded that HgU was slightly elevated in children with amalgam fillings, but there were no evidence of adverse effects on children's health.

However, genetic aspects and predispositions should be considered. Elimination of Hg involves glutathione-s-transferase (GST), and depends on enzymes related to glutathione synthesis and degradation. Selenium is structurally incorporated into selenoproteins, and it acts as an antioxidant, protecting against mercury toxicity. However, many glutathione-related enzymes are highly polymorphic, and the polymorphism may be related to disturbances in antioxidant action and to modulation of the detoxification system.[34,35] Woods *et al.* (2008)[11] evaluated urinary concentrations of biomarkers of renal proximal and distal tubular integrity in subjects (8–18 years old) who were treated with amalgam or composite. Biomarkers were annually measured for 7 years after the dental treatment. GST-π is the biomarker for distal tubular integrity, and its levels increased, especially in females.[11] Genetics vary for the heme pathway enzymes coproporphyrinogen oxidase (CPOX), metallothionein (MT), and catechol-O-methyltransferase (COMT), which have important roles in mercury metabolism and elimination, as well as in regulating dopamine and other neurotransmitter availability. In addition, polymorphism in the serotonin transporter may interfere with the limbic system that is associated with mood and behavior, as well as neuromotor function and visual perception.[36–40]

4.2. *Amalgam Safety for Dentists and Dental Staff*

The "mad-hatter syndrome" is the earliest occupational risk that was associated with using mercury, and it is characterized by symptoms such as tremors, irritability, and mental instability. In the 19th century, felt for hats was obtained from small animals' furs that was separated from the skin using mercuric nitrate. The felt was repeatedly immersed in boiling water to shape the hat, followed by drying. In this process, the room was saturated with mercury vapor causing a high level of chronic poisoning. The disease was generally represented as the eccentric "Mad Hatter" character seen in the book *Alice's Adventures in Wonderland*, written by Lewis Carroll in 1865.

Currently, those who work in chloralkali plants, with fluorescent lamps, switches, sphygmomanometers, and in the thermometer industry, as well as dentists, who work on placing or replacing amalgam restorations, are daily occupationally exposed. These people can be exposed to long-term low-dose mercury poisoning for years. Neuropsychological impairment is the main symptom seen in those workers, but psychological disorders encompass a wide array of social, behavioral, and physiological conditions with different etiologies, thus making it difficult to diagnose the condition earlier. Thus, workers exposed to a potentially hazardous environment must be examined periodically to monitor the chronic occupational mercury exposure risk or to diagnose the syndrome as early as possible.

The chloralkali industry is the main industrial activity that uses mercury for the production of sodium hydroxide and chlorine gas from sodium chloride, and this process involves electrolysis in which liquid mercury is used as cathode. Electrolysis separates the sodium and chlorine gas, but it results in the escape of high amounts of mercury vapor and chlorine gas into the air. Because of the intense mercury vapor generated during that activity, the parameters for occupational risk were usually based on the chloralkali plant working conditions. Fortunately, mercury vapor action is reduced in an environment where chlorine gas exists concomitantly, once mercury vapor (Hg^0) converts to $Hg^{+2}Cl_2^{-1}$. Hg^{+2} is not able to cross the BBB. Therefore, the mercury concentration limit that is acceptable for chloralkali workers may not be safe for other occupations.[16]

The maximum amount of mercury vapor suspended in the air at an ambient temperature of 24°C is 18 mg/m^3 before condensing. Regulatory agencies establish limits for mercury vapor in the air to which a worker can be exposed at any time. According to the Occupational Safety and Health Administration (OSHA), United States, the air concentration permissible exposure limit (PEL) is 0.1 mg/m^3. Canadian law determines that 0.15 mg/m^3 is an occupational exposure limit (ceiling exposure value). Other agencies established the time-weighted for hour/workday or hour/workweek. For the National Institute for Occupational Safety and Health (NIOSH), United States, the recommend exposure limit (REL) is 0.05 mg/m^3

for a 10-hour workday and a 40-hour work week. On the other hand, the European Scientific Committee on Occupational Exposure Limit Value determined 0.02 mg/m^3 for an eight-hour workday.

The concern about the impact of mercury vapor on dental staff is an important part of the mercury debate because dentists and dental assistants are exposed to mercury vapor during manipulation, insertion, carving, finishing, and polishing procedures to make an amalgam restoration, as well as exposure during removal of an old restoration. When amalgam is cut with dental burs, small particles are produced increasing the surface area and facilitating mercury vaporization. In addition to the immediate vapor generated to restore teeth or remove amalgam restorations, the rest of the liquid mercury and amalgam residue may increase the mercury vapor concentration in the dental office. Warwick *et al.*[41] measured mercury vapor levels released in the air during amalgam removal, using simultaneous water spray and suction, using suction only, and using neither suction nor water spray. The authors concluded that when water spray and suction were used, the arithmetic mean of mercury vapor was 0.008 mg/m^3, which is below the Occupational Health and Safety threshold limit value for an eight-hour time-weighted period (0.025 mg/m^3).[41] However, amalgam removal can produce particles in the range of 1–3 μm to submicron size that are fully respirable, and may be lodged in the lungs or ingested.[42] Therefore, the use of masks to block particles and to reduce vapor inhalation must be used during all procedures. However, the usual masks are not able to filter these particles and vapor. To be effective, a "half-mask" respirator with a pre-filter that is capable of removing particles as small as 0.3 microns is advisable.

In addition to the mercury vapor in air measurements, the urinary mercury levels should be tested periodically to identify occupational risks. The threshold limit of the biological exposure index (BEI) has been set to 35 μg Hg/g creatinine. Values above this limit reflect low mercury exposure, but impairments in neurological functions have been related to concentrations below 25 μg Hg/g creatinine.[43] Studies have shown that the HgU level is not directly related to health impairment of dental professionals. Symptoms of diseases that are typical of long-term chronic mercury poisoning have been reported, even for dentists and dental assistants who have HgU levels close to the general population.

Ritche *et al.*[44] compared health and cognitive function of dentists to a control group with a similar university education. The mercury vapor in the air at different places in the dental office related to the clinical procedure (amalgam insertion or removal) was also measured, and 68% of dental offices were shown to have mercury levels higher than the OES stated by the Health and Safety Executive (0.025 mg/m^3 for an eight-hour day). Among the psychological evaluation, there is significant difference in memory disturbance only, but it was not possible to correlate this result to mercury exposure. Dentists showed HgU levels over four times higher than that for the control group, but the average of HgU of dentists was below the biological exposure index (BEI).[44] In other study, Moen *et al.*[45] compared neurological symptoms of dental assistants to assistant nurses and concluded that, in the dental assistants group, the occurrence of neurological symptoms, psychosomatic symptoms, memory, concentration, fatigue, and sleep disturbance were significantly higher than the reference group, particularly with regard to memory deficit. No difference was found concerning mood, anxiety, and perception of health status.

For removing old amalgam restorations, dentists and dental assistants must use personal protective equipment (EEP). It is advisable to use a rubber dam to help contain the amalgam grinding debris. The restoration has to be cut by slicing with an efficient dental bur under a constant water spray and a high volume evacuation. To overcome uncertainty about dental staff safety regarding dental amalgam, the FDI[46] (2007) published a Mercury Hygiene Guidance, with the following recommendations: avoid direct skin contact with mercury or freshly mixed dental amalgam and exposure to potential sources of mercury vapor; train all personnel evolved with amalgam manipulation; install impervious, easy-to-clean surfaces including continuous seamless-sheet flooring extending up the walls; and work in well-ventilated areas, with fresh air exchanges and outside exhaust. If the work areas are air-conditioned, replace the air-conditioning filter periodically; use pre-capsulated amalgam; use an amalgamator with a completely enclosed arm that complies with international standard

ISO 7488; and recap single-use capsules after use, if feasible. Store them in a closed container and dispose of them through a mercury reclamation company that handles amalgam waste; use high-volume evacuation systems (fitted with traps or filters) when finishing or removing amalgam; clean amalgam contaminants from instruments before heat sterilization or heat disinfection; avoid heating mercury or amalgam or any equipment used with amalgam; and follow best management practices for amalgam waste.

Other dangerous sources of mercury vapor exposure are related to improper clean-up of the dental office, lack of ventilation and air-conditioner cleaning; porous and/or floors with cracks, such as carpet or wood, making it difficult to remove the mercury. Moreover, even an apparently insignificant amount of spilled mercury can produce high concentration of mercury vapor indoors.[1] In case of a mercury spill, the FDI recommends the following protocol: pick up the droplets using adhesive tape or a hypodermic syringe; mix small mercury spills (less than 10-g) with an alloy powder to form amalgam and add the resultant scrap to the scrap container; use a commercial mercury spill clean-up kit to manage larger spills (10-g or more); never use a vacuum cleaner of any type; do not use household cleaning products; do not pour or allow mercury to go down the drain; do not use a broom or a paintbrush to clean up mercury; and prevent people whose shoes may be contaminated with mercury from walking around or leaving the spill area until the mercury-contaminated items have been removed. Handling and use of bulk mercury is to be strongly discouraged. Check the dental surgical area for mercury vapor, preferably annually or after a spill clean-up.[46]

4.3. *Environmental Issues Related to Dental Amalgam*

Mercury into the atmosphere comes back to the surface via wet and dry atmospheric deposition. When mercury reaches the surface, its vapor may return to the atmosphere in a reemission cycle between the air, soil, and water, which gradually increases the accumulation, mainly in aquatic ecosystems. Elemental or inorganic mercury can convert to the organic form by anaerobic bacteria in natural settings.

Water with high mercury levels is the main environmental concern because it can potentially affect crops, drinking water, and particularly the aquatic food chain, causing bioaccumulation.

There is much uncertainty about estimating new emission and reemission of mercury into the atmosphere from natural and anthropogenic sources. In 2013, the United Nations Environment Programme (UNEP)[47] published a report on global mercury assessment, where the current annual mercury release from natural sources was estimated to be up to 600 t/y, from anthropogenic emissions, it was approximately 2,000 t/y, and from reemission, it was more than 4,000 t/y. Mercury emission from natural and anthropogenic sources has increased after the industrial age, and in the last 100 years, emission increased 300–500%, while reemission increased 200%. The data suggest that human activities are mainly responsible for the global increase of mercury in the environment.[48]

Approximately 84% of the mercury load related to anthropogenic activities is from combustion of fossil fuels. Among the other anthropogenic sources, dental amalgam has an important role in the environmental accumulation, but the real impact of dental amalgam is not known. A European Commission report estimated that dentistry accounts for approximately 75 t/y, of which about 45 t/y is attributed to dental office effluent. This waste reached the impressive mark of up to 13% of the overall European emissions into surface water.

A concern about the effect of dental amalgam on the environment is the mercury released as result of human cremation; it is estimated that each human body has an average 2.5 g of mercury from dental restoration, amounting at 3.6 t/y globally. Regardless of pollution control devices, cremation remains an important source of mercury vapor.[47]

The main source of mercury in dentistry is from restorative procedures and removal of old amalgam restorations. To make an amalgam restoration 15–50% of the prepared amalgam is lost as amalgam scrap — a non-contact waste from surplus of trituration and carving, and the remaining amount in used capsules. If this solid waste, as well as the extracted teeth with amalgam restoration and waste that has contact with human fluids such as rubber dams, cotton rolls, and particles retained in the filters, is sent for incineration, it will produce mercury vapor emission.[49] On the other hand, if those residues are sent to landfill sites, the mercury may become volatile by leaching from the landfill.[50]

During an old amalgam restoration removal, a sludge constituted by a heterogeneous mixture of liquids and particles of amalgam and dental tissues is trapped into the drain. This sludge has a wide range of macroscopic to submicron size particles, which may reach the sewerage systems. Inorganic mercury from amalgam waste can be converted to MeHg by a biochemical mechanism resulting from sulfate-reducing bacteria, which are common in the patient's mouth. MeHg has been found in dental wastewater in significantly higher concentrations than in natural settings. Even taking into account the mercury removal efficiency by wastewater treatment facilities, 4% of mercury is released into the environment.[51] As a complicating factor, oxidizing substances that are usually applied as a vacuum disinfectant may release mercury from amalgam waste.[49]

Amalgam separators were developed to reduce emission of amalgam particles into the waste water. This equipment can be based on centrifugation, sedimentation, and filtration principles. A 95% efficacy in preventing amalgam particles is expected, according to the international standard organization (ISO 11143), but there is a large variation in removal efficiency among the working methods in the separators. Despite the recommendation, installing amalgam separators is not mandatory in most countries, even though there is increasing environmental concern.

General procedures to be followed by dental clinics can be summarized according to the amalgam waste management adopted by the FDI: "Dental offices should collect, store safely and forward for recycling as much of the amalgam waste as possible, regardless of whether or not it has been in contact with a patient. Such waste includes used amalgam capsules, excess amalgam and amalgam waste retained in chair side traps, vacuum pump filters and amalgam separators. Extracted teeth restored with amalgam can also be recycled with other types of amalgam waste. If amalgam separators are to be installed in the dental clinic, they should comply with ISO 11143."

The Minamata Convention on Mercury, a multilateral environment agreement to help reduce global mercury pollution by anthroponogenic activities, was signed in 2013, and this agreement expects to reduce or eliminate the use of mercury where it is feasible. For dental amalgam, it was agreed to phase-down and create initiatives to reduce its use, focusing rather on the caries prevention and health promotion, on research for developing new and effective dental restorative materials, and on sound lifecycle waste management.[52,53]

5. Final Remarks and Recommendations

(1) Dental amalgam is considered safe for most patients, including children, but sensitive people who have genetic polymorphisms may be at higher toxicological risk. It is recommended that decisions for amalgam placement or replacement of any other restorative material be made on an individual basis.
(2) Dentists and dental assistants may be subject to long-term, low-level chronic mercury exposure, and although most professionals are minimally affected, the mercury concentration in the air, urine, and biological markers must be monitored in workers, in case some are sensitive to the mercury toxicity.
(3) Dental amalgam is an important source of wastewater mercury pollution, and best practices of waste management are required to protect the environment.

References

1. WHO. *Exposure to Mercury: A Major Public Health Concern. Preventing Disease through Healthy Environments*, **2006**, 4. Available at: http://www.who.int/phe/news/Mercury-flyer.pdf (Accessed 29 May 2018).
2. Heyer, N. J.; Echeverria, D.; Martin, M. D.; Farin, F. M., Woods, S. *J. Toxicol. Environ. Health* **2010**, *72* (9), 599–609.
3. FDI. World Dental Federation. *Statement on Dental Amalgam*, **1999**. Available at: https://www.fdiworlddental.org/sites/default/files/media/documents/WHO-consensus-statement-on-dental-amalgam-1997.pdf (Accessed 29 May 2018).

4. Scientific Committee on Emerging and Newly Identified Health Risks (SCENIHR). *The Safety of Dental Amalgam and Alternative Dental Restoration Materials for Patients and Users* (San Francisco: May **2008**).
5. ADA. *Statement on Dental Amalagam.* Available at: http://www.ada.org/en/about-the-ada/ada-positions-policies-and-statements/statement-on-dental-amalgam (Accessed 29 May 2018).
6. Zamm, A. V. *J. Orthomol. Med.* **1991**, *6*, 2.
7. Bernhoft, R. A. *J. Environ. Public Health* **2012**, *2012*, 460–508.
8. Clarkson, T. W.; Magos, L. *Crit. Rev. Toxicol.* **2006**, *36* (8), 609–662.
9. Ng, D. K. K.; Chan, C. H.; Soo, M. T.; Lee, R. S. Y. *Pediatr. Int.* **2007**, *49* (1), 80–87.
10. Nuttall, K. L. *Ann. Clin. Lab. Sci.* **2004**, *34* (3), 235–250.
11. Woods, J. S.; Martin, M. D.; Leroux, B. G. *Environ. Res.* **2008**, *108*, 393–399.
12. Mutter, J. *BioMed. Central Ltd.* **2011**, *6* (1), 2.
13. U.S. Food and Drug Administration. *Appendix I: Summary of Changes to the Classification of Dental Amalgam and Mercury.* Available at: http://www.fda.gov/MedicalDevices/ProductsandMedicalProcedures/DentalProducts/DentalAmalgam/ucm171120.htm#ifu.
14. Guzzi, G.; Grandi, M.; Cattaneo, C.; Calza, S.; Minoia, C.; Ronchi, A. *et al. Am. J. Forensic Med. Pathol. Off. Publ. Natl. Assoc. Med. Exam.* **2006**, *27* (1), 42–45.
15. Björkman, L.; Lundekvam, B. F.; Laegreid, T.; Bertelsen, B. I.; Morild, I.; Lilleng, P. *et al. Environ. Health* **2007**, *6* (1), 30.
16. Richardson, G. M.; Brecher, R. W.; Scobie, H.; Hamblen, J.; Samuelian, J.; Smith, C. *Regul. Toxicol. Pharmacol.* **2009**, *53* (1), 32–38.
17. Weiner, J. A.; Nylander, M. *Sci. Total Environ.* **1993**, *138* (1–3), 101–115.
18. Skare, I.; Engqvist, A. *Arch. Environ. Health* **1994**, *49* (5), 384–394.
19. Homme, K. G.; Kern, J. K.; Haley, B. E.; Geier, D. A.; King, P. G.; Sykes, L. K. *et al. BioMetals.* **2014**, *27* (1), 19–24.
20. Bailer, J.; Rist, F.; Rudolf, A.; Staehle, H. J.; Eickholz, P.; Triebig, G.; *et al. Psychol. Med.* **2001**, *31* (2), 255–263.
21. Björkman, L.; Brokstad, K. A.; Moen, K.; Jonsson, R. *Toxicol. Lett.* **2012**, *211* (2), 120–125.
22. Gottwald, B.; Traenckner, I.; Kupfer, J.; Ganss, C., Eis, D.; Schill, W-B. *et al. Int. J. Hyg. Env. Heal.* **2001**, *204*, 223–229.

23. Sjursen, T. T.; Lygre, G. B.; Dalen, K.; Helland, V.; Lægreid, T.; Svahn, J. *et al. J. Oral Rehabil.* **2011**, *38* (11), 835–848.
24. Melchart, D.; Vogt, S.; Köhler, W.; Streng, A.; Weidenhammer, W.; Kremers, L.; Hickel, R.; Felgenhauer, N.; Zilker, T.; Wühr, E.; Halbach, S. *J. Dent. Res.* **2008**, *87* (4), 349–353.
25. Weidenhammer, W.; Bornschein, S.; Zilker, T.; Eyer, F.; Melchart, D.; Hausteiner, C. *Commun. Dent. Oral Epidemiol.* **2010**, *38* (2), 180–189.
26. Gundacker, C.; Gencik, M.; Hengstschlger, M. *Rev. Mutat. Res.* **2010**, *705* (2), 130–140.
27. Holmes, A. S.; Blaxill, M. F.; Haley, B. E. *Int. J. Toxicol.* **2003**, *22* (4), 277–285.
28. Zahir, F.; Rizwi, S. J.; Haq, S. K.; Khan, R. H. *Environ. Toxicol. Pharmacol.* **2005**, *20* (2), 351–360.
29. Al-Saleh, I., Al-Sedairi, A. A. *Sci. Total Environ.* **2011**, *409* (16), 3003–3015.
30. Vahter, M.; Akesson, A.; Lind, B.; Björs, U.; Schütz, A.; Berglund, M. *Environ. Res.* **2000**, *84* (2), 186–194.
31. Bellinger, D. C.; Trachtenberg, F.; Barregard, L.; Tavares, M.; Cernichiari, E.; Daniel, D. *et al. JAMA* **2006**, *295* (15), 1775–1783.
32. DeRouen, T.; Woods, J.; Leroux, B.; Martin, M., *Hum. Exp. Toxicol.* **2015**, *34*(3), 330–2.
33. Ye, X.; Qian, H.; Xu, P.; Zhu, L.; Longnecker, M. P.; Fu, H., *Int. J. Hyg. Environ. Health.* **2009**, *212*(4), 378–86.
34. Gundacker, C.; Wittmann, K. J.; Kukuckova, M.; Komarnicki, G.; Hikkel, I.; Gencik, M. *Environ. Res.* **2009**, *109* (6), 786–796.
35. Goodrich, J. M.; Wang, Y.; Gillespie, B.; Werner, R.; Franzblau, A.; Basu, N. *Toxicol. Appl. Pharmacol.* **2011**, *257* (2), 301–308.
36. Woods, J. S.; Heyer, N. J.; Echeverria, D.; Russo, J. E.; Martin, M. D.; Bernardo, M. F. *et al. Neurotoxicol. Teratol.* **2012**, *34* (5), 513–521.
37. Woods, J. S.; Heyer, N, J.; Russo, J. E.; Martin, M. D.; Pillai, P. B.; Farin, F. M. *Neurotoxicol. Teratol.* **2013**, *39*, 36–44.
38. Woods, J. S.; Heyer N. J.; Russo, J. E.; Martin, M. D.; Farin, F. M. *Neurotoxicology* **2014**, *44*, 288–302.
39. Guzzi, G.; La Porta, C. A. M., *Toxicology* **2008**, *244* (1), 1–12.
40. Echeverria, D.; Woods, J. S.; Heyer, N. J.; Martin, M. D.; Farin, F. M. *et al. J. Toxicol. Environ. Health A* **2010**, *73* (15), 1003–1020.

41. Warwick, R.; Connor, A. O.; Lamey, B. *J. Occup. Med. Toxicol.* **2013**, *8* (27), 1–7.
42. Mark, G. *Hum. Ecol. Risk. Assess.* **2003**, *9*, 6.
43. Meyer-Baron, M.; Schaeper, M.; Seeber, A. *Arch. Toxicol.* **2002**, *76* (3), 127–136.
44. Ritchie, K. A.; Burke, F. J. T.; Gilmour, W. H.; Macdonald, E. B.; Dale, I. M.; Hamilton, R. M. *et al. Br. Dent. J.* **2004**, *197* (10), 625–632, discussion 621.
45. Moen, B.; Hollund, B.; Riise, T. *J. Occup. Med. Toxicol.* **2008**, *3*, 10.
46. FDI. *FDI Policy Statement: Mercury Hygiene Guidance*, **2007** (October), 6–8. Available at: https://www.fdiworlddental.org/sites/default/files/media/documents/Mercury-hygiene-guidance-2007.pdf (Accessed 29 May 2018).
47. United Nations Environment Programme (UNEP). *Arctic Monitoring and Assessment Programme (AMAP). Technical Background Report for the Global Mercury Assessment*, **2013**, 263. Available at: http://www.amap.no/documents/doc/technical-background-report-for-the-global-mercury-assessment-2013/848 (Accessed 29 May 2018).
48. Mason, R. P.; Choi, A. L.; Fitzgerald, W. F.; Hammerschmidt, C. R.; Lamborg, C. H.; Soerensen, A. L. *et al. Environ. Res.* **2012**, *119*, 101–117.
49. Hiltz, M. *J. Can. Dent. Assoc.* **2007**, *73* (1), 59–64.
50. Vandeven, J. A.; McGinnis, S. L. *Water Air Soil. Pollut.* **2005**, *164* (1–4), 349–366.
51. Stone, M. E.; Cohen, M. E.; Liang, L.; Pang, P. *Dent. Mater.* **2003**, *19* (7), 675–679.
52. UNEP. *Minamata Convention on Mercury — Text and Annexes*, **2013**, 69. Available at: http://www.mercuryconvention.org/Portals/11/documents/Booklets/Minamata%20Convention%20on%20Mercury_booklet_English.pdf (Accessed 29 May 2018).
53. Homme, K. G.; Kern, J. K.; Haley, B. E.; Geier, D. A.; King, P. G.; Sykes, L. K. *et al. BioMetals.* **2014**, *27* (1), 19–24.

Chapter 6

Zirconia in Dentistry

Paulo Francisco Cesar*, Susana Salazar-Marocho, Erick de Lima, Lucas Hian da Silva, Karen Fukushima, and Ranulfo Benedito de Paula Miranda

Department of Biomaterials and Oral Biology, University of Sao Paulo, Av. Prof. Lineu Prestes, 2227 — Cidade Universitária, São Paulo, Brazil

**paulofc@usp.br*

This chapter intends to present information regarding many aspects of the use of zirconia in dentistry. First, the composition, microstructure, and mechanical properties are discussed. The second part deals with the problem of chipping of dental porcelains applied over Y-TZP structures, its causes, and possible solutions for the problem. The third part presents the innovations related to translucent zirconia, explaining how manufacturers managed to increase light transmittance by means of tailoring the microstructure. The fourth part explains how zirconia reacts to the aging phenomenon that occurs in the oral cavity. The fatigue mechanisms and laboratory chewing simulation works are discussed. Finally, the fifth and last part presents the advantages and disadvantages of zirconia implants in comparison to titanium implants.

1. Introduction

Zirconium dioxide (ZrO_2) or zirconia is used in dentistry to fabricate frameworks for anterior and posterior fixed dental prostheses (FDP) and abutments for dental implants because of its excellent properties such as high strength, high biocompatibility, and high chemical stability.

The 3 mol% yttria-stabilized tetragonal zirconia polycrystal (3Y-TZP) material was first applied in restorative dentistry in 1995.[1] From this year on, 3Y-TZP ceramics stood out among all other types of dental ceramics due to the superiority of its mechanical properties such as high fracture toughness (from 4.4 to 15.0 $MPa \cdot m^{1/2}$) and flexural strength (1,100 MPa) compared with feldspathic porcelains, glass ceramics, alumina, and glass-infiltrated ceramics.[2–4] The superior mechanical properties of Y-TZP result from the toughening mechanism (phase transformation); however, its almost purely crystalline composition also improved its mechanical properties as opposed to materials with amorphous phases in their composition.

Zirconia is a material with polymorphic crystal structure that has three crystalline forms: monoclinic (m), tetragonal (t), and cubic (c). At room temperature, the material is stable in the monoclinic form until 1170°C. When heated at higher temperatures, the transformation to the tetragonal phase occurs, and subsequently to cubic phase at about 2370°C, which exists up to the melting temperature of 2680°C. During cooling, at temperatures below 1070°C, the transformation from the tetragonal to the monoclinic phase ($t \rightarrow m$) takes place accompanied by a volumetric expansion of 3–4.5%.

The addition of dopant oxides or stabilizers to the zirconia, such as calcium oxide (CaO), magnesium oxide (MgO), yttrium oxide (Y_2O_3), aluminum oxide (Al_2O_3), or ceria (CeO_2). promote the formation of

(i) fully stabilized zirconia (FSZ) in the cubic form by adding sufficient amounts of stabilizing oxides (16 mol% MgO, 16 mol% CaO, or 8 mol% Y_2O_3);

(ii) partially stabilized zirconia (PSZ) formed by nanoscale particles in the monoclinic or tetragonal phase immersed in the cubic zirconia matrix. The stabilizers added are CaO, MgO, or also Y_2O_3 (in smaller proportion than that used for TZP);

(iii) tetragonal zirconia polycrystals (TZP) consist predominantly of the tetragonal phase stabilized at room temperature with Y_2O_3 (usually 3 mol%), leading to the Y-TZP (stabilized tetragonal zirconia polycrystals). Small amounts of secondary cubic phase have also been reported in TZP.[5,6]

As stated before, the Y-TZP is the most commonly used zirconia-based dental material. The transformation from tetragonal to monoclinic phase in Y-TZP restorations can be induced by usual procedures such as the adjustment with diamond burs and sandblasting, which incorporate surface defects as scratches and grinding flaws. The phase transformation results in volume expansion with the generation of compressive stresses with an approximate depth of 30 μm,[7] which hinders crack propagation,[8] thus increasing the fracture toughness of the material.

Highly crystalline ceramic materials such as Y-TZP have no vitreous phase in the microstructure, and therefore their translucency is lower than that observed for materials with high glass content, such as feldsphatic ceramics. Therefore, restorations built with Y-TZP need to be veneered with a more aesthetic and compatible ceramic material. Feldspathic porcelains and glass ceramics are the most used veneering materials for this purpose.[9] Recently, more translucent Y-TZPs have been developed to fabricate monolithic fixed partial dentures.

The basic microstructure of 3Y-TZP consists of equiaxed grains with an average diameter ranging from 0.2 to 0.5 μm. The sintering temperature has a great influence on the final grain size as sintering the material at lower temperatures results in smaller grains.

Restorations obtained from 3Y-TZP can be machined in the partially sintered (soft machining) or fully sintered (hard machining) states. The latter processing method is more time consuming, involves high wear of the milling instruments, and can cause unwanted phase transformation and irreversible damage to the ceramic surface. Thus, soft machining is the preferred processing method for dental Y-TZPs due to its higher efficiency in producing dental prostheses. On the other hand, the fully sintered zirconia has a smaller fraction of pores, higher hardness, and better resistance to hydrothermal aging. Y-TZP is presented commercially in the form of plates, cylinders, or partially sintered discs that are milled in a computer-aided design/computer-aided machining (CAD/CAM system) to achieve the final shape of the dental restoration.

2. The Bilayer Porcelain/Zirconia

Due to aesthetic limitations, Y-TZP restoration need to be veneered with a porcelain layer with relatively low mechanical properties. Although clinical follow-ups have shown low failure rates for single crowns produced with Y-TZP frameworks, a high failure probability of the veneering porcelain has been reported in these studies.[10] This type of failure is called chipping of the porcelain veneer layer and varies according to the size of the chipped area, from small porcelain fractures (which can be repaired by polishing the restoration) to more extensive fractures that require remaking the FPD entirely.[11]

2.1. *Causes of Porcelain Chipping*

One of the causes of chipping of the veneering ceramic applied to Y-TZP frameworks is the association between thermal residual stresses existing within the restoration and the mechanical stresses generated by masticatory cycles. Thermal residual stresses are generated during rapid cooling of the restoration in the furnace for porcelain sintering.

During the preparation of an all-ceramic restoration using the traditional method for porcelain application, both materials (infrastructure and veneering layer) are submitted to a series of thermal cycles to apply the different porcelain layer and reproduce the anatomy of a particular tooth. At the end of each cycle, the restoration is cooled to room temperature.[12]

Studies showed that the thermal residual stresses are developed during the cooling stage of the ceramic restoration,[13] and two main factors are described as being responsible for the development of these thermal stresses: the differences in the coefficient of thermal expansion (CTE) between the porcelain and Y-TZP and the temperature gradient created during cooling.[14,15] The last sintering cycle performed is the most important since it determines the final residual stress profile in the ceramic restoration.

The coefficient of thermal expansion (CTE) mismatch between the Y-TZP framework ($\alpha_{\text{infrastructure}}$) and the veneering porcelain ($\alpha_{\text{porcelain}}$) results in different contraction rates for these two materials during cooling of the ceramic piece. The resulting thermal residual stress profile in the restoration will depend on the porcelain layer exhibiting a higher or lower CETL than that of the Y-TZP used as framework.

When the porcelain veneering layer has a much higher CTE compared to that of the infrastructure ($\alpha_{\text{infrastructure}} < \alpha_{\text{porcelain}}$), pre-existing cracks in the porcelain layer will propagate more easily during the application of chewing mechanical loads due to the accumulation of tensile residual stresses in the porcelain. On the other hand, an opposite situation ($\alpha_{\text{infrastructure}} > \alpha_{\text{porcelain}}$) will result in the development of compressive stresses in the porcelain. These compressive stresses will make it more difficult for small flaws or defects present in the material to propagate during the clinical performance of the restoration, thus reducing the risk of material failure.

The thermal gradient generated along the ceramic restoration occurs because both the Y-TZP and the veneering porcelain have very low thermal diffusivity when compared to metal alloys. During fast cooling of the ceramic restoration, low thermal diffusivity generates a temperature difference between deeper regions (near the Y-TZP infrastructure) and the outer surface of the veneering porcelain layer. This fact is critical because the outer surface solidifies first, while the inner layers remain liquid (above the glass transition temperature, Tg). This thermal gradient between the deeper layers and the outer surface of the veneering porcelain influences the appearance of thermal residual stresses along the restoration.

A solution found by researchers during the production of an all-ceramic restoration to reduce the formation of thermal residual stresses resulting from the thermal gradient was to perform a porcelain sintering cycle associated with a slow cooling protocol in order to ensure a temperature homogenization in the various thicknesses of the porcelain veneering layer.[16,17]

In addition to the thermal residual stresses, studies also pointed out the design of the Y-TZP framework, the mechanical properties, and processing method of the porcelain layer as possible factors related to the occurrence of porcelain chipping. The zirconia framework design is considered a risk factor for chipping in situations in which the porcelain is left without the framework support.[17] The cusps and interproximal regions are the areas with highest chipping rates due to the larger volume of porcelain applied in these places to reproduce the dental anatomy. It is recommended to individualize the design of the infrastructure according to each clinical case, in order to ensure the greatest support possible for the porcelain layer that is applied on the Y-TZP framework.

The fact that dental porcelains have the lowest mechanical properties compared to all dental ceramic materials also influences the chipping rate of the porcelain layer. In addition to this, the presence of defects in the veneering layer related to the processing method may favor the porcelain chipping.[18,19]

The application of porcelain by the traditional or stratification technique, in which a porcelain slurry is applied to the Y-TZP infrastructure with the aid of a brush, generates a veneering layer with high porosity, which reduces the mechanical properties of the structure. Thus, new processing techniques have been developed in order to obtain a coating layer with improved mechanical properties.

One of these techniques is the so-called press-on technique, in which porcelain pellets are pressed over a Y-TZP framework (previously milled and sintered). The process is conducted in a special furnace under high temperature, resulting in a porcelain layer with lower porosity and better mechanical resistance compared to porcelain layers built by the traditional method.[20]

Two techniques have been recently introduced in the market with the objective of reducing the risk of chipping of the veneering porcelain layer. In one of these systems, a layer of Y-TZP (infrastructure) and a veneering porcelain layer are produced via CAD-CAM and then bonded together by means of a cementation step. This system aims to avoid the appearance of thermal residual stresses generated during the cooling of the restoration. The porcelain used in the veneering layer is produced in ideal industrial conditions that ensure a material with less defects, resulting in a more homogeneous and mechanically resistant porcelain layer. The other system uses CAD-CAM blocks of a lithium disilicate glass-ceramic to produce the veneering layer. This material has a higher crystalline content and better mechanical properties when compared to feldspathic porcelain. The bond of the veneering layer with Y-TZP infrastructure is made by means of a low fusion temperature glass-ceramic, using a sintering cycle that promotes fusion of the two layers (veneering and framework) and final crystallization of the veneering layer.

3. Monolithic Zirconia

In 2011,[21–22] dentistry started using monolithic restorations of Y-TZP, and consequently the chipping problem presented by veneering ceramics was eliminated. However, in the beginning, these monolithic restorations offered only a satisfactory aesthetic result due to lower translucency of Y-TZP and its use was restricted to molars.[21,23] With the development of novel processing methods, more translucent Y-TZPs were developed for monolithic restorations in the anterior area.[23,24]

3.1. *Microstructure and Optical Properties*

Currently, the microstructure and the composition of monolithic zirconia are significantly different from those of conventional Y-TZP. The first attempt to reduce the opacity of the Y-TZP involved a decrease in the amount of sintering additives in its composition.[25] Sintering additives have different refractive indexes compared to zirconia (ZrO_2) and therefore increase the opacity of the Y-TZP due to high light scattering.

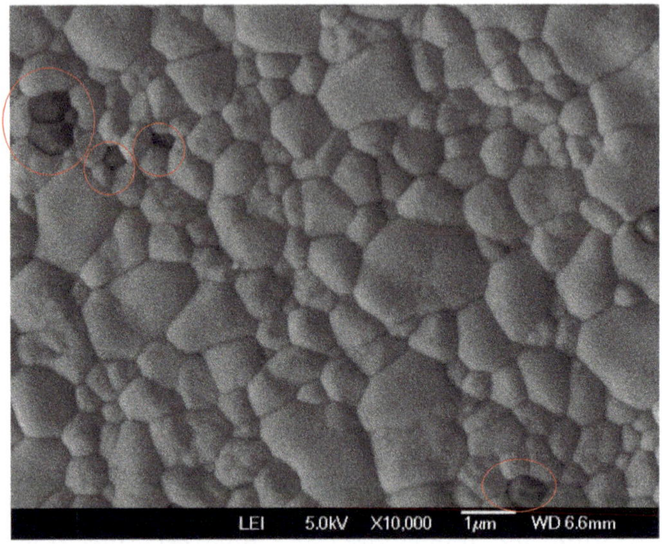

Figure 1. Photomicrograph by scanning electron microscopy of the conventional Y-TZP microstructure. Red ellipses show the presence of crystalline grains of alumina previously identified by energy dispersive spectroscopy

An additive frequently used in Y-TZP is aluminum oxide (alumina; Figure 1), which inhibits the growth of zirconia grains during sintering and increases the ceramic resistance to low-temperature degradation (LTD). A smaller alumina content (0.1 mass%) is present in the microstructure of the Y-TZP for monolithic restorations in comparison to the conventional Y-TZP (0.43 mass%),[26] resulting in higher translucency for the first.

The increase in translucency observed for monolithic Y-TZP restorations is also related to smaller crystalline grain sizes, which are associated to higher density and a reduced number of impurities, flaws, and porosities. Among these, the factor that contributes the most for the increased translucency of Y-TZP is the crystalline grain size.

Grain size is the microstructural property that is more directly related to the control of translucency and opacity of polycrystalline ceramics. Initially, the creation of ceramic materials with high translucency was possible by promoting the increase of the crystalline grain

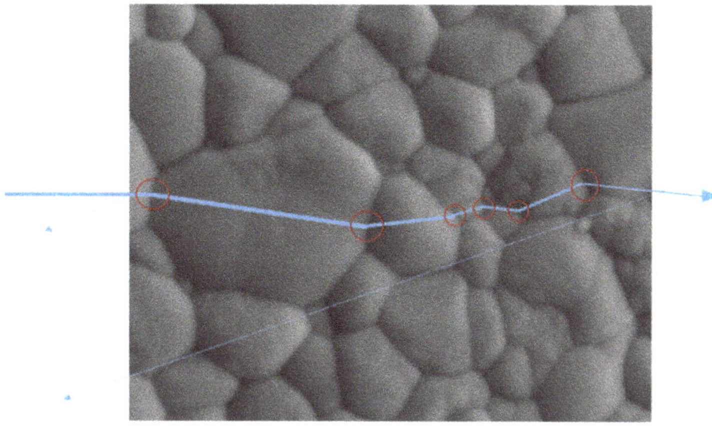

Figure 2. Image representing the interaction of light with the Y-TZP microstructure. The light path is represented by the blue arrows, and red ellipses show the regions of grain boundaries where refraction and scattering of light occur. The final light intensity is lower due to reflections and scatterings suffered during transmission

size during sintering.[27] Larger grains lead to a reduction in the number of grain boundaries, and consequently less scattering (Figure 2). However, for Y-TZP, it is known that a larger crystal grain size directly reflects a decrease of its mechanical properties and loss of the stability of the tetragonal phase. Therefore, increasing the grain size of Y-TZP is not a viable option to improve its translucency.

An alternative to increase the translucency of Y-TZP is to decrease the grain size down to a level that can mitigate the influence of the birefringence phenomenon and thus generate a less opaque material.[28] Birefringence occurs in Y-TZP due to the large amount of tetragonal crystal phase (>90%), which is a crystal that has different refractive indexes according to space orientation in the microstructure. This anisotropic behavior of the refractive index causes significant scattering of the light when it is transmitted through the material.

Studies have shown that decreasing the grain size also decreases the birefringence influence of anisotropic structures, thus increasing the translucency.[23,24] This technique is still under development, since there is no ideal mathematical model for Y-TZP to define the correct grain size that eliminates the large birefringence of the tetragonal crystals of zirconia. However, it is believed that to achieve a translucency close to the one presented by feldspathic porcelain, the grain size should be around 120 nm.[29] Currently, it is not possible to obtain a Y-TZP piece with such a small grain size using conventional furnaces. Nevertheless, by reducing as much as possible the grain size of the Y-TZP for monolithic restorations (Table 1) and decreasing the amount of sintering additives, it is possible to achieve a significant improvement in the translucency. Figure 3 shows photomicrographs obtained by scanning electron microscopy of the microstructures of monolithic restorations by Y-TZP and conventional Y-TZP, showing the size of the crystalline grain of each material.

One of the most accepted ways to measure the translucency of a material is by means of the translucency parameter.[30] The translucency parameter is the color difference measured for one material when it is placed first on a white background and then on a black background; to calculate this difference, the color of the material is measured based on reflected light (reflectance). Hence, the translucency parameter indicates the influence of a background color (black or white) on the final color of a material. A material that is highly opaque will show small values of color difference in the above-mentioned condition,

Table 1. Mean diameter (Feret) of the crystalline grains of conventional and monolithic restorations Y-TZP[a]

Material	**Mean ± Standard deviation (nm)**
Conventional Y-TZP (Cercon Zircônia, Dentsply)	700 ± 270
Y-TZP for monolithic restoration (Lava Plus, 3M ESPE)	550 ± 210

Note: [a]Values obtained based on 800 crystalline grains measured on three specimens of each material.

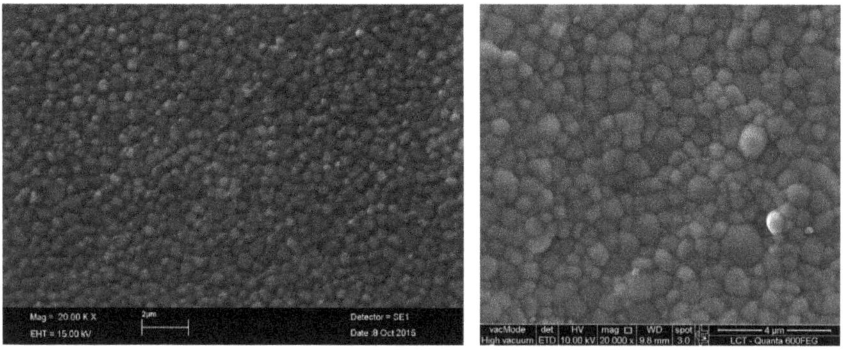

(a) (b)

Figure 3. Photomicrographs obtained by scanning electron microscopy of the microstructure of Y-TZP suitable for monolithic restorations (a) and conventional Y-TZP (b), showing the size of the crystal grain at a magnification of 20,000×

i.e. the material has a high masking ability. When the material is very translucent, the color difference will be large, indicating that the background color has greater influence on the final color of the material. Knowing this concept, it is expected that higher values of translucency parameter will be observed for monolithic Y-TZPs than for conventional Y-TZPs. In pieces with thicknesses close to that used in monolithic prosthetic restoration (1 mm), the translucency parameter values measure in conventional Y-TZPs are approximately three units higher than those measured for monolithic Y-TZPs.[31] This difference of three units may seem insignificant on a scale from 0 (fully opaque material) to 18.1 (translucency parameter of human tooth enamel).[32] However, scientific studies on optical properties showed that the human eye can see variations of translucency (i.e. color differences) in dental ceramics restorations when differences in the range of two units are obtained.[33] Table 2 shows approximate values of translucency parameter measured for thicknesses of 1 mm of dentin and enamel, a Y-TZP brand suitable for monolithic restorations, and two Y-TZP brands indicated for fabrication of fixed dental prostheses infrastructure.[31]

In addition to Y-TZP for monolithic restorations, other materials are emerging in the market as a result of the association of tetragonal

Table 2. Translucency parameters of human teeth structures in comparison with different types of Y-TZPs[31,32]

Material	Translucency parameters
Dental enamel	18.1
Dentin	16.4
Y-TZP for infrastructures (Cercon Base, DeguDent GmbH)	5.5
Y-TZP for infrastructures (Lava Standard, 3M ESPE)	10.5
Y-TZP for monolithic restorations (Lava Plus, 3M ESPE)	13.5

zirconia with cubic zirconia crystalline phase. Such material cannot be called yttria-stabilized tetragonal zirconia polycrystals (Y-TZP), because a most of its microstructure is composed of cubic zirconia (>25%).[34] Cubic zirconia provides aesthetic advantages for monolithic restorations because it has an isotropic refractive index. In other words, its cubic crystal shape keeps the same refractive index regardless of its spatial orientation in the structure. However, if on one hand the cubic zirconia promotes an aesthetic advantage to the material, on the other hand it promotes a decrease in mechanical properties.

3.2. *Mechanical Properties*

As mentioned earlier, Y-TZP has excellent mechanical properties when compared to other ceramics. The most clinically relevant properties to be considered are: flexural strength, fracture toughness, and hardness. The flexural strength of conventional Y-TZP is one of the highest amongst all dental ceramics.[35] The Y-TZP for monolithic restorations also has a good flexural strength, which is similar to that of conventional Y-TZP.[36] Table 3 shows the main mechanical properties for the two kinds of Y-TZP.

As shown above, the Y-TZP has high hardness compared to enamel (~3.2 GPa)[38] or feldspathic porcelain (~4.5 GPa),[39] and this

Table 3. Main mechanical properties of conventional and suitable-for-monolithic restorations Y-TZP[a,37]

Material	Flexural strength (MPa)	Fracture toughness ($MPa \cdot m^{1/2}$)	Hardness (GPa)
Y-TZP for infrastructures	990	3.63	12.88
Y-TZP for monolithic restorations	1,416	3.24	13.11

Note: [a]Values obtained for pieces manufactured using ceramic powders from Tosoh Corporation. Large variations in these properties can occur between among the brands available.

property along with others is directly related to the potential of the material to wear the opposing tooth. In general, all ceramic prostheses are not indicated for patients with parafunctional habits, such as bruxism, because these restorations have a high potential for antagonist tooth wear.[40] An exacerbated antagonist tooth wear can compromise the entire occlusion balance of a person and cause serious future complications.[41] Nevertheless, despite the high wear potential of Y-TZP, the scientific literature shows that monolithic restorations with good surface finishing do not cause significant wear of the antagonist dentition.

Other factors that have direct influence on the wear process are: the type of food being processed, the individual chewing pattern, the salivary properties (e.g. acidity), and the surface roughness of the restorative material. The property that proved to be more directly linked to antagonist wear was the restoration surface roughness.[37,38] A monolithic Y-TZP restoration has good surface finishing and probably will not wear significantly the antagonist element. However, following up these Y-TZP restorations is important because if there is a surface quality loss their wear potential will increase due to its high hardness.

4. Fatigue of Dental Ceramics

Despite the excellent mechanical properties of Y-TZP, there were many doubts regarding the possibility of achieving success with this material in dentistry, as it showed a high failure rate in the medical field. A literature review published in 2006 showed that, in 2001, approximately 400 femoral head prostheses (hip joint implant) fractured in a short period of time, causing a drop of more than 90% in Y-TZP implants sales for a specific brand (Prozyr) between 2001 and 2002.[42]

When zirconia is applied in an organism, i.e. exposed to temperatures near to 37°C and to moisture, aging occurs by slow transformation of the tetragonal superficial grains to monoclinic phase due the presence of water or water vapor and this phenomenon is called low temperature degradation (LTD). The transformation starts on isolated grains at the surface by a stress corrosion mechanism, and this initial transformation of a specific grain may be related to its lower yttria content, a specific surface orientation, the presence of residual stresses, or the presence of cubic phase. This transformation is induced by the reaction of water molecules with zirconium oxide, leading to the formation of hydroxides on the crack surface. The T-M grain transformation leads to an increase in volume, inducing stresses around it and resulting in the microcrack formation. These cracks allow more water to penetrate into the material structure, leading to additional grain transformation, and generating more cracks with subsequent increase in surface roughness and degradation of the mechanical properties.[42]

An important aspect to be considered when studying the fracture phenomenon in dental ceramics is the fact that clinical failures are usually related to a fatigue process. The fatigue failure occurs after the material has been subjected to stresses of lower magnitude than those related to the static fracture strength of the material. Fatigue is a process involving nucleation, propagation, and coalescence of cracks.[43,44]

An important phenomenon that is observed in ceramic materials subjected to fatigue is the subcritical or slow crack growth (SCG). This phenomenon is caused by the interaction of water with the ceramic material on the tip of cracks that are under stress. In the presence of stresses below a critical level, the water causes hydrolysis of the metal oxide of the material, resulting in a stable growth of these cracks.[45] SGC is extremely sensitive to the load applied to the structure and also depends on the ambient humidity, temperature, and other external variables, which means that under suitable conditions, defects can grow for some time until they reach a critical size, leading to catastrophic failure.[46,47] The oral environment presents many elements that favor SGC in ceramic restorations, such as water present in saliva, mastication forces that generate subcritical stresses, temperature around 37°C, and pH variations. SCG can be characterized by the stress corrosion coefficient (n), which is dimensionless and indicates the susceptibility of the material to the growth of defects that lead to failure. Once the value of n is known, it is possible to predict the degradation in strength of the materials subjected to SCG. Therefore, high values of n indicate less susceptibility to SCG.[43]

The fatigue behavior of ceramic material can be characterized using direct or indirect laboratorial tests. Direct methods are not very popular for testing dental materials due to their complexity and the necessity of using large specimens. For these reasons, the indirect methods are the most used, and they are based on classic flexural strength tests.[43] The most used techniques are the dynamic fatigue, static fatigue, and cyclic fatigue tests.[48]

A widely used method to determine SCG parameters in ceramic materials, without performing direct measurement of crack growth is the dynamic fatigue test. This is the preferred test method because it allows an estimation of lifetime in a less subjective way than those obtained by the measurement of the crack; in addition, the defects and fractures simulated by this method are more clinically relevant.[43] Using the dynamic fatigue test, it is possible to determine the SGC parameters. The cyclic fatigue test allow the determination of SCG parameters, the fatigue resistance, the lifetime, and the fatigue limit of the material.

In general, in cyclic fatigue tests, stresses are applied repeatedly and regularly. The generated stresses can be axial (tension-compression), flexural, or torsional. There are three types of cyclic stresses. The reverse cycle is represented schematically by a regular sinusoidal time-dependent curve, which has a symmetric amplitude, i.e. the alternation of maximum tensile stress values to the minimum compression is of equal magnitude. When repeated stress cycles are applied, maximum and the minimum stresses are asymmetric in relation to zero.[44]

Another way to study the dental ceramic fatigue behavior is using chewing simulators to assess the strength degradation of these materials after mechanical cycling. During simulation of mastication, the application of low loads in a 100% humidity environment may trigger subcritical growth of defects similar to what occurs in the restoration function in the oral cavity.

Reproducing the factors involved in the chewing process is relatively difficult, and the first simulators had as main objective to reproduce the chewing dynamics, but they were not designed to test dental materials under fatigue. In 1968, a device comprising a number of steel wires was developed, in which the load was applied to simulate the muscular strength generated during mastication. The machine was activated by an electric engine that moved two antagonistic stone models. In this device, the direction of force application was a major concern, as the objective was to recreate the jaw opening and closing dynamic.[49] Another study used a dry human skull instead of stone models to analyze the influence of stresses generated during chewing on bone growth.[50] The introduction of computerized finite element models represented an evolution in this field, as it allowed the simulation of the dynamics involved in chewing for various purposes, such as analysis of the influence of muscle stresses caused by chewing on the bone surface growth, distribution of masticatory forces on the jaw and muscle movements during mastication.[51–53]

With the evolution of chewing simulators, scientists developed machines that allowed the mechanical cycling of dental restorations *in vitro* with the ultimate goal of aging dental materials. These devices were seeking to recreate the oral environment by using parameters such as masticatory loads, direction of applied forces, cycles frequency, presence of moisture, and temperature around 37°C. An example of such a simulator is the ACTA equipment, developed at the Dental College of Amsterdam (ACTA Academisch Tandheelkunde Centrum Amsterdam), which is composed of two wheels that rotate in opposing directions, one that contains the specimens and the other acts as the antagonist.[54]

There are more sophisticated simulators that allow both wear, due to sliding between two surfaces, and the application of loads in the vertical axis. Thus, antagonist pistons will apply the load, while a lower support, which contains the specimen, performs horizontal movements, compatible with sliding surfaces during mastication.[55–57] These simulators also allow adjustments in its structure in order to make the most accurate simulation of the elements present in the oral cavity, such as use of natural teeth as antagonists and use of materials that simulate the periodontal tissue during loading.

The "Alabama machine" (University of Alabama, USA) can generate localized or generalized wear. This machine uses springs for load application (maximum 200 kg). The Munich Artificial Mouth developed in the Ludwig Maximilians University Munich, is a machine driven by pneumatic cylinders that apply sliding force (linear distance of 8 mm) between specimens and antagonists. The OHSU machine, developed at Oregon Health and Science University in Portland (USA), uses human molars cusps that are processed to acquire the shape of spheres with 10 mm diameter. These cusps are pressed against the specimens with a slurry composed of a mixture of poppy seeds with PMMA beads (polymethyl methacrylate). First, a 50 N load is applied on the specimen, with a linear sliding of 8 mm, yielding an abrasive wear and after a static load of 80 N is applied to cause localized wear. Another machine developed by Zurich University also uses cusps of maxillary molars as antagonists and applies loads of 50 N with a frequency of 1.7 Hz. In this case, the cusps are pressed against the specimen surfaces, which are mounted over a rubber base, with an angulation of 45°, allowing sliding between the surfaces.

Some chewing simulators models do not promote sliding of antagonists or samples, and therefore were not initially designed for wear tests. In these machines, the specimens are attached to a base and the load is applied by pistons that perform vertical movement by pneumatic system. These devices allow adjustments for cycling with or without load impact between the piston and the specimen.[58] The use of chewing simulators may be considered a great resource to evaluate the strength degradation of ceramic materials after *in vitro* aging.

5. Y-TZP for Dental Implants

5.1. *Tissue/Implant Interfaces*

Biomaterials used as implants should interact with the human body, and this interaction will promote a response from the body. The interaction depends on factors associated with tissue (type, age, health, blood circulation) and factors associated with the implant (composition, surface morphology, porosity). Thus, there are four different types of response to the interaction/interface/reaction implant tissue[59]:

✓ *Toxic*: cells that are nearby and touch the implant die.
✓ *Biologically inert*: a fibrous capsule is developed around the implant. The fibrous tissue formed has the objective of isolating the implant from the rest of the body. Metals, ceramics, and polymers can produce this type of response.
✓ *Bioactive*: a bond occurs at the interface between the implant and the tissue. This type of interaction prevents the implant from moving and mimics the type of interface that is formed when natural tissues are repaired.[59]

Another important concept is the biocompatibility. A biocompatible biomaterial is one that has the ability to obtain an appropriate host response in a specific application. This definition emphasizes that biocompatibility is not only the lack of toxicity, but is also related to the fact that the biomaterial should perform its function properly. Depending on the application, the same biomaterial may or may not be considered biocompatible.[59,60] For example, feldspathic porcelain is biocompatible when applied as a laminate veneer. But if it is used as a dental implant material, it would not be considered biocompatible, since its mechanical properties are not sufficient for this function.

5.2. *Titanium Implants*

Dental treatments involving implants have brought many solutions for the oral rehabilitation of edentulous patients and also a considerable improvement in their psychosocial characteristics.[61] The success of an implant can be influenced by several factors, such as its diameter, length, surgical technique, patient health, and biomaterial.[62]

In implantology, the biomaterial most commonly used to replace the lost tooth root is titanium (commercially pure titanium or titanium alloy, Ti-6Al-4V), which has excellent biocompatibility and high mechanical properties.[61,63] There is a very large number of clinical studies that followed this biomaterial for periods that exceed 10 years and showed a success rate higher than 90%.[61,64,65]

Despite the good results in these clinical trials, in some clinical situations titanium implants cannot yet fully satisfy the patients' aesthetic expectations. This is due to an inherent characteristic of titanium, which is its grayish color. The dentist must evaluate each clinical case carefully, and during planning of the oral rehabilitation he should discuss with the patient about this topic. The grayish color of titanium implants may compromise the final aesthetic result in two ways: (a) with time, due to gingival recessions, the implant can be exposed and dark areas start to appear, and (b) change of gingival color, since the darkened color of the implant may appear by transparency through the peri-implant tissues in patients with thin gingival biotype. This problem is more serious in treatments involving anterior teeth and in patients who show a large area of the gum in their smiles.[66–68]

Another disadvantage of using titanium is related to allergic responses reported in the literature. The descriptions of these cases show that hypersensitivity to titanium is a possible reason for the failures observed in some rehabilitations. However, there is a lack of epidemiological data on the incidence of hypersensitivity to titanium, and it is known that millions of patients have been rehabilitated with titanium implants and had no allergic reaction.[69,70]

5.3. *Y-TZP Implants*

Yttria-stabilized tetragonal zirconia polycrystals (Y-TZP) have white coloration, and is one of the main alternatives to titanium for treatments involving implants with great aesthetic requirement. The feature that allows the application of Y-TZP in implantology is its relatively high fracture toughness (K_{Ic}), which is greater than those of all other dental ceramics and is associated with the toughening mechanism known as martensitic transformation.

Companies that produce Y-TZP implants try to convince clinicians of the fact that patients are increasingly demanding more aesthetic treatments, and that this growing demand would be fulfilled by ceramic implants. Research carried out in Europe shows that more than half of the patients (53%), when asked what biomaterial they would prefer for rehabilitation with dental implants, responded that they do not know which biomaterial is the best. But among those who have a preference for a biomaterial, the number that prefer a ceramic implant (35%) is 3.5 times higher than the number of patients who prefer metallic implants (10%).

Studies *in vitro* and *in vivo* showed that the surface of the Y-TZP is less susceptible to adhesion of bacteria from the oral flora when compared with titanium.[71–73] However, some studies have recently shown that Y-TZP and titanium have similar responses in relation to bacteria colonization.[74–75]

It should be emphasized that the Y-TZP is classified as a bioinert material. A bioinert material has a weak interaction with the surrounding living tissues.[76] In implantology, low bioactivity adversely affects the osseointegration process and can lead to implant failure. Surface modifications are used to overcome this feature and may be performed in different ways, such as acid etching, lasers, coating with calcium phosphate ceramics, or micropatterned silica thin films. The goal is to promote better and faster osseointegration.[77–80] In fact, Y-TZP implants with different surface treatments showed similar levels of osseointegration compared to titanium implants.[81]

There are few studies in the literature using the Y-TZP implants, and they did not follow-up patients for more than 5 years. One study followed 831 Y-TZP implants for a period of 5 years, observing a success rate of 95%.[8] Another study followed 170 Y-TZP implants for 3 years and showed a success rate of 82%.[83]

One work followed 20 implants in aesthetic areas for a period of 4 years and had a success rate of 100%.[67] There is clearly a lack of long-term scientific evidence to justify the use of ceramic oral implants. The existing studies show that Y-TZP has a great potential to be a very interesting alternative to titanium for selected clinical cases. Therefore, clinicians must wait for additional clinical trials that can bring more long-term results regarding Y-TZP implants.[84]

References

1. Meyenberg, K. H.; Luthy, H.; Scharer, P. *J. Esthet. Dent.* **1995**, *7* (2), 73–80.
2. Pittayachawan, P.; McDonald, A.; Petrie, A.; Knowles, J. C. *Dent. Mater.* **2007**, *23* (8), 1018–1029.
3. Luthardt, R. G.; Holzhuter, M.; Sandkuhl, O.; Herold, V.; Schnapp, J. D.; Kuhlisch, E.; Walter, M. *J. Dent. Res.* **2002**, *81* (7), 487–491.
4. Harada, K.; Shinya, A.; Gomi, H.; Hatano, Y.; Shinya, A.; Raigrodski, A. J. *J. Prosthet. Dent.* **2016**, *115* (2), 215–223.
5. Denry, I.; Kelly, J. R. *Dent. Mater.* **2008**, *24* (3), 299–307.
6. Kelly, J. R.; Denry, I. *Dent. Mater.* **2008**, *24* (3), 289–298.
7. Kosmac, T.; Oblak, C.; Jevnikar, P.; Funduk, N.; Marion, L. *Dent. Mater.* **1999**, *15* (6), 426–433.
8. Garvie, R. C.; Nicholson, P. S. *J. Am. Ceram. Soc.* **1972**, *55*, 303–305.
9. Manicone, P. F.; Rossi Iommetti, P.; Raffaelli, L. *J. Dent.* **2007**, *35* (11), 819–826.
10. Sailer, I.; Feher, A.; Filser, F.; Gauckler, L. J.; Luthy, H.; Hammerle, C. H. *Int. J. Prosthodon.* **2007**, *20* (4), 383–388.
11. Heintze, S. D.; Rousson, V. *Int. J. Prosthodont.* **2010**, *23* (6), 493–502.
12. Swain, M. V. *Acta Biomater.* **2009**, *5* (5), 1668–1677.
13. Al-Amleh, B.; Waddell, J. N.; Lyons, K.; Swain, M. V. *Dent. Mater.* **2014**, *30* (3), 271–280.
14. Meira, J. B. C.; Reis, B. R.; Tanaka, C. B.; Ballester, R. Y.; Cesar, P. F.; Versluis, A.; Swain, M. V. *Dent. Mater.* **2013**, *29* (5), 594–601.
15. Tholey, M. J.; Swain, M. V.; Thiel, N. *Dent. Mater.* **2011**, *27* (11), 1102–1110.

16. Benetti, P.; Kelly, J. R.; Sanchez, M.; Della Bona, A. *Dent. Mater.* **2014**, *30* (5), 554–563.
17. Guess, P. C.; Bonfante, E. A.; Silva, N. R.; Coelho, P. G.; Thompson, V. P. *Dent. Mater.* **2013**, *29* (3), 307–316.
18. Tang, X.; Nakamura, T.; Usami, H.; Wakabayashi, K.; Yatani, H. *J. Dent.* **2012**, *40* (5), 372–380.
19. Scherrer, S. S.; Quinn, J. B.; Quinn, G. D.; Wiskott, H. A. *Dent. Mater.* **2007**, *23* (11), 1397–1404.
20. de Araujo, M. D.; Miranda, R. B.; Fredericci, C.; Yoshimura, H. N.; Cesar, P. F. *J. Mech. Behav. Biomed. Mater.* **2015**, *44*, 85–95.
21. Marchack, B. W.; Sato, S.; Marchack, C. B.; White, S. N. *J. Prosthet. Dent.* **2011**, *106* (3), 145–152.
22. Christensen, G. J. *J. Am. Dent. Assoc.* **2011**, *142* (6), 668–671.
23. Rinke, S.; Fischer, C. *Quintessence Int.* **2013**, *44* (8), 557–566.
24. Holt, L. R.; Boksman, L. *Dent. Today* **2012,** *31* (12), 78, 80–81.
25. Zhang, H.; Li, Z.; Kim, B.-N.; Morita, K.; Yoshida, H.; Hiraga, K.; Sakka, Y. *J. Nanomater.* **2012**, *2012*, 5.
26. Fathy, S. M.; El-Fallal, A. A.; El-Negoly, S. A.; El Bedawy, A. B. *Acta Biomater. Odontol. Scand.* **2015**, *1* (2–4), 86–92.
27. Cheng, J.; Agrawal, D.; Zhang, Y.; Roy, R. *Materials Letters* **2002**, *56* (4), 587–592.
28. Zhang, Y. *Dent. Mater.* **2014**, *30* (10), 1195–1203.
29. Klimke, J.; Trunec, M.; Krell, A. *J Am. Ceram. Soc.* **2011,** *94* (6), 1850–1858.
30. Barizon, K. T. L.; Bergeron, C.; Vargas, M. A.; Qian, F.; Cobb, D. S.; Gratton, D. G.; Geraldeli, S. *J. Prosth. Dent.* **2013**, *110* (5), 397–401.
31. Wang, F.; Takahashi, H.; Iwasaki, N. *J. Prosth. Dent.* **2013**, *110* (1), 14–20.
32. Xiong, F.; Chao, Y.; Zhu, Z. *J. Prosthet. Dent.* **2008**, *100* (1), 11–7.
33. Ghinea, R.; Pérez, M. M.; Herrera, L. J.; Rivas, M. J.; Yebra, A.; Paravina, R. D. *J. Dent.* **2010**, *38* (Suppl 2), e57–e64.
34. Casolco, S. R.; Xu, J.; Garay, J. E. *Scripta Mater.* **2008**, *58* (6), 516–519.
35. Garvie, R. C.; Hannink, R. H.; Pascoe, R. T. *Nature* **1975**, *258* (5537), 703–704.
36. Vichi, A.; Sedda, M.; Fabian Fonzar, R.; Carrabba, M.; Ferrari, M. *J. Esthet. Restor. Dent.* **2016**, *28* (Suppl 1), S32–S39.

37. Tong, H.; Tanaka, C. B.; Kaizer, M. R.; Zhang, Y. *Ceram. Int.* **2016**, *42* (1 Pt B), 1077–1085.
38. Chuenarrom, C.; Benjakul, P.; Daosodsai, P. *Mater. Res.* **2009**, *12*, 473–476.
39. Kontonasaki, E.; Kantiranis, N.; Papadopoulou, L.; Chatzistavrou, X.; Kavouras, P.; Zorba, T.; Sivropoulou, A.; Chrissafis, K.; Paraskevopoulos, K. M.; Koidis, P. T. *Dent. Mater.* **2008**, *24* (10), 1362–1373.
40. Mahalick, J. A.; Knap, F. J.; Weiter, E. J. *J. Am. Dent. Assoc.* **1971**, *82* (1), 154–159.
41. Oh, W. S.; Delong, R.; Anusavice, K. J. *J. Prosthet. Dent.* **2002**, *87* (4), 451–459.
42. Chevalier, J., *Biomaterials* **2006**, *27* (4), 535–543.
43. Baran, G.; Boberick, K.; McCool, J. *Crit. Rev. Oral Biol. Med.* **2001**, *12* (4), 350–360.
44. Callister, W. D. *Materials Science and Engineering: An Introduction*, Vol. 7 (Hoboken: John Wiley & Sons, Inc., **2007**).
45. Anusavice, K. J.; Lee, R. B. *J. Dent. Res.* **1989**, *68* (6), 1075–1081.
46. Gonzaga, C. C.; Yoshimura, H. N.; Cesar, P. F.; Miranda, W. G., Jr. *J. Mater. Sci.* **2009**, *20* (5), 1017–1024.
47. Morena, R.; Beaudreau, G. M.; Lockwood, P. E.; Evans, A. L.; Fairhurst, C. W. *J. Dent. Res.* **1986**, *65* (7), 993–997.
48. Thompson, J. Y.; Anusavice, K. J.; Naman, A.; Morris, H. F. *J. Dent. Res.* **1994**, *73* (12), 1824–1832.
49. Molnar, S. *J. Dent. Res.* **1968,** *47* (4), 559–563.
50. Usui, T.; Maki, K.; Toki, Y.; Shibasaki, Y.; Takanobu, H.; Takanishi, A.; Hatcher, D.; Miller, A. *Orthodont. Craniofac. Res.* **2003,** *6* (Suppl 1), 163–167, discussion 179–182.
51. Caroena, G.; Mori, M.; Gesualdi, M. R.; Liberti, E. A.; Ferrara, E.; Muramatsu, M. *J. Biomech.* **2010**, *43* (4), 680–686.
52. Hannam, A. G. *Orthodont.Craniofac. Res.* **2003**, *6* (Suppl 1), 59–65.
53. Hannam, A. G.; Stavness, I.; Lloyd, J. E.; Fels, S. *J. Biomech.* **2008**, *41* (5), 1069–1076.
54. Heintze, S. D.; Faouzi, M.; Rousson, V.; Ozcan, M. *Dent. Mater.* **2012**, *28* (9), 961–973.
55. Durner, J.; Glasl, B.; Zaspel, J.; Kunzelmann, K. H.; Hickel, R.; Reichl, F. X. *Dent. Mater.* **2010**, *26* (7), e197–e204.

56. Kohal, R. J.; Wolkewitz, M.; Mueller, C. *Clin. Oral Implants Res.* **2010**, *21* (12), 1345–1352.
57. Kohorst, P.; Dittmer, M. P.; Borchers, L.; Stiesch-Scholz, M. *Acta Biomater.* **2008**, *4* (5), 1440–1447.
58. Itinoche, K. M.; Ozcan, M.; Bottino, M. A.; Oyafuso, D. *Dent. Mater.* **2006**, *22* (11), 1029–1034.
59. Hench, L. L.; Wilson, J. *An Introduction to Bioceramics*, Vol. 1 (Singapore: World Scientific, **1993**).
60. Williams, D.; Black, J.; Doherty, P. *Adv. Biomater.* **1992**, *10*, 525–533.
61. Adell, R.; Lekholm, U.; Rockler, B.; Brånemark, P.-I. *Int. J. Oral Surg.* **1981**, *10* (6), 387–416.
62. Takamiya, A. S.; Goiato, M. C.; Gennari Filho, H. *Biomed. Pap. Med. Fac. Univ. Palacky Olomouc. Czech. Repub.* **2014**, *158* (4), 650–653.
63. Depprich, R.; Ommerborn, M.; Zipprich, H.; Naujoks, C.; Handschel, J.; Wiesmann, H.-P.; Kübler, N. R.; Meyer, U. *Head Face Med.* **2008**, *4*, 29.
64. Fugazzotto, P. A.; Vlassis, J.; Butler, B. *Int. J. Oral Maxillofac. Implants* **2003**, *19* (3), 408–412.
65. Buser, D.; Mericskestern, R.; Bernard, P.; Pierre, J.; Behneke, A.; Behneke, N.; Hirt, H. P.; Belser, U. C.; Lang, N. P. *Clin. Oral Implants Res.* **1997**, *8* (3), 161–172.
66. Heydecke, G.; Kohal, R.; Gläser, R. *Int. J. Prosth.* **1998**, *12* (2), 184–189.
67. Borgonovo, A. E.; Censi, R.; Vavassori, V.; Arnaboldi, O.; Maiorana, C.; Re, D. *Int. J. Dent.* **2014**, *2015*, 415029.
68. Eric Van Dooren, D.; Calamita, M.; Calgaro, M.; Coachman, C.; Ferencz, J. L.; Silva, N. R. **2012**, *7*, 396–417.
69. Egusa, H.; Ko, N.; Shimazu, T.; Yatani, H. *J. Prosth. Dent.* **2008**, *100* (5), 344–347.
70. Siddiqi, A.; Payne, A. G.; De Silva, R. K.; Duncan, W. J. *Clin. Oral Implants Res.* **2011**, *22* (7), 673–680.
71. Al-Radha, A. S. D.; Dymock, D.; Younes, C.; O'Sullivan, D. *J. Dent.* **2012**, *40* (2), 146–153.
72. Scarano, A.; Piattelli, M.; Caputi, S.; Favero, G. A.; Piattelli, A. *J. Periodont.* **2004**, *75* (2), 292–296.
73. Nascimento, C. D.; Pita, M. S.; Fernandes, F. H. N. C.; Pedrazzi, V.; de Albuquerque Junior, R. F.; Ribeiro, R. F. *Clin. Oral Implants Res.* **2014**, *25* (3), 337–343.

74. Kim, H.-Y.; Yeo, I.-S.; Lee, J.-B.; Kim, S.-H.; Kim, D.-J.; Han, J.-S. *Int. J. Art. Org.* **2012**, *35* (10), 773–789.
75. Salihoğlu, U.; Boynueğri, D.; Engin, D.; Duman, A. N.; Gökalp, P.; Baloş, K. *Int. J. Oral Maxillofac. Implants* **2011**, *26* (1), 101–107.
76. Pardun, K.; Treccani, L.; Volkmann, E.; Li Destri, G.; Marletta, G.; Streckbein, P.; Heiss, C.; Rezwan, K. *Clin. Implant Dent. Rel. Res.* **2015**, *17* (1), 186–198.
77. Wenz, H. J.; Bartsch, J.; Wolfart, S.; Kern, M. *Int. J. Prosth.* **2007**, *21* (1), 27–36.
78. Hao, L.; Ma, D.; Lawrence, J.; Zhu, X. *Mater. Sci. Eng. C* **2005**, *25* (4), 496–502.
79. Marchi, J.; Amorim, E. M.; Lazar, D. R.; Ussui, V.; Bressiani, A. H. A.; Cesar, P. F. *Dent. Mater.* **2013**, *29* (9), 954–962.
80. Pelaez-Vargas, A.; Carvalho, A.; Gallego-Perez, D.; Hansford, D.; Monteiro, F.; Arismendi, J.; Grenho, L.; Fernandes, M.; Ferraz, M.; Higuita-Castro, N. *Micropatterned Coatings for Guided Tissue Regeneration in Dental Implantology* (INTECH Open Access Publisher, **2012**).
81. Manzano, G.; Herrero, R.; Montero, J. *Int. J. Oral Maxillofac. Implants* **2014**, *29* (2), 311–320.
82. Oliva, J.; Oliva, X.; Oliva, J. D. *Int. J. Oral Maxillofac. Implants* **2009**, *25* (2), 336–344.
83. Gahlert, M.; Burtscher, D.; Pfundstein, G.; Grunert, I.; Kniha, H.; Roehling, S. *Int. J. Oral Maxillofac. Implants* **2012**, *28* (3), 896–904.
84. Hashim, D.; Cionca, N.; Courvoisier, D. S.; Mombelli, A. *Clin. Oral Invest.* **2016**, *20* (7), 1–15.

Chapter 7

Lithium Disilicate-Based Glass-Ceramics

Rodrigo França

Department of Restorative Dentistry, University of Manitoba, 780 Bannatyne Ave., Winnipeg, Canada

Rodrigo.franca@umanitoba.ca

Among dental ceramic restorations, the glass-ceramics group has been improving the quality of the services provided by dentists. Within this group, lithium disilicate-based glass ceramic has gained much popularity in recent years. The focus of this chapter is to discuss the contribution of lithium disilicate-based glass-ceramics for dental applications. The goal is to provide fundamental information to dental researchers about chemical composition, nucleation and crystallization mechanisms, and microstructure. In addition, physical and chemical properties and biocompatibility issues are reviewed.

1. Introduction

The development of glass-ceramics in the second half of the 20th century brought a great benefit to several areas of the ceramics field, dentistry included. Different from a normal glass, which has an amorphous structure, or conventional sintered ceramics, which undergo spontaneous crystal growth, glass-ceramics display a glassy matrix where a controlled crystallization process can convert about 99.5% of the glassy phase into crystalline phase.[1–3] This crystallization process provides several properties that explain the success of glass-ceramics, such as a very low amount of porosity (sometimes 0% porosity), workability (they can be molded as glass, pressed, milled, or sintered), and their final physical structure can be fully engineered for a particular application.[3]

1.1. *Historical*

This elegant class of materials was discovered accidentally by Dr. Stanley. D. Stookey, in 1953, when he worked in the field of photosensitive glasses at Corning Glass, Inc.[4] According to him, his intention was to produce a lithium silicate glass able to carry a photographic image. By accident, he permitted the oven temperature to reach 850°C instead of 450°C. To his surprise, inside the oven he saw a solid white material that had not melted, as expected. When this sample was removed from the furnace, it fell on the ground. The sample not only did not break like glass, but produced a "metallic sound". He called this new material Fotoceram and latter Pyroceram. Since then, more than 2,000 patents were granted on glass-ceramics only in the USA, and many products were produced using glass-ceramics, such as cookware, telescope mirrors, and missile's noisecones.[3,5]

In dentistry, several glass-ceramics compositions have been used for dental restorations, as shown in Table 1. The first glass-ceramics were leucite-based sintering ceramics, used for veneering metallic structures, and mica used for inlays and crowns. Both materials brought advances to the restorative technique. First, the leucite crystal formation ($KAlSi_2O_6$) permitted feldspathic porcelains to achieve a coefficient of thermal expansion (CTE) compatible to the metal core, and also improved optical and mechanical properties. Second, mica-based ceramics ($KMg_{2.5}Si_4O_{10}F_2$), like the Dicor systems, launched new concepts to produce monolithic all-ceramic restorations using either centrifugal casting technique or machining technologies (CAD/CAM).[5,6]

Table 1. Some glass-ceramics materials used in dentistry

Crystalline phase	Chemical formula	Commercial brand
Mica	$KMg_{2.5}Si_4O_{10}F_2$	Dicor*
Leucite	$KAlSi_2O_6$	
Lithium Disilicate	$Li_2Si_2O_5$	IPS e.max Press, Celtra Press
Lithium Meta/Disilicate	Li_2SiO_3 / $Li_2Si_2O_5$	IPS-e.max CAD, Suprnity

Note: *No longer available in the dental market.

Subsequently, lithium disilicate systems have provoked the interest of many researchers. Dr. George V. Beall, a leader in this field, conducted several projects at Corning Inc.[7–9] In the early 1990s, his team developed a lightweight and strong lithium disilicate glass-ceramic, using compositions in the SiO_2–Li_2O–Al_2O_3–K_2O–P_2O_5 system. At about the same time, Dr. Wolfram Höland and collaborators,[10] from Ivoclar Vivadent AG, developed a similar composition, now called IPS e.max Press,[11] a glass-ceramics with blade-like crystals, which could produce dental restorations by molding process.[5,9] Subsequently Dr. Höland's team[12] produced an improved lithium disilicate glass-ceramic with rod-like crystals and excellent mechanical properties. This product, called IPS e.max® CAD, can be easily machinable (using CAD/CAM techniques) when it is in the lithium metasilicate phase, and subsequently transformed to lithium disilicate on additional heat treatment. More recently, other companies have launched their glass-ceramics using: a) Zirconia-reinforced lithium silicate systems: Celtra® Duo and Celtra® Press from Dentsply Sirona,[13–14] and Vita Suprinity® from Vita Zahnfabrik.[15]; b) Lithium aluminosilicate ceramic reinforced with lithium disilicate: Straumann n!ce™, from Straumann.

Figure 1 displays fracture toughness values (SEVNB) from the groups of glass-ceramics in Table 1. Lithium disilicate-based glass-ceramics appear to satisfy most of the requirements for a metal-free dental crown or small bridge, with more than 90% of success rate. This fact may explain, for example, the success of lithium disilicate glass-ceramics (Empress® 2/ IPS e.max® systems), which produced more than 45 million dental restorations since 1991.[3,6,9,16]

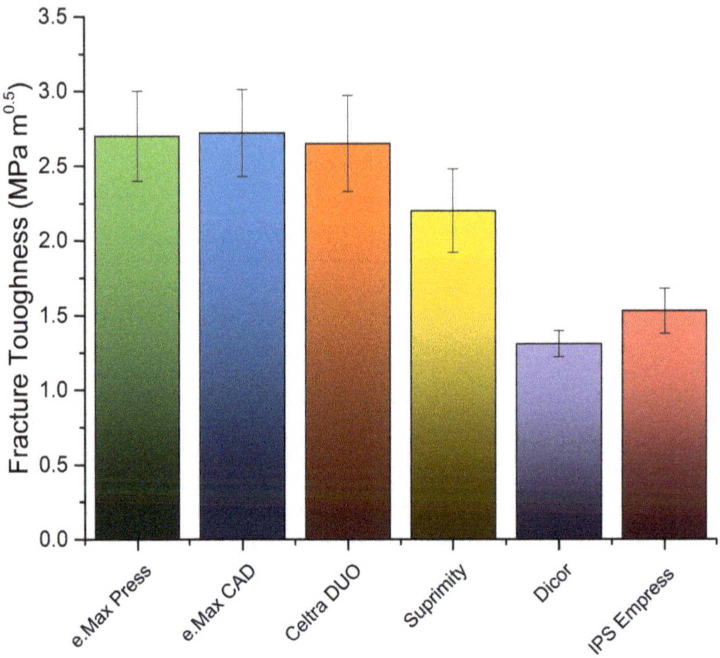

Figure 1. Fracture toughness values (SEVNB) for dental glass-ceramics listed in Table 1. Values according to the manufacturer

1.2. *Classification*

ISO 6872:2015 classify dental ceramics into two types[17]:

Type I: Ceramic products that are provided as powders, pastes, or aerosols.
Type II: All other forms of ceramic products.

This standard furnishes a classification according to the clinical use and the minimal flexural strength needed. Class 3 contains the monolithic ceramic for single-unit anterior or posterior prostheses and three-unit prostheses not involving molar restoration adhesive or non-adhesive restorations.

According to this norm, all lithium disilicate-based glass-ceramics available on the dental market fit in Type II, because they are monolithic, and Class 3, because their flexural strength reaches more than 300 MPa but not 500 MPa (as Class 4).

Lithium disilicate-based glass-ceramics can also be categorized according to the processing to create dental restorations.

(a) *Pressing*: In this technique, a ceramic ingot is put into an oven, where it reaches a viscous stage at ~850–920°C, and then is forced to flow into a cavity in a refractory mold.[5,18] Normally, the ingot is composed of highly crystalline LS2 glass-ceramics, and this procedure occurs in a dental technician's lab, using the well-known lost-wax technique.

(b) *CAD/CAM*: In this process, a ceramic ingot (partially or fully sintered) is ground to shape the desired dental structure. The computer-aided design (CAD) method is used to create a digital model of the restoration, and a computer-aided milling (CAM) machine transforms the ingot into the final dental restoration. This procedure simplifies the work of the dentist and the dental technician, and saves time for patients. Normally, the procedure takes place chairside, and just one appointment is needed. Restorations from partially sintered ingots (lithium metasilicate) must be annealed to achieve the final crystalline stage (LS2).

Lithium disilicate-based glass-ceramics can be ranked by their compositions. The manufacturer and some authors have pointed out that high percentage of zirconia (ZrO_2) and or alumina (Al_2O_3) have a major impact on the microstructure and, consequently, on the properties of dental restorations. Currently, there are the conventional lithium disilicate glass-ceramics, with ~2% ZrO_2, the so-called zirconia-reinforced lithium silicate ceramics, with ~10% ZrO_2, and the alumina-reinforced lithium silicate ceramics, with ~11% Al_2O_3. Table 2 displays the commercial brand names, according to the processing and the chemical composition.

Table 2. Classification of commercial products according to processing and the chemical composition

Composition	Pressing	CAD/CAM
Low Zr and Al (%)	e.Max Press	e.Max CAD
High Zr (%)	Celtra Press	Celtra Duo Suprinity
High Al (%)		n!ce

2. Physicochemical Characterization

2.1. *Chemical Composition*

The chemical compositions of lithium disilicate-based glass-ceramics can vary according to technical processing and manufacture formulation. In Table 3, an approximate composition (Wt.%), from manufacturer's scientific reports are given for some products.

These amounts provide little information on the chemical composition. To obtain a more accurate analysis, our research group has analyzed those materials, using X-ray photoelectron spectroscopy (XPS) for the surface atomic composition, and laser ablation ion coupled plasma mass spectroscopy (LA-ICP-MS) for bulk atomic composition. The XPS results (%) are displayed in Table 4.

2.2. *Mineral Properties*

It is important to notice that, in the composition provided by manufacturers, oxygen appears combined with other atoms, meaning that silicon is the major component of glass-ceramics. Silicon has been known to humans since pre-historical times, probably because it is the second most abundant element on earth (indeed, with oxygen, it represents 4 out of every 5 atoms present on earth's crust). Silicon, in the pure state, is very rare, and silicate is its more frequent compound (~95%). Important crystalline silicates include nesosilicates, sorosilicates, cyclosilicates, inosilicates, phyllosilicates,

Table 3. Chemical composition (Wt.%) according to the manufacturer

	IPS e.max® CAD	Vita suprinity®	Celtra DUO	Straumann n!ce®
SiO_2	57–80	56–64	58	64–70
Li_2O	11–19	5–21	18.5	10.5–12.5
K_2O	0–13	1–4	—	0–3
P_2O_5	0–11	3–8	5	3–8
ZrO	0–8	8–12	10.1	0–0.5
Al_2O_3	0–8	1–4	1.9	10.5–11.5
MgO	0–5	—	—	—
CaO	—	—	—	0–0.5
CeO_2	—	0–4	2	—
Tb_4O_7	—	—	1	—
Pigments	—	0–6	—	0–9

Table 4. Atomic composition by XPS for CAD/CAM ceramics

	e.Max CAD	Celtra Duo	Suprinity CAD	Straumann n!ce
O 1s	51.5	44.4	45.1	49.1
Si 2p	26.4	17.8	19.7	25.5
Li 1s	11.8	27.4	24.1	11.6
C 1s	2.5	0.6	1.5	5.6
Al 2p	1.4	1.2	1.3	5.0
P 2p	2.1	0.5	0.7	0
Ca 2p	0.3	1.6	1.7	0.2
K 2p	0.7	0.3	0.3	—
Zn 2p	0.2	—	—	—
Y 3p	0.3	—	—	0.2
Zr 3p	0.1	1.6	1.7	—
Sr 3p	0.3	0.2	—	—
Ce 3d	0.1	0.3	0.2	0.3
Yb 4d	—	1.5	1.5	—
N 1s	—	—	—	2.2
F 1s	—	—	—	0.2

and tectosilicates. In lithium disilicate-based glass-ceramics, the main silicate forms are:

(1) Lithium disilicate ($Li_2Si_2O_5$ or LS2), a phyllosilicate form, a layered silicate where Si shares three oxygen atoms with its neighbors (Figure 2).[19,20]
(2) Lithium metasilicate (Li_2SiO_3 or LM), an inosilicate, single-chain silicate (also called pyroxene). In this form, Si shares only 2 oxygen atoms. It is a metastable phase present at a temperature between 500°C and 800°C (Figure 2).
(3) Cristobalite (SiO_2), a stable form of silica that is a tectosilicate, also known as framework silicates. In this form, Si shares all 4 oxygen atoms.[5,21]

Lithium was first isolated from the sheet silicate mineral petalite, $LiAlSi_4O_{10}$, and afterward, from spodumene, $LiAlSi_2O_6$.[19] This alkali metal was originally used as a flux in porcelain formulations and in toughened glass production, as a Na ion exchange-strengthening agent. Besides the types already mentioned, other lithium compounds found on lithium disilicate-based glass-ceramics include lithia (LiO_2), present in the initial glass, and lithium orthophosphate (Li_3PO_4), an inductor for LM and LS2 growth.[22]

Aluminum is frequently found in natural silicates (e.g. kyanite, andalusite, mullite, sillimanite, and kaolinite). Kaolinite rocks produce the well-known china clay or kaolin ($Al_2Si_2O_5(OH)_4$). Sillimanite and mullite are also found in porcelain, as a refractory material, due to their high melting points and chemical stability.[5] Lithium aluminosilicates (LAS) can have two crystalline phases, b-spodumene and b-eucryptite, and these phases have a low coefficient of thermal expansion.[9]

Another compound that plays an important role includes phosphorus pentoxide (P_2O_5), which is added as the main nucleating agent.[21,22] Other nucleating agents include ZrO_2, CaO_2, and ZnO_2.[23] Ceria (CeO_2) can work as a nucleation agent, and also produces fluorescence, a desirable feature to mimic natural tooth.[5]

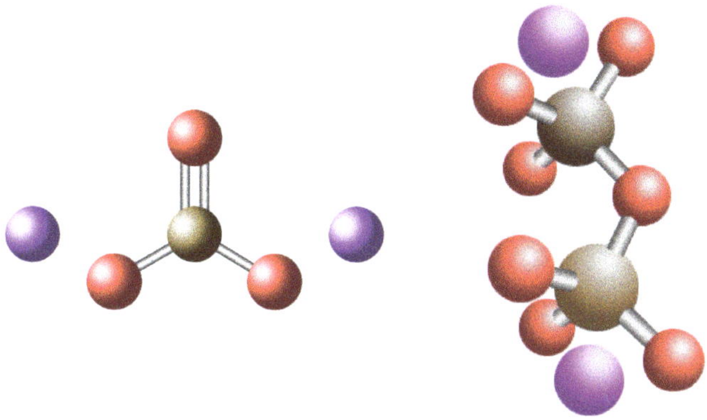

Figure 2. Molecular representation of Li_2SiO_3 and $Li_2Si_2O_5$

3. Fabrication

3.1. *Nucleation Process*

The control of the crystallization mechanism permits manufacturers to design and produce glass-ceramics with desirable properties. The main factor that rules crystal formation and growth is the nucleation process. Figure 3 schematizes the procedure (temperature/time cycle) to obtain a glass-ceramic body.[1]

In the first step, a *base glass* is produced at high temperature by melting the components. Then, the material is cooled to room temperature. At this point, normally, the base glass is very homogeneous; it can be completely amorphous or can contain very small crystals. In the next step, the material is heated to a holding temperature, at which the nucleation phase occurs. This phase can last 2 or 5 h. In the final step, the nucleated glass is heated even more, to permit crystal growth. The maximum temperature and the duration of this phase are controlled by the manufacturer to increase the kinetics of growth of all crystalline phases. This process can crystallize more than 90% of the original glass. For instance, in dentistry, manufacturers provide LS2 glass-ceramics for the pressing procedure, with approximate 70% crystallinity.[1,7,24,25]

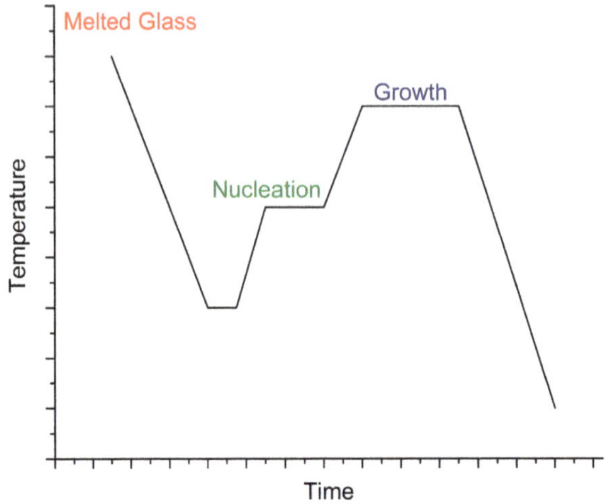

Figure 3. Schematic temperature–time for the controlled crystallization of a glass ceramic body. Adapted from Ref. [1]

Nucleation and crystallization processes are complex and have been studied for several decades. Nevertheless, a mathematical model able to describe the nucleation process is not yet available. Very often, this process can result in various kinds of crystals and glasses instead of only one kind of each. For that reason, it is very important to understand the thermodynamics of the first nuclei, also called *critical nuclei*, to determine how crystals are formed and how they were grown. The mechanism of nucleation is often divided into two kinds: homogeneous or heterogeneous. Nucleation can be initiated either at the surface or into the volume of the glass. In the next sections, a synthesis of all of these concepts is provided for dental researchers. For further information, see Refs. [6–7, 25–33].

3.1.1. *Homogeneous Nucleation*

The formation of the critical nuclei in the base glass depends on the formation of an interface between the two phases. Glasses are normally thermodynamically unstable. When the base glass is heated, and the temperature reaches the glass transition range, the devitrification process starts. The kinetics are very complex, but the thermodynamic driving force involves the increase of the Gibbs free energy of a very small region (including its surface energy) for interface boundary formation. In this mechanism, critical nuclei can be formed on the surface or in the volume of the glass.[1,5,8]

3.1.2. *Heterogeneous Nucleation*

This kind of nucleation can be associated to foreign substrates, catalytic agents, or grain boundaries different from the base glass.[5] It is the most frequent technique used for controlling crystal growing in glass-ceramics, especially LS2 systems. Basically, it is expected that the foreign nucleation agent produces a high interfacial energy with the base glass. This can be obtained in different ways as detailed below:

(1) When the nucleating agent is a metallic substance with a different coefficient of thermal expansion, a mechanical stress is produced in the interphase, during the hitting process, with the base glass increasing its Gibbs free energy. Ag, Au, Ce, and Pt have been used as metallic nuclei in Li–Si systems.[5,8]
(2) Another technique for heterogeneous nucleation is the microimmiscilibity approach, where oxides from Ti, Zr, P, Ta, W, and Fe can form a microphase inside the base glass, promoting phase separation. The increasing temperature provides the kinetic energy for a primary crystal phase formation, which will lead to the formation of additional crystal phases, including the main crystalline phase.[4–8,22,26]

An example of using microimmiscility to achieve crystal growing in lithium disilicate glass-ceramics is that described by Iqbal *et al.*[30]:

$$6(\text{Si-O}^{-}\ {}^{+}\text{Li}) + P_2O_5 = 2Li_3PO_4 + 3(\text{Si–O–Si}). \quad (1)$$

When a lithium disilicate glass, containing > 2 mol% of P_2O_5, reaches 500–560°C, the reaction described in Eq. (1) takes place, forming lithium orthophosphate (Li_3PO_4) and cristobalite. Li_3PO_4

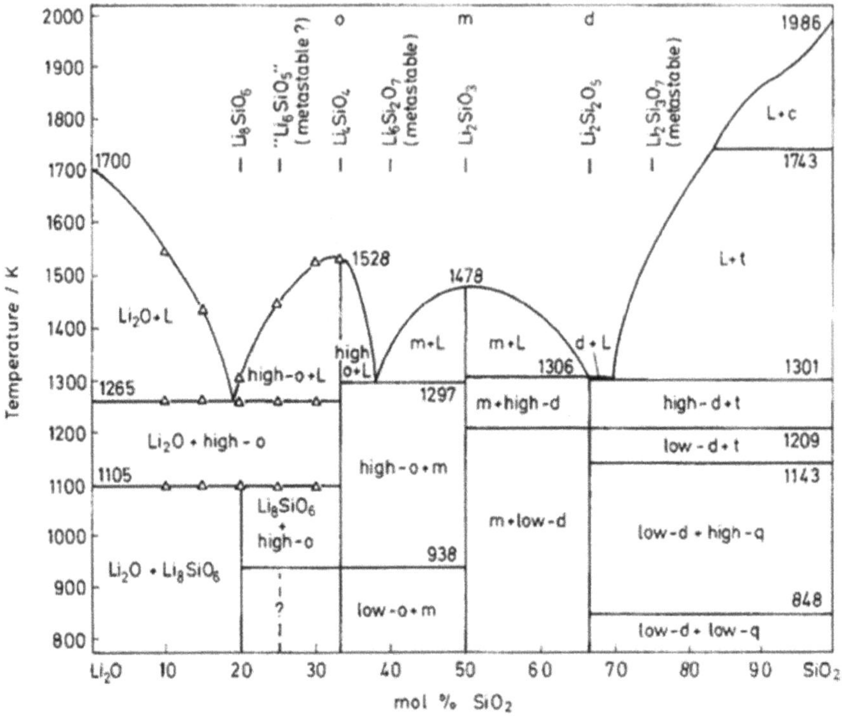

Figure 4. The phase diagram of the Li_2O–SiO_2 system according to Ref. [35]. Reprinted with the permission of Elsevier Science Publishers B.V

acts as heterogeneous nuclei and LM (metastable α') and LS2 (b') start to form on its surface. These primary and intermediary phases will subsequently contribute to the transformation of a stable crystalline phase of LS2 (Figure 4). Further, the addition of P_2O_5 provides a volume nucleation process, which permits controlling of the crystallization mechanism.[22,30,34]

3.2. *Crystallization Process*

Crystal growth process: Controlling the crystal growth of a multicompositional glass-ceramic such as lithium disilicate system is not simple. Indeed, all steps must be well managed by the manufacturer to produce a glass-ceramic with intended properties. The mechanism depends on the temperature and the degree of supersaturation. The thermodynamics of the nuclei/glass matrix interface will control the kinetic and morphological development of the process.

There are different models to describe crystal growth. Lithium disilicate glass-ceramic has a volume crystallization model, different from the surface crystallization used in leucite glass-ceramics.[34,36] As shown in Figure 5, the volume model provides not only a high level of lithium disilicate glass-ceramic crystallization but also a highly interlocked crystal network. This crystalline pattern results in great toughness and other desirable mechanical properties of the lithium disilicate-based glass-ceramics systems.

Crystal growth with the deposition of crystalline overlayers on foreign nucleation agents, called *epitaxy*, depends on several factors. The most important of them is the close relations between the lattices of the foreign nuclei and the forming crystal. The mismatch should not be more the 15%.[5,25] It also explains the fast LS2 crystallization process, since Li_3PO_4 and Li_2SiO_3 are both orthorhombic crystals with very similar lattice parameters.[20]

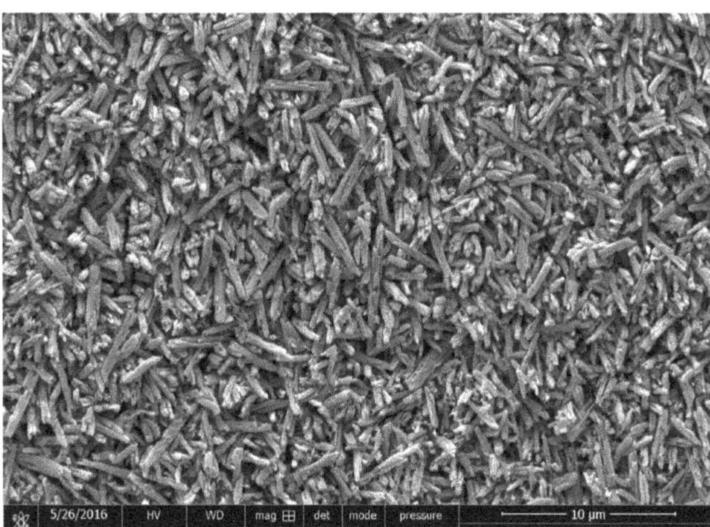

Figure 5. SEM image of e.Max press after etching with 5% HF

The epitaxy of glass-ceramics with composition SiO_2–Li_2O–K_2O–Al_2O_3–ZrO_2–P_2O_5 (IPS e.Max CAD) was well explained by Holand *et al.*[34] and other researchers.[29,37–39] After the heterogeneous nuclei formation described in Eq. (1), nanophases of Li_2SiO_3 and $Li_2Si_2O_5$ begin to precipitate on the Li_3PO_4 crystal surface. Between 530°C and 590°C, lithium metasilicate crystals grow with a dendritic shape, but LS2 nanophase sites do not show any crystallization in this temperature range. Li_2SiO_3 has maximum crystal growth above 750°C. Above 780°C and until 820°C, the Li_2SiO_3 phase completely decomposes, and $Li_2Si_2O_5$, the main phase, undergoes a rapid growth. Furthermore, cristobalite undergoes a decomposition process below 820°C, as described in Eq. (2).

$$\begin{aligned} &SiO_2 \text{ (crystal)} + Li_2SiO_3 \text{ (metastable phase)} \\ &\quad = Li_2Si_2O_5 \text{ (main crystal phase)}. \end{aligned} \tag{2}$$

4. Microstructure

4.1. *Lithium Disilicate Glass-Ceramics*

Lithium metasilicate (Li_2SiO_3), as an inosilicate, have a single chain structure. In addition, Li_2SiO_3 epitaxial growth produces a dendritic structure, with an orthorhombic crystal shape.[5,22] Figure 6 displays a SEM image from an IPS e.Max CAD ingot sample (blue block) after etching with 5% HF.

In this intermediary stage, the Li_2SiO_3 ingot can be easily milled by a CAD/CAM machine because its mechanical strength is lower than the final LS2 phase.

After thermal treatment at 820°C, Li_2SiO_3 undergoes a transformation to $Li_2Si_2O_5$ (Eq. (2)), which provokes a structural modification of the crystalline phase. This transformation was well explained by Zhang *et al.*[39] and the mechanism is illustrated in Figure 7. According to these authors, after the temperature reaches 820°C, the dendritic structure of LM decomposes to rod-like crystals. As the Li/Si molar ratio becomes lower than the base glass, Li^+ ions migrate from LM crystal to the glassy matrix and react with the silicate framework, forming LS2. In addition, the LM structure probably tends to

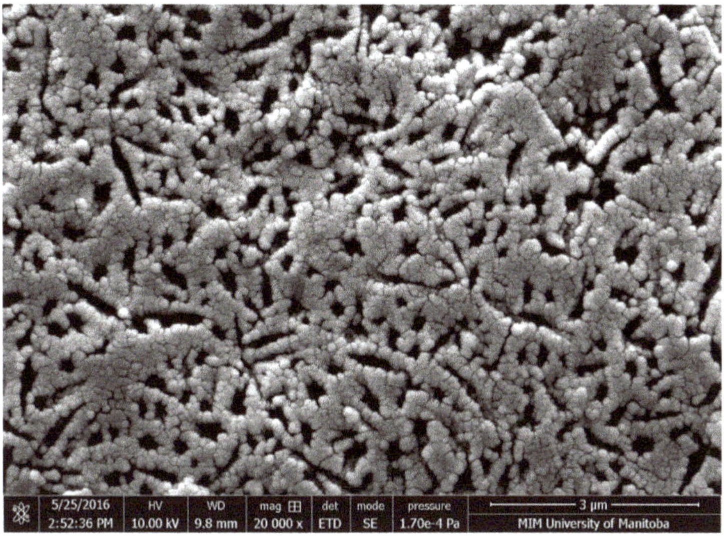

Figure 6. SEM image of e.Max CAD (blue stage) after etching with 5% HF

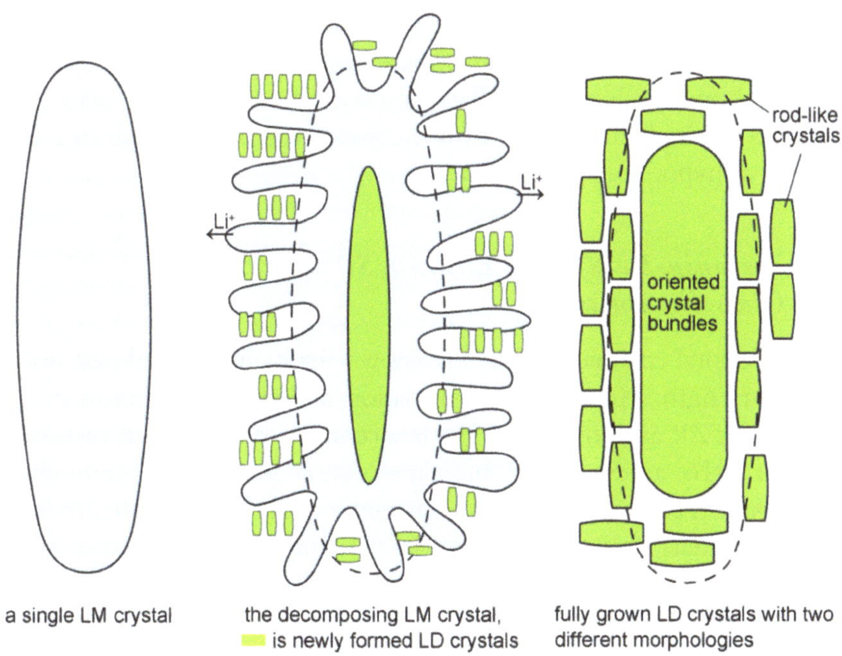

Figure 7. Mechanism transformation of LM to LS2 according to Ref. [39]. Reprinted with the permission of Elsevier Science Publishers B.V

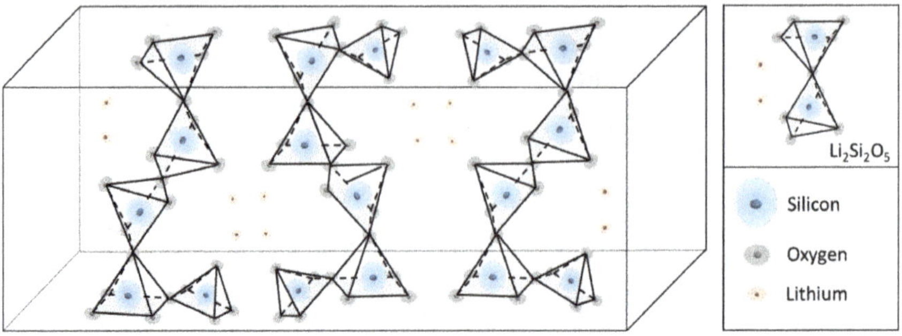

Figure 8. Phyllosilicate structure of the lithium disilicate crystal

reorient from the single chain structure to a phyllosilicate structure, to become electrically neutral.

Figure 8 shows the final phyllosilicate structure of the lithium disilicate crystal. It has a sheet structure, as in 2 monoclinic cell, with a mass of 105.05 Da.[5,20,40]

Our research group found that, at the nanolevel, after the thermal transformation, the LS2 crystal presents a "corn-like" shaped structure, as shown in Figure 9. The presence of rod-like LS2 crystals, about 60 nm in diameter, confirms the formation of two kinds of LS2 crystals, as hypothesized by Zhang *et al.*[39]

4.2. *Zirconia-Reinforced Lithium Silicate Glass-Ceramics*

Zirconia dental ceramic (Y-TZP) is known for its high toughness and flexural strength. However, the formation and the cementation processes of YTZP are not simple as glass-ceramics-based dental restorations. In 2016, a new monolithic glass-ceramic was released onto the dental market, claiming to be zirconia-reinforced lithium silicate (ZLS). These products were developed by Degudent GmbH and the Fraunhofer Institute for Silicate Research ISC, and they go by the brand names Suprinity (Vita) and Celtra (Dentsply).[13–15,41,42] Suprinity is a CAD/CAM monolithic glass-ceramics with a fabrication process similar to IPS e.Max CAD. Celtra presents two different products;

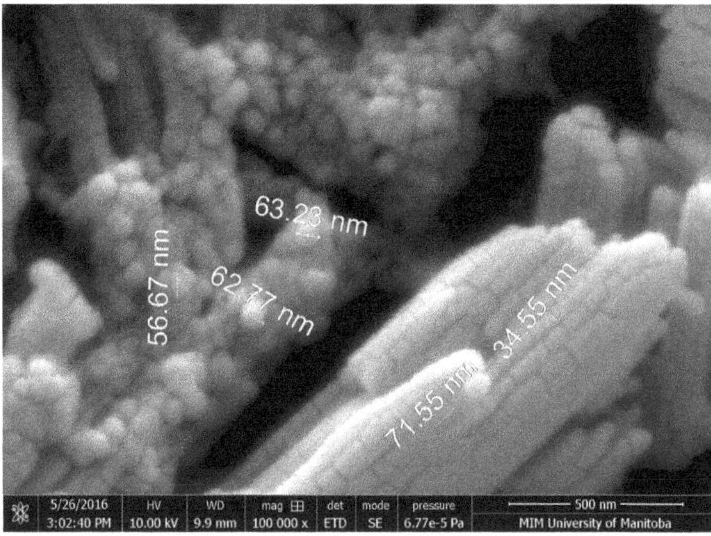

Figure 9. SEM image, high magnification of e.Max press after etching with HF 5%. (100,000×). "Corn-like" structure of LS2 crystals

one can produce dental restorations by a molding process (Celtra Press) and another, a machinable one (Celtra Duo). Different from Suprinity and e.Max CAD, Celtra Duo does not need an additional thermal treatment after being milled in a CAD/CAM machine.[14,37]

There are few data available on the physicochemical characterization, nucleation process, and microstructure of these new products. However, manufacturers advertise that ZLS glass-ceramics contain approximately 10% ZnO_2 by weight. According to them, zirconia works as a nucleating agent to produce four to eight times smaller crystals than LS2.[13] These small crystals would create an "ultra-fine" microstructure, responsible for optimal mechanical and optical properties.[13–15,42] Figures 10 and 11 present SEM images of Celtra Duo and Suprinity, respectively.

Belli *et al.*[37] using Raman spectrometry and XRD, reported the presence of Li_3PO_4, Li_2SiO_3, and $Li_2Si_2O_5$ in Celtra DUO and Suprinity. They suggested that ZrO_2 is present only dissolved in the glass matrix and is not present in the crystal structure.[37] Another

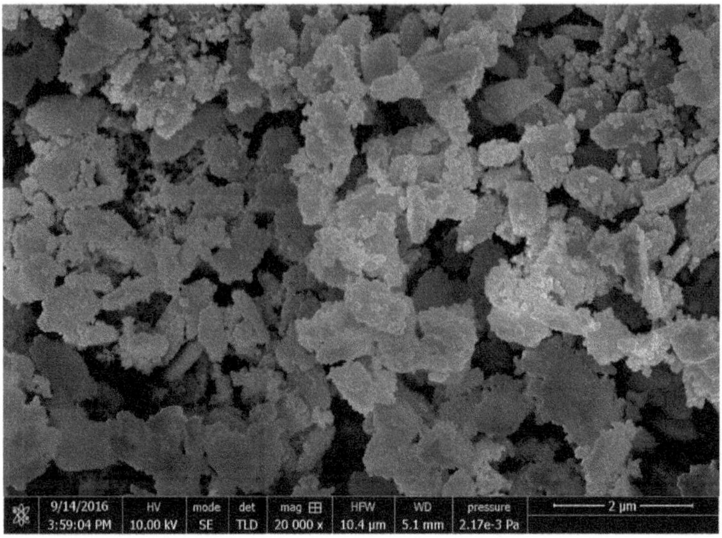

Figure 10. SEM image of Celtra DUO after etching with 5% HF

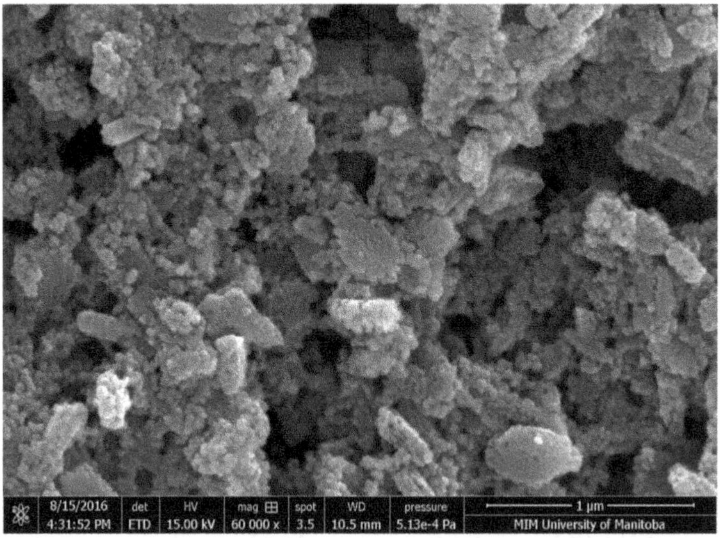

Figure 11. SEM image of Suprinity after etching with 5% HF

study,[43] using XRD, showed Suprinity also has aluminum silicate and tetragonal zirconia.

Related to the crystallization process of ZLD glass-ceramics, Belli *et al.*[37] noticed an increase of peak intensity for Li_3PO_4 and Li_2SiO_3 after thermal treatment at 840°C for Suprinity. This finding may indicate a crystal growth of these phases that would contrast with the process of conventional lithium disilicate glass-ceramics (IPS e.Max CAD). They also detected a decreased intensity of the $Li_2Si_2O_5$ peak for Suprinity and Celtra Duo, compared with IPS e.Max CAD.

SEM images showed that after etching with 5% HF acid, Suprinity and Celtra Duo display rod-like crystals, different from the needle-like crystals found in LS2 samples.[37,43] Apel *et al.*[44] demonstrated that a content of about 4% wt ZrO_2 can prevent $Li_2Si_2O_5$ crystal growth. Our XPS and LA-ICP-MS results (Table 4) confirm a high content of ZrO_2 in both ZLS glass ceramics but no crystalline zirconia structure was found by XRD.[37]

5. Properties of Lithium Disilicate-Based Glass-Ceramics

In this section physical, chemical, and biological properties will be discussed. The mechanical properties of lithium disilicate-based glass-ceramics have been very well investigated. However, relatively few data are available related to other important physical properties, such as thermal, electrical, and optical. Even in some manufacturers' scientific documentation, essential information is not available, which underlines the importance of having independent dental scientists do research on these issues.

5.1. *Mechanical Properties*

In Dentistry, the analysis of mechanical properties plays a major role in selecting restorative materials.[45] From the general practitioner's standpoint, having high fracture strength is considered fundamental in dental ceramics. One reason for that is because a catastrophic failure of a ceramic restoration, under masticatory loading, could be interpreted as malpractice by the lay patient. However, for a dental material researcher, there are many other important mechanical properties which should be investigated, such as Young's modulus, a Weibull modulus, fracture toughness, hardness, tribological features, and others.[45,46] Only an analysis of the complete set of these properties will bring a deeper understanding of the behavior of a dental ceramic.

The 6872:2015 ISO standard brings recommendations for mechanical testing. For flexural test methods, only three-point bending, four-point bending, and biaxial flexure (piston-on-three-balls) are accepted. According to this norm, the preferable number of 30 samples, with the requirement that all samples must be from the same lot, should be observed.[17]

5.1.1. *Fracture Strength*

As brittle materials, glass-ceramics exhibit little or no plastic deformation before fracture. Different from ductile materials such as metals, this ceramic never experiences necking or fatigue fracture by cold working. A fracture of a glass-ceramics dental restoration is always a result of the production and the propagation of a crack. The origin of a crack can be explained according to Griffith[47]: "flaws in the materials can act as stress concentrators and that the separation of surfaces in fracture takes place sequentially rather than simultaneously across the cross section".[1,48] In consequence of this theory, the fracture failure of a glass-ceramic depends on the probability of a Griffith flaw initiating the crack under the specific stress. This probability could explain why the spread range of fracture strength results from lithium disilicate-based glass-ceramics found in the literature.[16,45,49–57] Figure 12 displays the flexural strength of lithium disilicate-based glass-ceramics from different research groups.

Static load-bearing test results are not easily correlated with the clinical performance of ceramic restorations. The particularity of oral environmental conditions is a major factor to contribute for the mismatch between *in vitro* and clinical results. The effect of water, temperature pH fluctuations, and cyclic loading can have a negative impact in the mechanical behavior of glass-ceramics.

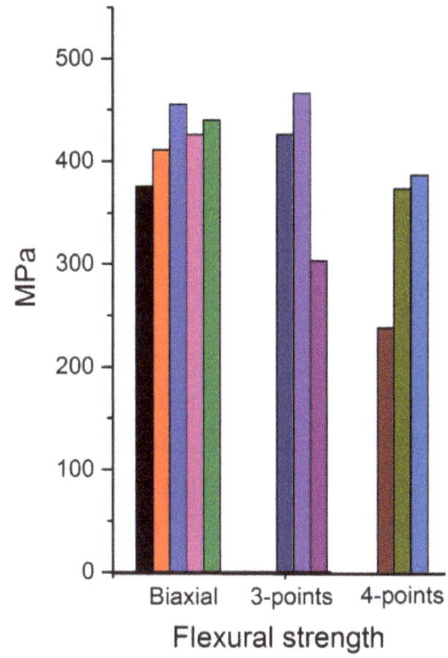

Figure 12. Flexural strength of e.Max press using different testing methods. Adapted from Ref. [11]

In vitro cyclic fatigue tests have been introduced to fill this gap because they try to reproduce intraoral conditions. However, the lack of standards for cyclic fatigue testing and the different setups preclude the possibility of comparing results from different articles. Nawafleh *et al.*[57] reviewing several studies on the fatigue resistance of LS2 dental restorations, concluded that the range of loadings (30–1400 N), the frequency of cycles (10.000–3.6 million), and thermocycling (4–60°C) do not reproduce the normal mastication or the thermo-fluctuations inside the mouth. For more details about cyclic fatigue tests, consult the following references.[53,57–61]

5.1.2. *Young's Modulus*

The elastic modulus of a ceramic material connotes the force capable of resisting the variations in the interatomic spacing when the structure is under loading. For one-phase ceramics, the elastic modulus can also be correlated with the lattice energy.[1] However, for two-phase ceramics, such as glass-ceramics, the elastic modulus reflects the interrelationship of the elastic moduli of both phases.[62] The following equations may be used to calculate the upper and the lower bounds on the elastic moduli:

$$E_u = V_2E_2 + (1 - V_2)E_1, \tag{3}$$

$$1/E_l = V_2/E_2 - (1 - V_2)/E_1, \tag{4}$$

where E_u is the upper bond, and E_l is the lower bond, V_2 is the volume fraction of the phase with modulus E_2, and E_l is the modulus of the other phase. The first model, E_u, assumes that the strain is the same in each phase, and the second model, E_l, assumes that the stress is the same in each phase.[1]

Several studies have assessed Young's modulus of lithium disilicate-based glass-ceramics.[37,38,43,54,58,63,64] As shown in Table 5, the mean can fluctuate from 95 to 107 GPa. Some of these articles present standard deviation values, such as those of Ivoclar Vivadent for e.Max systems.[11] Nevertheless, more studies are needed to determine the elastic moduli accurately for multiphase ceramics, such as the LS2 and ZLS systems.

Table 5. Mechanical properties of lithium disilicate-based glass-ceramics

	e.Max Press	**e.Max CAD**	**Celtra Duo**	**Suprinity**
Young's modulus (GPa)	95 (± 5)	95 (± 5)	107.9¥	104.9¥
Weibull modulus (MPa $m^{1/2}$)	2.64*	1.9*	5.5¥	5.5¥
Fracture toughness (SEVNB) (MPa $m^{1/2}$)	2.5–3	2.0–2.5	2.65	2.0
Hardness (GPa)	5.5			7
Flexural strength (MPa)	400 (± 40)			

Sources: Adapted From *Ref. [49] and ¥Ref. [37].

5.1.3. *Fracture Toughness* (K_{IC})

The fracture toughness of a material indicates the ability of its structure to resist crack propagation. A dental ceramic with high fracture toughness envisages good clinical performance.[38,49,50,65] ISO 6872: 2015 and ASTM E1820-16 describe the standard test methods for measuring fracture toughness. Diverse approaches have been used to assess fracture toughness, among them the most common methods are indentation strength, indentation fracture, single-edge V-notched beam (SEVNB), compact tension, and chevron-notched short rod (CNSR).[50,65–67] Each method has advantages and limitations, and some are technique-sensitive. Probably for that reason, the literature reports different K_{IC} values for the same lithium disilicate-based glass-ceramics, as shown in Figure 13. (For further information about crack propagation, fracture toughness, and Weibull modulus consult the chapter on Fractography.)

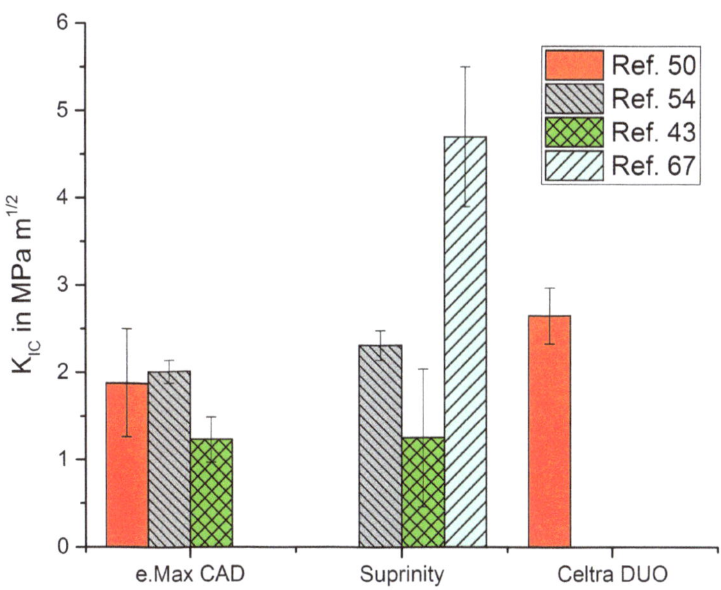

Figure 13. Fracture toughness of CAD/CAM glass-ceramics from different research groups

5.1.4. *Hardness*

In lithium disilicate-based glass-ceramics, hardness testing is frequently used to determine the resistance to deformation, densification, and fracture.[68] The measurement techniques commonly employed in the dental literature are those of Vickers[52,58,66,69] and Knoop.[70,71] These hardness tests can have many pitfalls, especially when testing polycrystalline materials, such as like glass-ceramics. Factors such as crystal size, grain boundaries, the hardness of the glassy phase, and the hardness of the crystalline phase may be responsible for the large scatter of results.[68,72] Nanoindentation testing has been introduced, in the ceramic research field, as a powerful tool for providing more accurate results.[73,74] The small indentations used in this technique may be on the order of 10 nm to 1 μm, and the loads may be 10–100 mN. The nanoindentation technique can provide the Young's modulus and the hardness values continuously, along different crystalline phases of lithium disilicate-based glass-ceramics.[38,63,74] Figure 14 shows nanoindentation results for some commercial products. For more information, please consult the chapter on Nanoindentation.

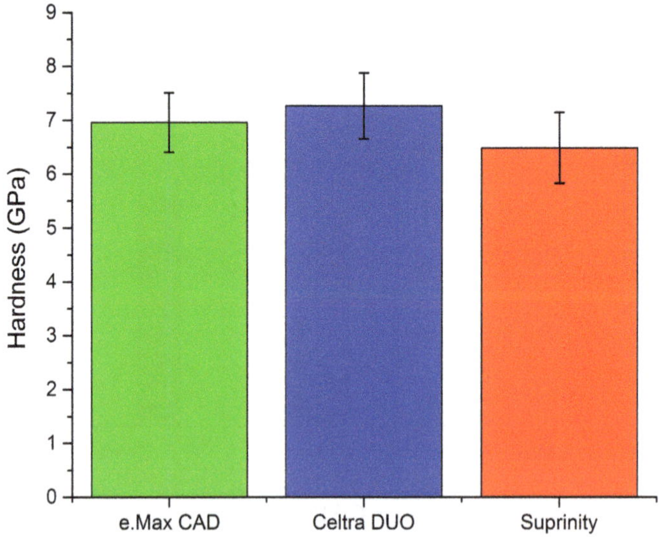

Figure 14. Hardness values from nanoindentation tests

5.1.5. *Wear*

Wear and other tribological properties are directly related to hardness. Ideally, it is expected that restorative ceramic materials have wear rates as low as that of natural enamel. Further, it is not suitable that they cause attrition and abrasion of opposing teeth.[58,75,76] In one study,[75] the results of which are found in Figure 15, the wear rates of LS2 and ZLS glass-ceramics showed no statistical difference from that of dental enamel after 120,000 cycles. However, the author called attention to a detectable reduction in the wear rates when Celtra DUO undergoes the optional glaze step. Another *in vitro* study[76] showed that LS2 glass-ceramics increased the wear rate 1.7 times when the pH of the solution decreased from pH 7 to pH 3. In another study, the abrasion of LS2 glass-ceramic by toothbrushing was studied.[77] The authors pointed out that all the glass-ceramics studied had a reduction of the superficial gloss by the high abrasivity of the toothpaste slurry.

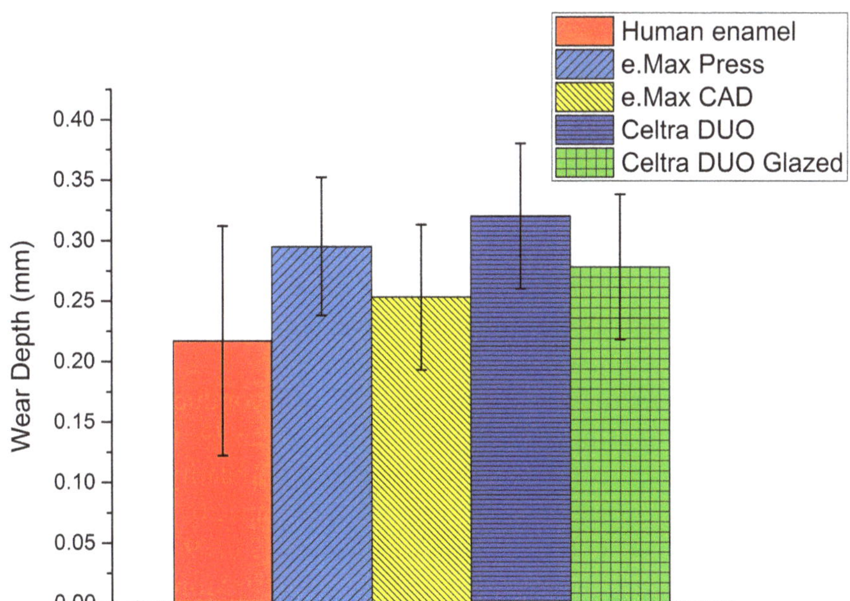

Figure 15. Wear rate of lithium disilicate-based glass-ceramics compared with enamel. Adapted from Ref. [75]

5.2. *Other Physical Properties*

5.2.1. *Density*

The density of a glass-ceramic is mainly determined by the atomic packing of the crystalline structure. A close-packed structure with oxygen ions has a high density of atomic packing, and thus more atoms per volume. In contrast, structures with simple cubic packing of the oxygen atoms, e.g. SiO_2, have low densities.[1,5] Density of LS2 and ZLS glass-ceramics are ~2.6 g/cm^3, and these values are less than half, compared with 3Y-TZP materials (6 g/cm^3).[37] The Ultrasonic Pulse Echo method or Density Functional Theory are normally used for density characterization.[37,64] However, the Archimedes method is still used. This method consists of obtaining the mass the sample and then dividing by the volume of water displaced. One study showed lower density values for LS2 and ZLS when the Archimedes method was used.[43]

5.2.2. *Thermal Properties*

Heat capacity, thermal conductivity, and the coefficient of thermal expansion (CTE) are crucial properties of a dental ceramic. Heat capacity, or thermal capacity, measures the amount of thermal energy necessary to raise the temperature of the material by 1°C.[78] ASTM E1269-11 details the standard test method for determining specific heat capacity, using differential scanning calorimetry. The measurement of this property permits examining the difference between vitreous and crystalline phases of glass-ceramics.[78,79]

Thermal conductivity is the amount of heat conducted through the body per unit temperature gradient.[1,5,8] It can be measured by several techniques; one method that has gained popularity is the Laser Flash Technique, which can also provide heat capacity and thermal diffusivity data.[80] The LiO_2–SiO_2 glass system (21–79 wt.%) has a thermal conductivity ~0.901 Wm^{-1} k^{-1} at 30°C.[81] More research is needed to characterize the heat capacity and thermal conductivity of the LS2 and ZLS dental glass ceramics, because these properties are important in understanding thermal stresses in materials that need to be annealed to obtain high mechanical strength.

Table 6. Physicochemical properties of lithium disilicate-based glass-ceramics

	e.Max Press	e.Max CAD	Celtra DUO	Suprinity
CTE (100–500°C) (10^{-6} K^{-1})	10.55 ± 0.35	10.45 ± 0.4		12.3
Density (g/cm^3)	2.5 ± 0.1	2.5 ± 0.1	2.62 ± 0.01¥	2.58 ± 0.06¥
Linear shrinkage during tempering (%)		0.2		
Chemical solubility (mg/cm^2)	40 ±10	40 ±10		40
Poisson's ration	2.3	0.215¥	0.222¥	0.208¥

Notes: Data from manufacturer's reports.
¥ Ref. [37].

The CTE expresses the amount of dimensional changing (volume or linear) per degree of temperature change. It is expressed in the follow equation:

$$\alpha = \frac{\Delta l}{l \Delta T} \tag{5}$$

In a ceramic structure, the specific volume of any given crystal increases with temperature. As the vibrations of atoms increase, the lattice energy increases, corresponding to a lattice expansion. Thermodynamically, the internal energy in the ceramic lattice increases but the entropy decreases.[1,5,7] Lithium disilicate glass-ceramics may have very different CTE values; depending on their composition, the CTE can be near zero for cookware tools or near 10×10^{-6} k^{-1} for dental applications, as shown in Table 6.[3,5,8,9]

5.2.3. *Optical Properties*

Ceramic dental restorations were introduced in dentistry mainly because they mimic the aesthetic features of natural teeth. Nowadays, cosmetic properties are as important as mechanical properties, and they are the principal demand and the first feature remarked on by patients. On this issue, glass-ceramics for all ceramic restorations

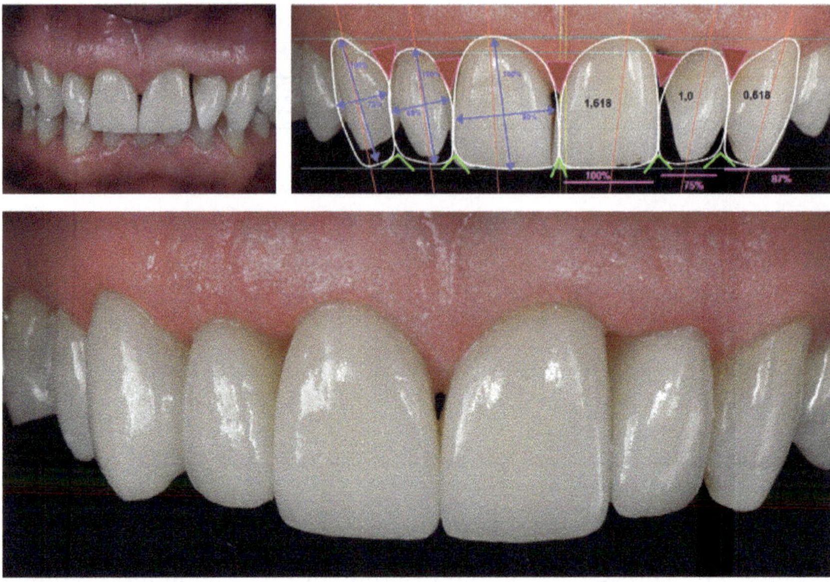

Figure 16. Clinical case showing six anterior laminates using lithium disilicate-based glass-ceramics (Courtesy Dr. Carlos Francci, University of Sao Paulo.)

were able to copy or even "outperform natural tooth structure" (Figure 16).[5] Nevertheless, optical properties, such as opacity, translucence, absorption, refractive index, dispersion, surface gloss, and color have been barely studied for LS2 systems[82–90] and minimally for ZLS systems.[91]

5.3. *Chemical Properties*

Dental ceramics are considered more chemically stable than other dental materials. However, they are not insoluble in oral fluids.[92–94] The broad range of pH values (e.g. fruit juices at pH 2.0, soy beans at pH 12) to which a dental ceramic is exposed can result in surface corrosion.[93] This chemical corrosion can increase surface roughness, staining and biofilm attachment, and affect fracture strength.[95]

ISO 6872:2015 recommends a chemical solubility test in 4% acetic acid at 80 ± 3°C for 16 h.[17] The maximal chemical solubility permitted for a class 3 ceramic is < 100 $\mu g/cm^2$. Table 6 shows that the chemical solubility of the lithium disilicate-based glass-ceramic assessed is < 50 $\mu g/cm^2$, far below the standard limit. However, clinical reports have mentioned patients' complaints due to overglaze degradation.[93,96–98]

5.4. *Biocompatibility Issues*

Nowadays, lithium has been used in several applications in engineering (e.g. glass-ceramics for cooking utensils, battery systems, etc.) and medicine (e.g. as a drug for neurological disorders) besides dental restorations. Issues related to the biosafety of these lithium-based products have been raised in the literature.[99–101] Further, the number of cases of lithium-related diseases has increased over the last decades. In Dentistry, some researchers have pointed out the potential release of lithium ions from all ceramic restorations.[93,102–105]

The recommended daily intake of lithium is between 0.1 and 3.4 mg, but levels up 10 mg/day have shown no adverse effect on human health.[106] In medicine, drugs containing lithium salts have been used since the 1940s for psychiatric treatment, notably for cases involving bipolar disorder and depression.[107] For patients with mild bipolar disorder, the prescribed lithium dosage normally is between 200 and 400 mg/day but, in severe cases, it can reach 2000 mg/day.[108] Extensive research has been carried out on the collateral effects of lithium-based drugs in medicine; due to the narrow therapeutic index (0.6–1.5 meq/L), there is little space between therapeutic and toxic levels.[99,107,109] Neurological dysfunction is the most important potential sequela of lithium intoxication; however, in these cases, the lethal rate is lower than 1%.[99] Table 7 displays some of these systemic side effects for acute and chronic intoxication with lithium, according to Ref. [106, 109].

Probably due to the excellent biocompatible results obtained from feldspathic porcelains, dental researchers have presumed that the new ceramics are not hazardous.[102] Only a few studies have been published on ion release from lithium disilicate-based glass-ceramics, and *in vitro* cytotoxicity tests are even rarer.[102,110,111] Reports have detected

Table 7. Systemic effect of lithium intoxication according to Ref. [106, 109]

	Symptoms of lithium intoxication	
System	**Acute**	**Chronic**
Nervous	Tremor, weakness, hyperreflexia, muscle twitching, may lead to seizures or coma	
Renal	Urine concentrating defect	Nephritis, nephrogenic diabetes insipidus, renal failure
Digestive	Nausea, vomiting, diarrhea	
Cardiovascular	Prolonged QT interval and T-wave changes	Myocarditis

the following ions from LS2 glass-ceramics on acid immersion tests: potassium, silicon, aluminum, and lithium.[92,103,105] Messer *et al.* assessed the mitochondrial activity of fibroblasts in contact with dental ceramics; they reported severe cytotoxicity for LS2 pressable glass-ceramics.[102] However, the authors recognized that their results could not be extrapolated to clinical performance. Anusavice and Zang,[103] studying glass-ceramics from the Li_2O–Al_2O_3–CaO–SiO_2 system, detected a very low amount of lithium ion released, even under lengthy storage conditions (pH 11 and 80°C). They calculated that, even assuming that someone has all his teeth crowned, the amount of lithium ion released would be 1.2 mg/day.

Manufacturers recognized that dental technicians are those with highest biological risk potential.[11] Often, ceramic restorations need to be ground and polished in dental labs; as a consequence, the dental technician is exposed to the inhalation of fine dust that can contain lithium and other minerals. Using protective masks and suction equipment are a source of additional protection, which must be carried out to avoid health issues.

Acknowledgments

The author acknowledges Dr. Edgar D. Zanotto and Dr. Edward Sacher for reviewing this chapter. Also, thanks are due to the students

Muna Bebsh, Ana Carla Carvalho Fernades, and Miguel França for performing some of the experiments and for doing some of the art-work. Thanks to Elsevier Science Publishers B.V. for allowing to the use of some figures. This chapter was made possible due to the funding received from College of Dentistry Research Grant from the University of Manitoba.

References

1. Kingery, W. D.; Bowen, H. K.; Uhlmann, D. R. *Introduction to Ceramics*, 2nd ed. (Hoboken: Wiley, **1976**).
2. Holand, W.; Rheinberger, V. In: *Bioceramics and their Clinical Applications*, Kokubo, T., ed. (Swaston: Woodhead Publishing Limited, **2008**), pp. 548–568.
3. Zanotto, E. D. *Am. Ceram. Soc. Bull.* **2010**, *89* (8), 19–27.
4. Stookey, S. D. *Ind. Eng. Chem.* **1959**, *51* (7), 805–808.
5. Holand, W.; Beall, G. H. *Glass Ceramic Technology*, 2nd ed. (Hoboken: Wiley, **2012**), p. 440.
6. Holand, W.; Rheinberger, V.; Apel, E.; van't Hoen, C.; Holand, M.; Dommann, A.; Obrecht, M.; Mauth, C.; Graf-Hausner, U. *J. Mater. Sci. Mater. Med.* **2006**, *17* (11), 1037–1042.
7. Beall, G. H. In: *Advances in Nucleation and crystallization in Glasses*, Hench, L. L.; Freiman, S. W., eds. (Colombus, OH: American Ceramic Society, **1971**), pp. 251–261.
8. Beall, G. H. *A. Rev. Mater. Sci.* **1992**, *22*, 91–119.
9. Beall, G. H. *Int. J. Appl. Glass Sci.* **2014**, *5* (2), 93–103.
10. Schweiger, M.; Frank, M.; Rheinberger, V.; Hoeland, W. Sinterable Lithium Disilicate Glass Ceramic, US Patent, **1999**.
11. Bühler-Zemp, P.; Völkel, T.; Fischer., K. *Scientific Documentation IPS e.max® CAD*. Ivoclar Vivadent, A. G. ed. (Liechtenstein: e.max® Press, **2011**).
12. Schweiger, M.; Rheillberger, V. M.; Burke, H.; Holand, W. Lithium Silicate Materials, **2008**, US Patent 7,316,740 B2.
13. Celtra: Developed to Make a Difference Clinical Guide. Dentsply Sirona Prosthetics. Dentsply International Inc., www.celtra-dentsplysirona.com, **2016**.

14. Celtra® Duo: Developed to make a difference. Dentsply Sirona, International. Available at: http://www.degudent.com/Communication_and_Service/Download/Celtra/Celtra_Duo/CELTRA_DUO_BRO_EN_VFIN.pdf?Z_highmain=3&Z_highsub=2&Z_highsubsub=0, **2016**.
15. Virdi, S.; Schettini, A. C. T.; França, R. *Dent. Mater.* **2016**, *32*, e75.
16. Heintze, S. D.; Rousson, V. *Int. J. Prosthodont.* **2010**, *23* (2), 129–133.
17. Standardization, I. O. F. Dental Ceramics. DIN EN ISO 6872:2015, European Committee for Standardization. Technical Committee CEN/TC 55 "Dentistry", sponsoring body, **2015**, p. 35.
18. Anusavice, K. *Phillips' Science of Dental Materials*, 12th ed. (Philadelphia: W.B. Saunders Company, **2013**).
19. Greenwood, N. N.; Earnshaw, A. *Chemistry of the Elements*, 2nd ed. (Amsterdam: Elsevier, **1997**).
20. De Jong, B. H. W. S.; Super, H. T. J.; Spek, A. L.; Veldman, N.; Nachtegaalc, G.; Fischer, J. C. *Acta Cryst. B* **1998**, *58*, 568–577.
21. Wen, G.; Zheng, X.; Song, L. *Acta Mater.* **2007**, *55* (10), 3583–3591.
22. Headley, T. J.; Loehman, R. E. *J. Am. Ceram. Soc.* **1984**, *67* (9), 620–625.
23. Beall, G. H.; Karstetter, B. R.; Rittler, H. L. *J. Am. Ceram. Soc.* **1967**, *50* (4), 181–190.
24. Holand, W.; Beall, G. H. In: *Handbook of Advanced Ceramics: Materials, Applications, Processing, and Properties*, Kaneno M.; Shigeyuki Somiya eds. (Cambridge: Academic Press, **2013**), pp. 371–412.
25. Holand, W.; Rheinberger, V.; Schweiger, M. *Phil. Trans. R. Soc. Lond. A* **2003**, *361*, 575–589.
26. Bischoff, C.; Eckert, H.; Apel, E.; Rheinberger, V. M.; Holand, W. *Phys. Chem. Chem. Phys.* **2011**, *13* (10), 4540–4551.
27. Fokin, V. M.; Zanotto, E. D.; Yuritsyn, N. S.; Schmelzer, J. W. P. *J. Non-Cryst. Solids* **2006**, *352* (26–27), 2681–2714.
28. Granasy, L.; James, P. F. *J. Non-Cryst. Solids* **1999**, *253*, 210–230.
29. Huang, S.; Cao, P.; Li, Y.; Huang, Z.; Gao, W. *Cryst. Growth Des.* **2013**, *13* (9), 4031–4038.
30. Iqbal, Y.; Lee, W. E.; Holland, D.; James, P. F. *J. Mater. Sci.* **1999**, *34*, 4399–4411.
31. Karthika, S.; Radhakrishnan, T. K.; Kalaichelvi, P. *Cryst. Growth Des.* **2016,** *16* (11), 6663–6681.

32. Martis, V.; Nikitenko, S.; Sen, S.; Sankar, G.; van Beek, W.; Filinchuk, Y.; Snigireva, I.; Bras, W. *Cryst. Growth Des.* **2011**, *11* (7), 2858–2865.
33. Nascimento, M. L.; Fokin, V. M.; Zanotto, E. D.; Abyzov, A. S. *J. Chem. Phys.* **2011**, *135* (19), 194703.
34. Höland, W.; Apel, E.; van 't Hoen, C.; Rheinberger, V. *J. Non-Cryst. Solids* **2006**, *352* (38–39), 4041–4050.
35. Migge, H. *J. Nucl. Mater.* **1988**, *151* (2), 101–107.
36. Höland, W.; Frank, M.; Rheinberger, V. *J. Non-Cryst. Solids* **1995**, *180*, 285–291.
37. Belli, R.; Wendler, M.; de Ligny, D.; Cicconi, M. R.; Petschelt, A.; Peterlik, H.; Lohbauer, U. *Dent. Mater.* **2017**, *33* (1), 84–98.
38. Lien, W.; Roberts, H. W.; Platt, J. A.; Vandewalle, K. S.; Hill, T. J.; Chu, T. M. *Dent. Mater.* **2015**, *31* (8), 928–940.
39. Zhang, P.; Li, X.; Yang, J.; Xu, S. *J. Non-Cryst. Solids* **2014**, *392–393*, 26–30.
40. Soares, P. C.; Zanotto, E. D.; Fokin, V. M.; Jain, H. *J. Non-Cryst. Solids* **2003**, *331* (1–3), 217–227.
41. Dental glass ceramics. Available at: http://www.isc2.fraunhofer.de/focal-areas/dental/dental-glass-ceramics/?L=1: Fraunhofer Institute for Silicate Research ISC; 2013 (accessed on Feb. 2017).
42. Celtra® Press, Directions for use. Dentsply Sirona International. Available at: http://www.degudent.com/Communication_and_Service/Download/Celtra/Celtra_Press/Ansicht_Celtra_Press_Instructions_EN.pdf?Z_highmain=5&Z_highsub=3&Z_highsubsub=0, **2016**, p. 32.
43. Ramos Nde, C.; Campos, T. M.; Paz, I. S.; Machado, J. P.; Bottino, M. A.; Cesar, P. F.; Melo, R. M. *Dent. Mater.* **2016**, *32* (7), 870–878.
44. Apel, E.; van't Hoen, C.; Rheinberger, V.; Höland, W. *J. Eur. Ceram. Soc.* **2007**, *27* (2–3), 1571–1577.
45. Wendler, M.; Belli, R.; Petschelt, A.; Mevec, D.; Harrer, W.; Lube, T.; Danzer, R.; Lohbauer, U. *Dent. Mater.* **2017**, *33* (1), 99–109.
46. Danzer, R. *J. Eur. Ceram. Soc.* **2014**, *34* (15), 3435–3460.
47. Griffith, A. A. *Phil. Trans. R. Soc. Lond. A* **1921**, *A221*, 163–197.
48. Maugis, D. *J. Mater. Sci.* **1985**, *20* (9), 3041–3073.
49. Alkadi, L.; Ruse, N. D. *J. Prosthet. Dent.* **2016**, *116* (4), 591–596.

50. Badawy, R.; El-Mowafy, O.; Tam, L. E. *Dent. Mater.* **2016**, *32* (7), 847–852.
51. Belli, R.; Petschelt, A.; Hofner, B.; Hajto, J.; Scherrer, S. S.; Lohbauer, U. *J. Dent. Res.* **2016**, *95* (1), 67–73.
52. Deubener, J.; Holand, M.; Holand, W.; Janakiraman, N.; Rheinberger, V. M. *J. Mech. Behav. Biomed. Mater.* **2011**, *4* (7), 1291–1298.
53. Dhima, M.; Carr, A. B.; Salinas, T. J.; Lohse, C.; Berglund, L.; Nan, K. A. *J. Prosthodont.* **2014**, *23* (5), 353–357.
54. Elsaka, S. E.; Elnaghy, A. M. *Dent. Mater.* **2016**, *32* (7), 908–914.
55. Holberg, C.; Winterhalder, P.; Wichelhaus, A.; Hickel, R.; Huth, K. *Dent. Mater.* **2013**, *29* (12), 1244–1250.
56. Kang, S. H.; Chang, J.; Son, H. H. *Restor. Dent. Endod.* **2013**, *38* (3), 134–140.
57. Nawafleh, N.; Hatamleh, M.; Elshiyab, S.; Mack, F. *J. Prosthodont.* **2016**, *25* (2), 116–126.
58. Lawson, N. C.; Bansal, R.; Burgess, J. O. *Dent. Mater.* **2016**, *32* (11), e275–e283.
59. Takamizawa, T.; Barkmeier, W. W.; Tsujimoto, A.; Berry, T. P.; Watanabe, H.; Erickson, R. L.; Latta, M. A.; Miyazaki, M. *Dent. Mater.* **2016**, *32* (2), e9–e21.
60. Yassini, E.; Mirzaei, M.; Alimi, A.; Rahaeifard, M. *J. Mech. Behav. Biomed. Mater.* **2016**, *61*, 62–69.
61. Zhao, K.; Wei, Y. R.; Pan, Y.; Zhang, X. P.; Swain, M. V.; Guess, P. C. *Dent. Mater.* **2014**, *30* (2), 164–171.
62. Z. Hashin; Shtrikman, S. *J. Mech. Phys. Solids* **1963**, *11*, 127–140.
63. Alao, A. R.; Yin, L. *J. Mech. Behav. Biomed. Mater.* **2015**, *49*, 162–174.
64. Biskri, Z. E.; Rached, H.; Bouchear, M.; Rached, D. *J. Mech. Behav. Biomed. Mater.* **2014**, *32*, 345–350.
65. Scherrer, S. S.; Kelly, J. R.; Quinn, G. D.; Xu, K., *Dent. Mater.* **1999**, *15* (5), 342–348.
66. Traini, T.; Sinjari, B.; Pascetta, R.; Serafini, N.; Perfetti, G.; Trisi, P.; Caputi, S. *Dent. Mater. J.* **2016**, *35* (5), 748–755.
67. Strobl, S.; Rasche, S.; Krautgasser, C.; Sharova, E.; Lube, T. *J. Eur. Ceram. Soc.* **2014**, *34* (6), 1637–1642.
68. Quinn, J. B.; Quinn, G. D. *Key Eng. Mater.*, **1997**, *132–136*, 460–463.

69. Apel, E.; Deubener, J.; Bernard, A.; Holand, M.; Muller, R.; Kappert, H.; Rheinberger, V.; Holand, W. *J. Mech. Behav. Biomed. Mater.* **2008**, *1* (4), 313–325.
70. Pick, B.; Gonzaga, C. C.; Junior, W. S.; Kawano, Y.; Braga, R. R.; Cardoso, P. E. *Eur. J. Dent.* **2010**, *4* (3), 314–323.
71. Rizkalla, A. *Dent. Mater.* **2004**, *20* (2), 198–206.
72. Balog, M.; Šajgalík, P.; Hnatko, M.; Lenčéš, Z.; Monteverde, F.; Kečkéš, J.; Huang, J. L. *J. Eur. Ceram. Soc.* **2005**, *25* (4), 529–534.
73. Peng, Z.; Wen, T.; Gong, J.; Wang, C.; Fu, Z.; Miao, H. In: *Testing and Evaluation of Inorganic Materials II : Selected, Peer Reviewed Papers From the Second Annual Meeting on Testing and Evaluation of Inorganic*, Bao, Y. ed. (Changsha, China: Trans Tech Publications Ltd, **2012**).
74. Calahoo, C.; Zhang, X.; Zwanziger, J. W. *J. Phys. Chem. C* **2016**, *120* (10), 5585–5598.
75. D'Arcangelo, C.; Vanini, L.; Rondoni, G. D.; De Angelis, F. *J. Prosthet. Dent.* **2016**, *115* (3), 350–355.
76. Figueiredo-Pina, C. G.; Patas, N.; Canhoto, J.; Claudio, R.; Olhero, S. M.; Serro, A. P.; Ferro, A. C.; Guedes, M. *J. Mech. Behav. Biomed. Mater.* **2016**, *53*, 226–238.
77. Mormann, W. H.; Stawarczyk, B.; Ender, A.; Sener, B.; Attin, T.; Mehl, A. *J. Mech. Behav. Biomed. Mater.* **2013**, *20*, 113–125.
78. Tequi, C.; Grinspan, P.; Richet, P. *J. Am. Ceram. Soc.* **1992**, *75* (9), 2601–2604.
79. Labban, A.; Berg, R.; Zhou, J.; Johnson, D. A.; Westrum, E. F. *J. Chem. Thermodynam.* **2007**, *39* (7), 991–1000.
80. Gorinta, J.; Choudhary, A.; Bhattacharyya, S. Chaudhuri, P.; Mazumder, R. *Trans. Indian Ceram. Soc.* **2012**, *71* (4), 229–231.
81. Salman, S. M.; Ghoneim, N. A.; Gharib, S. *Thermochim. Acta* **1984**, *72* (3), 269–276.
82. Awad, D.; Stawarczyk, B.; Liebermann, A.; Ilie, N. *J. Prosthet. Dent.* **2015**, *113* (6), 534–540.
83. Barizon, K. T.; Bergeron, C.; Vargas, M. A.; Qian, F.; Cobb, D. S.; Gratton, D. G.; Geraldeli, S. *J. Prosthet. Dent.* **2017**; *118* (3), 430–436.
84. Botos, A.; Gasparik, C.; Colosi, H.; Badea, M.; Dudea, D. *Key Eng. Mater.* **2014**, *614*, 95–99.

85. Dos Santos, D. M.; da Silva, E. V.; Vechiato-Filho, A. J.; Watanabe, D.; Bitencourt, S. B.; Guiotti, A. M.; Goiato, M. C. *J. Prosthet Dent.* **2017**, *118* (3), 430–436.
86. Harada, K.; Raigrodski, A. J.; Chung, K. H.; Flinn, B. D.; Dogan, S.; Mancl, L. A. *J. Prosthet. Dent.* **2016**, *116* (2), 257–263.
87. Lawson, N. C.; Burgess, J. O. *J. Esthet. Restor. Dent.* **2016**, *28* (Suppl 1), S40–S45.
88. Pires, L. A.; Novais, P. M.; Araujo, V. D.; Pegoraro, L. F. *J. Prosthet. Dent.* **2017**, *117* (1), 144–149.
89. Stawarczyk, B.; Liebermann, A.; Eichberger, M.; Guth, J. F. *J. Mech. Behav. Biomed. Mater.* **2015**, *55*, 1–11.
90. Taskonak, B.; Sertgoz, A. *Dent. Mater.* **2006**, *22* (11), 1008–1013.
91. Aurelio, I. L.; Dorneles, L. S.; May, L. G. *Dent. Mater.* **2017**, *33* (2), 226–240.
92. Elshahawy, W.; Watanabe, I.; Koike, M. *Dent. Mater.* **2009**, *25* (8), 976–981.
93. Esquivel-Upshaw, J. F.; Dieng, F. Y.; Clark, A. E.; Neal, D.; Anusavice, K. J. *J. Dent. Res.* **2013**, *92* (5), 467–471.
94. Milleding, P.; Haraldsson, C.; Karlsson, S. *J. Biomed. Mater. Res.* **2002**, *61* (4), 541–550.
95. Pinto, M. M.; Cesar, P. F.; Rosa, V.; Yoshimura, H. N. *Dent. Mater.* **2008**, *24* (6), 814–823.
96. Esquivel-Upshaw, J. F.; Rose, W. F., Jr.; Barrett, A. A.; Oliveira, E. R.; Yang, M. C.; Clark, A. E.; Anusavice, K. J. *Dent. Mater.* **2012**, *28* (6), 615–621.
97. Esquivel-Upshaw, J. F.; Young, H.; Jones, J.; Yang, M.; Anusavice, K. J. *Int. J. Prosthodont.* **2006**, *19* (4), 391–396.
98. Esquivel-Upshaw, J. F.; Young, H.; Jones, J.; Yang, M.; Anusavice, K. J. *Int. J. Prosthodont.* **2008**, *21* (2), 155–160.
99. Gitlin, M. *Int. J. Bipolar Disord.* **2016**, *4* (1), 27.
100. Rossi, A.; Vignola, S.; Nason, F.; Boschetti, F.; Bramerio, M.; Bailini, A.; Pinarello, G. *J. Pediatr. Gastroenterol. Nutr.* **2017**, *65* (5), 496–499.
101. Zamani, N.; Paeezi, M.; Hassanian-Moghaddam, H. *Basic Clin. Pharmacol. Toxicol.* **2016**, *67*, 183–193.
102. Messer, R. L. W.; Lockwood, P. E.; Wataha, J. C.; Lewis, J. B.; Norris, S.; Bouillaguet, S. *J. Prosth. Dent.* **2003**, *90* (5), 452–458.

103. Anusavice, K. J.; Zhang, N. Z. *Dent. Mater.* **1997**, *13* (1), 13–19.
104. Richardson, G. M.; Clemow, S. R.; Peters, R. E.; James, K. J.; Siciliano, S. D. *J. Expo. Sci. Environ. Epidemiol.* **2016**, *26* (1), 70–77.
105. Kukiattrakoon, B.; Hengtrakool, C.; Kedjarune-Leggat, U. *J. Prosthet. Dent.* **2010**, *103* (3), 148–162.
106. Shahzad, B.; Mughal, M. N.; Tanveer, M.; Gupta, D.; Abbas, G. *Environ. Sci. Pollut. Res. Int.* **2017**, *24* (1), 103–115.
107. Zyoud, S. H.; Waring, W. S.; Sweileh, W. M.; Al-Jabi, S. W. *Basic Clin. Pharmacol. Toxicol.* **2017**, *121* (1), 67–73.
108. Gelenberg, A. J.; Kane, J. M.; Keller, M. B.; Lavori, P.; Rosenbaum, J. F.; Cole, K.; Lavelle, J. *N. Engl. J. Med.* **1989**, *321* (22), 1489–1493.
109. Timmer, R. T.; Sands, J. M. *J. Am. Soc. Nephrol.* **1999**, *10* (3), 666–674.
110. Brunot-Gohin, C.; Duval, J. L.; Azogui, E. E.; Jannetta, R.; Pezron, I.; Laurent-Maquin, D.; Gangloff, S. C.; Egles, C. *Dent. Mater.* **2013**, *29* (9), e205–e212.
111. Brunot-Gohin, C.; Duval, J. L.; Verbeke, S.; Belanger, K.; Pezron, I.; Kugel, G.; Laurent-Maquin, D.; Gangloff, S.; Egles, C. *J. Periodontal Implant Sci.* **2016**, *46* (6), 362–371.

Chapter 8

Fractography of Dental Ceramics

Susanne S. Scherrer

Division of Fixed Prosthodontics-Biomaterials,
University Clinic of Dental Medicine, University of Geneva,
1, rue Michel-Servet, 1204 Geneva, Switzerland

susanne.scherrer@unige.ch

Fractography has a tremendous potential in providing to the clinical and scientific community key information regarding failure analysis of dental ceramic materials with respect to design issues, processing, and handling. This chapter provides an overview of applied qualitative (descriptive) and quantitative fractography to dental ceramics. The most common fractographic features found in dental ceramics have been illustrated and described. Qualitative fractography is mainly shown for clinical fractured ceramic restorations, for which key fractographic features have been identified for determination of the crack propagation direction and the origin of failure. A systematic approach on how to analyze such clinical failures is further described, including the use of *in vivo* replicas for securing valuable fracture surface information of *in situ* remaining broken parts. Quantitative fractography is applied on *in vitro* strength-tested specimens, for which the critical crack is measured on the fractured surface providing useful information regarding processing issues and correlating with toughness estimates.

1. Introduction

Fractography is described by the ASTM C1322 as the means and methods for characterizing fractured specimens or components.[1] It involves a meticulous surface failure analysis, searching on its fractured surface specific crack features, indicating the overall crack propagation direction, the final breakthrough zone, and pointing back to the crack origin (flaw) or area in which fracture started.

It is applied to laboratory specimens with controlled fractured conditions as well as to in-service failures. Fractography is part of fracture mechanics and failure analysis to locate and characterize fracture origins, crack sizes, and surface crack pattern and has been documented in several key standards[1–3] and reference books.[4–8] The ability to read cracks and understand fractured surface are routinely used in the field of mechanical engineering and R&D laboratories. It however created an impact on the dental ceramic field only in the 1990 with the very first papers published using fractography for clinically failed ceramic parts.[9–11] The major breakthrough of using fractography in Dentistry occurred with the free e-book *NIST Recommended Practice Guide: Fractography of Ceramics and Glasses* by George Quinn,[5] for which a second edition is now available and downloadable from http://dx.doi.org/10.6028/NIST.SP.960-16e2. This book has provided the needed practical tools and guidance with a wealth of information (over 500 illustrations) to perform good fractographic failure analysis and includes many examples of dental ceramics.

Currently, a large variety of dental ceramic materials is available with different chemical compositions (K, Na alumina-silicates, lithium disilicates, alumina, zirconia), reinforcing microstructures (leucite, sanidine, mica, fluorapatite, lithium disilicate, alumina, zirconia), and fabrication process (i.e. porcelain-fused-to-metal, heat-pressing, glass-infiltration, polymer-infiltration, layering and sintering, CAD-CAM of ceramic blocs). Due to their chemical and microstructural differences, fracture surface analysis can be quite challenging, and thus a good knowledge of fracture surface features is needed. The type of ceramic, mode of failure, processing in the laboratory, sintering schedules, coefficients of thermal expansion (CTE), and ceramic surface treatments such as grinding or sandblasting, are important information when analyzing a fractured surface. Most clinical fractures are often due to a combination of negatively affecting factors which include ceramic processing flaws, grinding damage, inadequate design, thermal residual stresses in conjunction with mechanical loading, and localized excessive contact wear. The careful analysis of fracture surface using microscopy will reveal a topography which contains characteristic fracture surface features or patterns in relation to the fracture process helping in tracing back to a fracture origin, usually a critical flaw.

This chapter will provide an overview of *qualitative fractography* which identifies and describes fracture surface crack features tracing back to the fracture origin site, as well as *quantitative fractography,* based on critical flaw size measurements and fracture mechanics relationships for dental ceramics.

2. Qualitative Fractography

2.1. *Key Fractographic Features*

Qualitative fractography, also called descriptive fractography, is performed on the fracture surface of broken parts to identify all characteristic features regarding crack propagation and crack origin. There are many fractographic markings that have been described for ceramics and glasses.[1,5] A selection of the most common fracture surface features in dental ceramics is shown in Figures 1–11. The nomenclature and definitions of fracture surface features (or markings) used and described below are reproduced from the *NIST Recommended Practice Guide: Fractography of Ceramics and Glasses.*[5] Typical surface crack features seen in ceramic parts that failed clinically such as hackle, wake hackle, and twist hackle are radiating outward from an origin (usually a critical flaw), indicating the crack propagation direction (dcp). These features when closely monitored on the entire fractured part will trace back to the fracture origin.

By definition, ***Hackle*** is a line on the surface running in the local direction of cracking (dcp), separating parallel but non-coplanar portions of the crack surface (Figure 1).

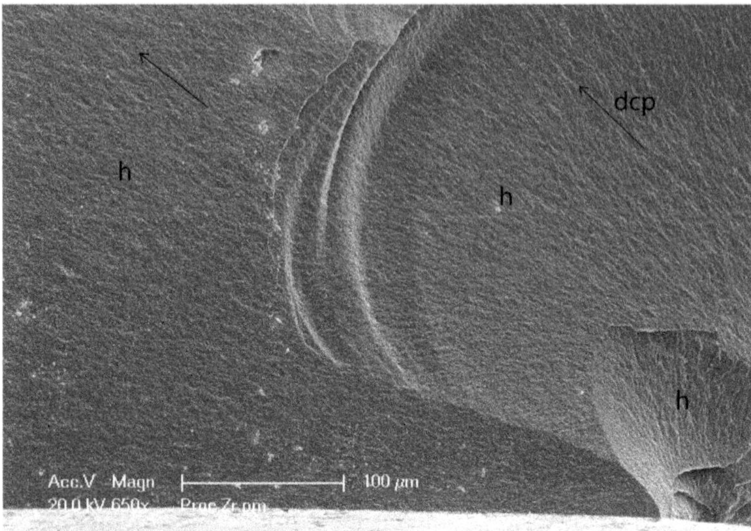

Figure 1. Hackle (h) in a 3Y-TZP ceramic. The direction of crack propagation (dcp) is indicated by arrows. A couple of arrest lines are temporarily stopping the crack front

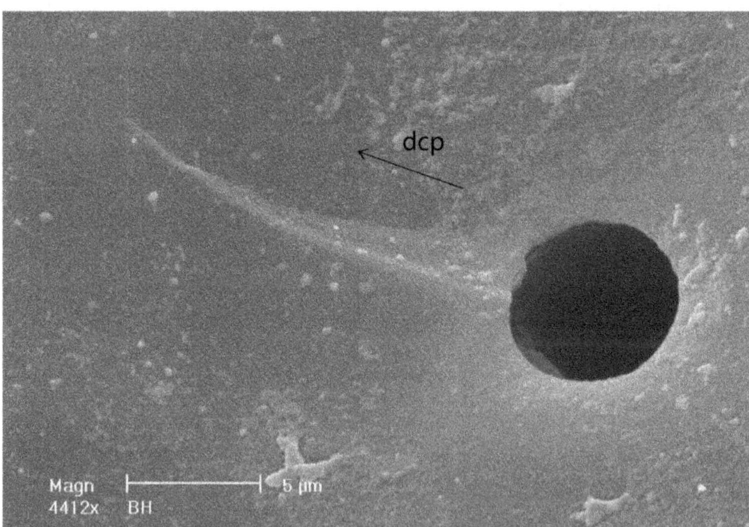

Figure 2. Wake hackle in a veneering ceramic. The direction of crack propagation (dcp) is indicated by an arrow

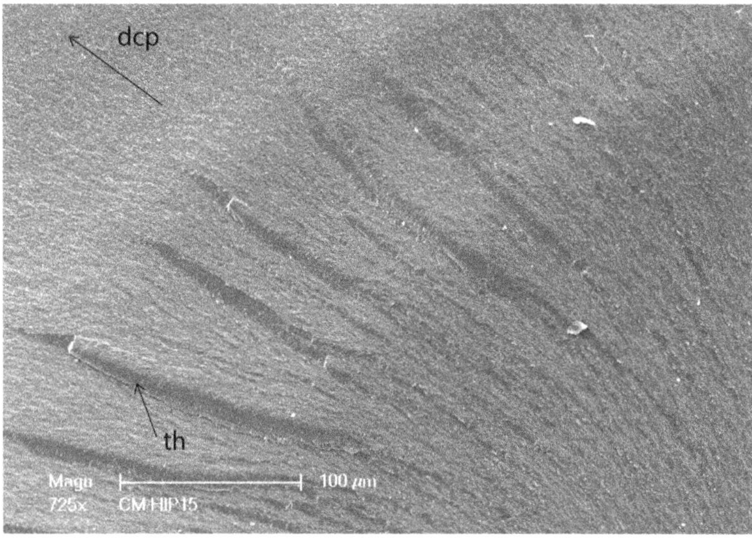

Figure 3. Twist hackle (th) and dcp on a 3Y-TZP

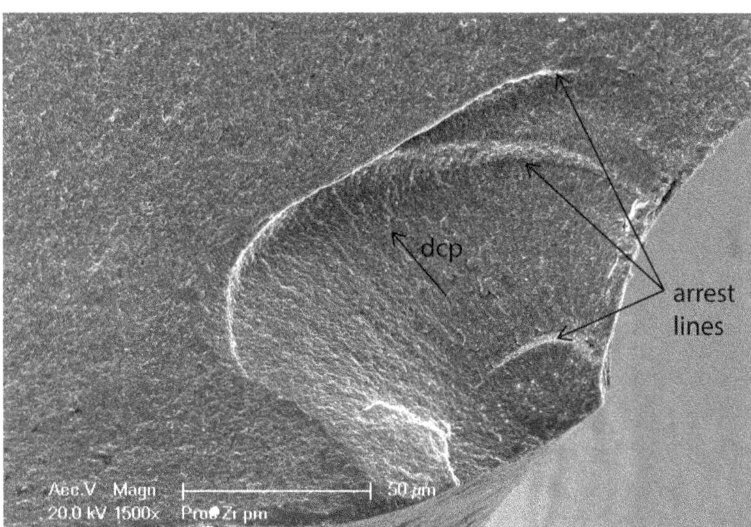

Figure 4. Arrest lines and dcp on a 3Y-TZP

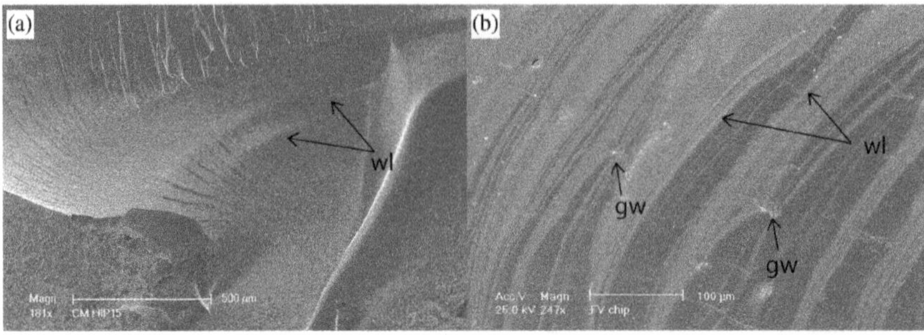

Figure 5. Wallner lines (wl) and Gull wings (gw) shown in two fractured surfaces of veneering ceramics. Figure (a) is a lower magnification of Figure 3 showing Wallner lines (wl) twist hackle and an arrest line above the Wallner lines. Figure (b) has many sequentially following ripples which are Wallner lines (wl) and a few gull wings, emanating from pores and often combined with a wake hackle

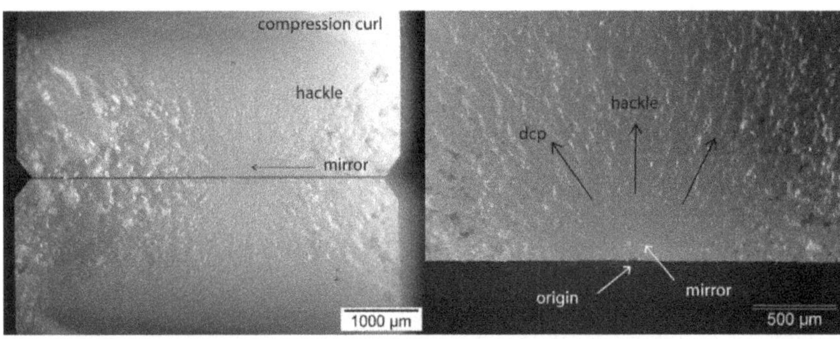

Figure 6. Fracture mirror centered around a surface flaw (origin) in a broken zirconia bend bar. Hackle are radiating from the mirror region outward toward the compression zone. The direction of crack propagation (dcp) is indicated by the black arrows

Wake hackle is a hackle mark extending from a singularity (i.e. a pore, an inclusion) at the crack front in the direction of crack propagation (Figure 2).

Twist hackle is a hackle that separates portions of the crack surface, each of which has rotated from the original crack plane in

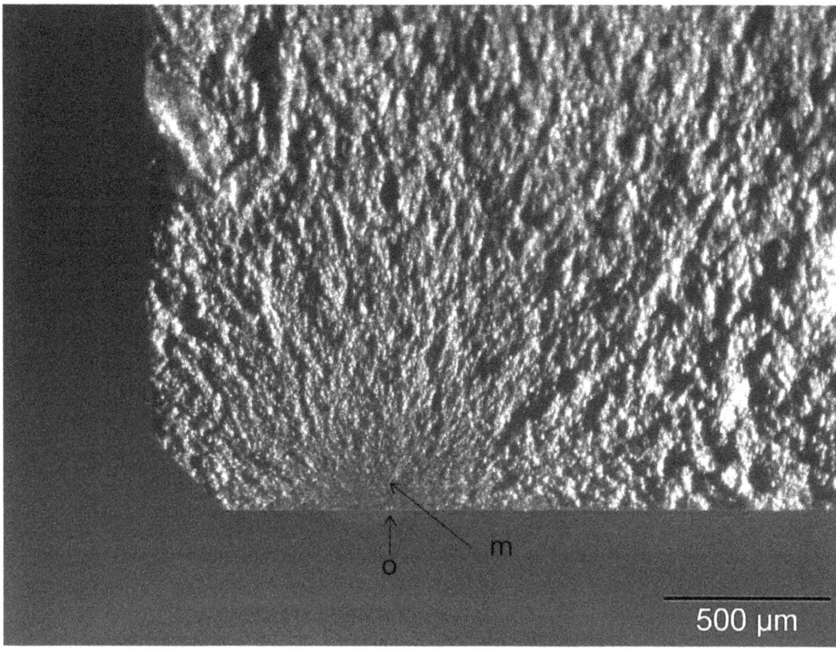

Figure 7. Gold-coated specimen. Fracture mirror (m) centered around an origin (o) which is a surface flaw in a broken zirconia bend bar. Hackle are radiating from the mirror region

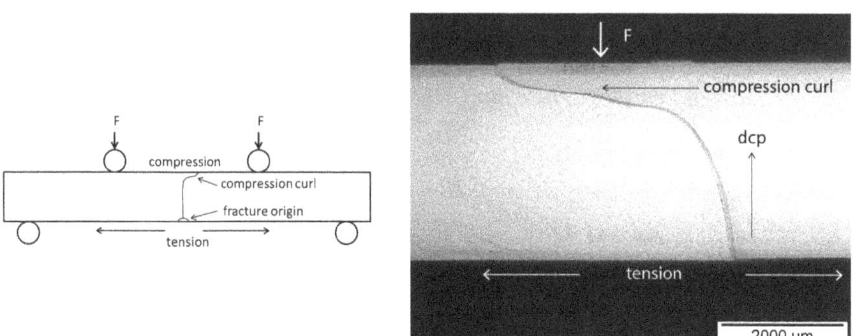

Figure 8. Load-to-fracture test and schematic of a zirconia bend bar broken in 3-point bending. A *compression curl* is easily recognizable as the crack path deviates from its direction of crack propagation (dcp) while entering the compression zone of the ceramic bend bar specimen

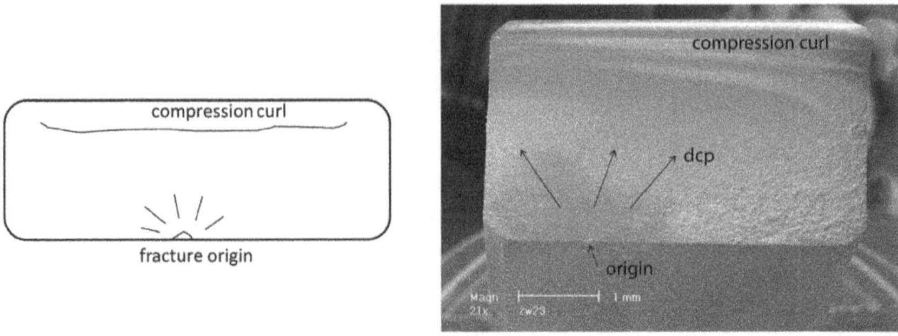

Figure 9. Schematic of a fracture surface in a zirconia bend bar broken in 3-point bending. A *compression curl* together with a few *arrest lines* is recognizable at the top. The direction of crack propagation (dcp) is indicated by the black arrows. The failure *origin* is located on the opposite side which is under tension

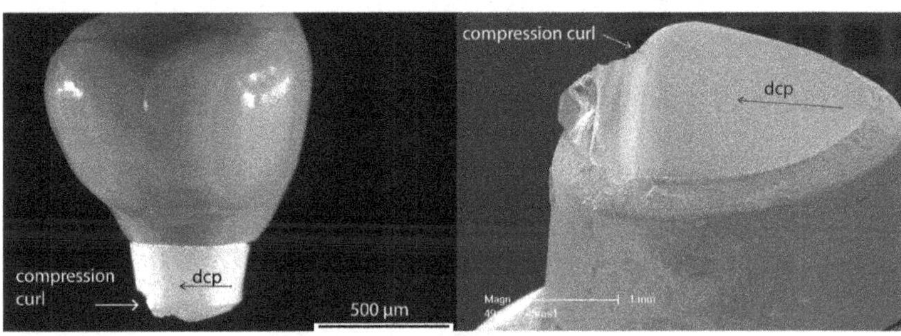

Figure 10. *Compression curl* in a clinically broken dental zirconia implant. The direction of crack propagation (dcp) goes from right to left

response to a lateral rotation or twist in the axis of principal tension (Figure 3). An ***arrest line*** is a sharp line on the fracture surface defining the crack front shape of an arrested or momentarily hesitated crack prior to resumption of crack propagation under a more or less altered stress configuration (Figure 4). ***Wallner line,*** which is a form of arrest line, is a rib-shaped mark with a wave-like contour caused by a temporary excursion of the crack front out of plane in response to a tilt in the axis of principal tension. It may also form from passage of the crack front through a region with a locally

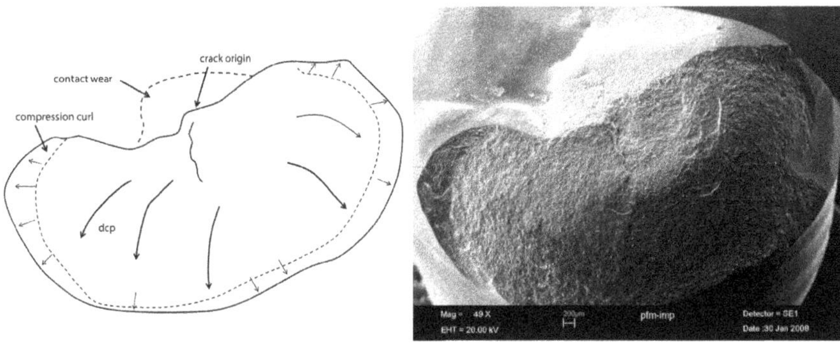

Figure 11. *Compression curl* in a chip fracture of a feldspar-based veneering ceramic in a porcelain-fused-to-metal crown. The *compression curl* is present around the periphery of fractured surface as indicated by the dotted line. The dcp goes from top to bottom, exiting at the compression curl. Excessive occlusal contact pressure visible on the worn surface was responsible for initiating and propagating the crack within the veneering ceramic

shifted stress field, as an inclusion, pore, or surface discontinuity (Figure 5 (a,b)). Among the most common Wallner lines seen in dental ceramics are *Gull wings* within glassy veneering ceramics (Figure 5(b)). An arrest line is very sharp, whereas a Wallner line is rather rounded in its contour. The crack origin is always located on the concave side of an arrest line. It may however not be the critical crack origin, which should be identified by mapping the crack propagation direction over the entire piece based on the recognition of key crack features as will be shown in clinical examples of fractured ceramic restorations.

A *fracture mirror* is a relatively smooth region surrounding and centered on the fracture origin (Figure 6). Although mirrors have been extensively documented for soda lime glass, they are more difficult to see in polycrystalline ceramics,[12] especially with coarser microstructure, and dental feldspar-based porcelains.[13] The inherent roughness of the microstructure is dictating the smoothness and light reflectivity of the mirror region surrounding the origin. Figure 6 illustrates a mirror region surrounding a surface flaw in a 3Y-TZP dental zirconia bend bar which has an average microstructure of 500 nm grain size. Both images are taken with a stereomicroscope and lateral illumination to bring out the surface roughness and the mirror smoothness. Gold-coated specimens may help in the identification of a mirror using lateral illumination[3,5] and optical microscopy. In Figure 7, an example of a broken bend bar after gold coating is given when viewed under a stereomicroscope. The mirror is centered around the origin, which is a surface flaw of the tensile side. Except for zirconia dental implants and round-shaped connectors in bridge frameworks, mirrors will however rarely be seen in broken clinical dental ceramic restorations. This is due to the 3D complex multilayered shape of the ceramic restoration and often thin margins, which implies that the size of a mirror would usually exceed the ceramic thickness at the fracture origin site.

If bending is involved in the fracture process, then a *compression curl* (also called cantilever curl) will be present in the form of a curl (curved surface) just prior to the breaking through of the ceramic component. An example is given in Figure 8 of a zirconia bend bar undergoing flexural testing. The crack moves from the origin on the tensile side to the compressive loaded surface, where it is slowed down and changes direction (curve) before breaking through the specimen. On the fracture surface (Figure 9), the compression curl is easily recognizable by a curvature and arrest lines, which are often visible next to a compression curl as the crack is slowed down when entering the compression zone.

Compression curls are rather frequently seen in clinical failures as a flexure component and is often part of the fracture process. Figure 10 illustrates the fracture of a zirconia implant reconstructed by a ceramic crown. The fracture surface as viewed under the SEM shows a bend just before final breakage.

Figure 11 shows a veneering ceramic chip fracture with the occlusal chewing side on top and a compression curl all the way around the periphery. The schematic indicates the direction of crack propagation based on an initial crack at the occlusal contact wear surface and the presence of the compression curl. Localized contact pressure was responsible for this premature ceramic fracture in a porcelain-fused-to-metal crown.

A *fracture origin* is the critical flaw from which fracture started. It may be an inherent population of defects (also called flaws) due to the processing parameters which include quality of the starting powder (impurities), chemical composition, phase composition, particle size distribution, state of agglomeration, granule forming (binders), powder compaction (pressing parameters), homogeneity of particle packing, granule friction (binders), sintering, green state machining, partially sintered state machining, hard (sintered) machining and handling (22). These defects vary in size, shape, distribution and orientation. They are either volume distributed from the fabrication process (pores, large grains, microstructure heterogeneity, inclusions) or surface distributed from surface treatment (precracks, edge chips, machining scratches or grooves) (22). The material will fail when the nominal strength is overcome by a defect concentrated stress peak.

Volume flaw origins are usually introduced during the processing steps of powder compaction and sintering. The most documented ceramic material in Dentistry is zirconia, as the fabrication route is quite sensitive. The choice of the powder (purity, granules size), pressing (compaction) procedure (static, isostatic in 2D or 3D, pressure), sintering (debinding, sinter schedule, temperature, and time), grinding steps in the partially sintered ceramic, and grinding post-sintering are all critical steps in the processing that may create defects that are more critical than the inherent material flaws. Examples of flaw origins encountered in dental zirconia bend bars after strength testing[14–15] are shown in Figures 12–17 and illustrate problems encountered in the processing steps. Such a flaw population has to be thoroughly documented and described before condemning a specific ceramic material. If these processing defects are also encountered in clinically failed parts, then the fabrication methods and quality control need to be improved.

Figure 12 shows volume defects which are the origin of failure in zirconia bend bars. Both volume flaws are pores resulting from green

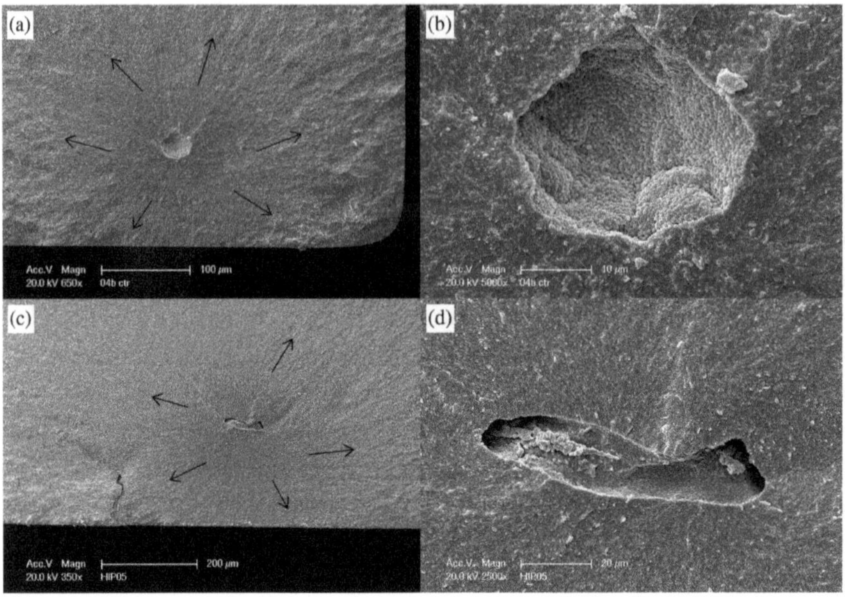

Figure 12. Critical ***volume flaws*** in 3Y-TZP bend bars tested in 4-point bending. The origin in (a) and (b) is a big void (35 μm) between agglomerates created during green compaction. The direction of crack propagation is indicated by the black arrows. The origin in (c) and (d) is a 70 μm elongated volume flaw 300 μm below the tensile surface and was more critical than its neighbor defect located near the surface

powder compaction problems. Inside the pore (Figure 12(b)), zirconia agglomerates are visible and the zirconia grains round in shape indicating free air sintering. In Figure 12 (c,d), the critical volume pore origin is rather elongated in shape and located 300 μm subsurface. Hackle is radiating outward from both volume pore origins as indicated by the arrows.

It is helpful to have within the SEM an option for EDAX to verify elemental composition of failure origins. For zirconia, sinter aids such as CaO are part of the chemical composition in very small mol%. If the distribution is not well controlled some localized concentration may lead to excessive grain growth. Figure 13 shows the failure

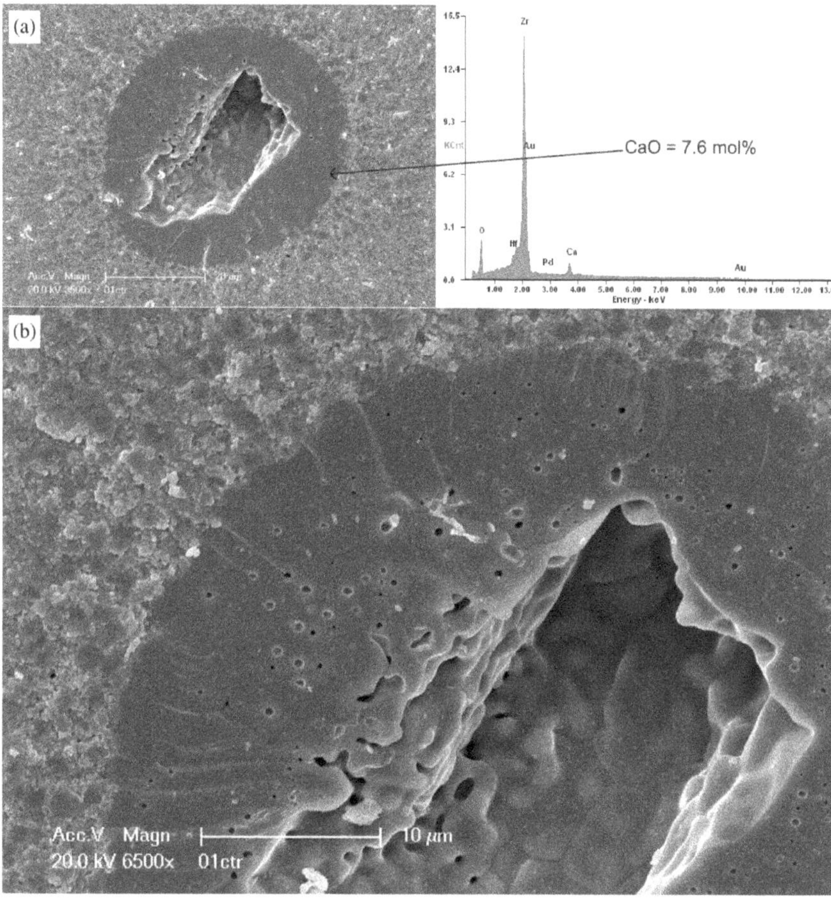

Figure 13. Fracture origin in 3Y-TZP. Volume pore surrounded by excessive grain growth due to a localized concentration of CaO used as sinter aid in the powder composition

origin, a volume pore surrounded by a smooth surface corresponding to localized excessive grain growth. Hackle and wake hackle are visible, emanating from the tiny pores on the fracture surface. Inside the pore, very large zirconia grains (~10 μm) are visible. EDAX measured 7.6 mol% of CaO, which exceeds by far the usual <1 mol%.

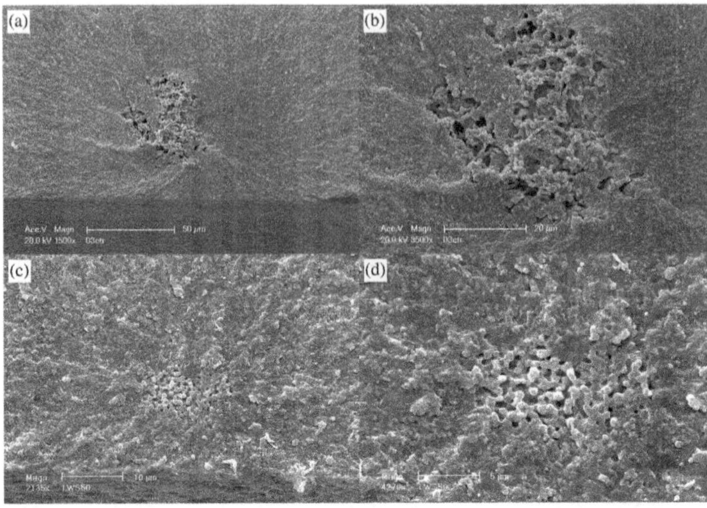

Figure 14. Failure origins are microporous regions located 10–20 μm below the tensile surface in two dental 3Y-TZP bend bars provided by different manufacturers

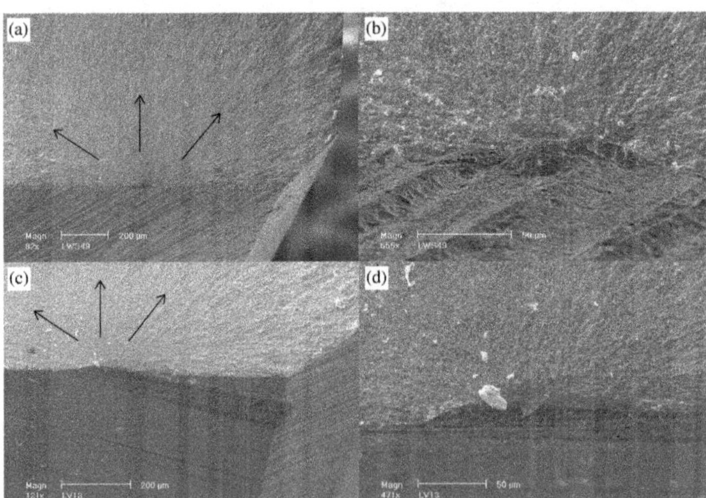

Figure 15. Critical surface flaws produced by machining during specimen preparation. Deep (coarse) grinding grooves at an angle to the tensile stress have created critical crack sizes from which the fracture started, as seen by fine hackle emanating from the origin and propagating along the black arrows toward the compression surface

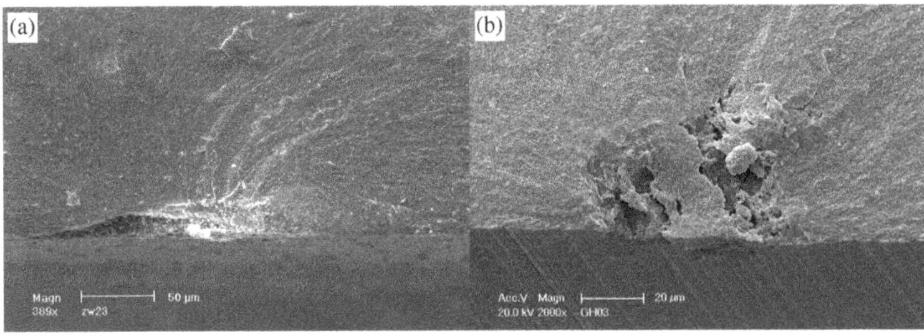

Figure 16. Critical surface flaws (pores) in 3Y-TZP bend bars introduced during the powder compaction step and reaching the surface after specimen shaping to the requested dimensions

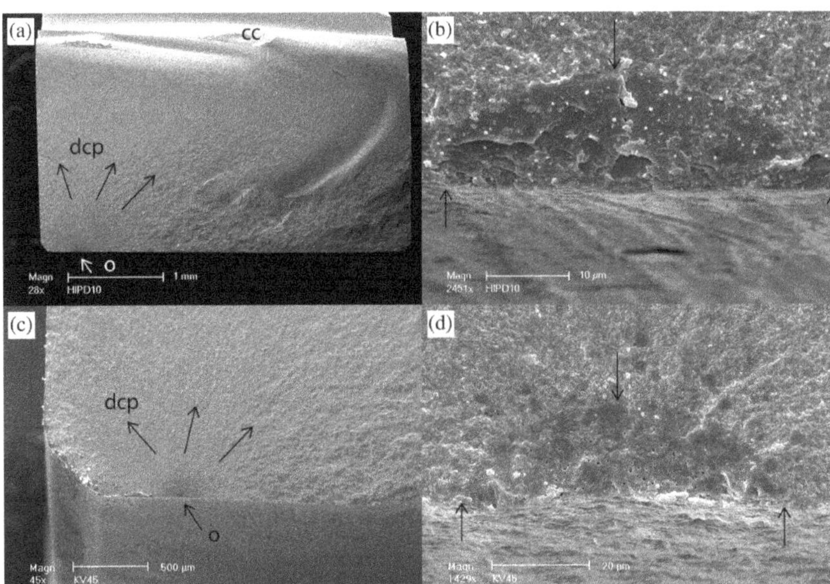

Figure 17. Surface flaw origins from compositional inhomogeneity in 3Y-TZP bend bars. The critical crack sizes for both semi-elliptical crack origins are delineated by the black arrows. Compositional inhomogeneity of CaO led to localized grain growth and micropores as seen by the difference in microstructure. A mirror region is surrounding the fracture origins (o) followed by hackle indicating the direction of crack propagation (dcp) and a compression curl (cc) before final breakthrough

Volume flaws may also be located very close to the tensile surface and are then described as *near the surface* (or subsurface) volume flaws.[1] Examples are given in Figure 14 which shows two fracture origins corresponding to microporous regions of respectively 50×40 μm (Figure 14 (a,b)) and 15×5 μm (Figure 14 (c,d)) located 10–20 μm below the tensile surface. Hackle is radiating outward from the origins. Fracture and tensile surfaces are viewed at an angle in Figure 14 (a,c), which helps in distinguishing it from origins located on the tensile surface. The zirconia bend bars were provided by different manufacturers for research purposes[14–15] demonstrating similar problems arising from processing.

Surface origins are often related not only to machining or grinding of specimens (Figure 15) but can also result from critical pores (Figure 16) or compositional inhomogeneity (Figure 17). In bend bars, the grinding should be smooth (below the critical flaw size of the material) and parallel to the stress direction which corresponds to the long axis in a bend specimen in order to avoid machining defects to be activated during mode I loading rather than the material's inherent flaws. Examples of specimen preparation machining defects activated during flexural strength testing are shown in Figure 15 for zirconia. Deep (coarse) grinding grooves at an angle to the tensile stress have created critical crack sizes from which the fracture started, as seen by fine hackle emanating from the origin and propagating along the black arrows toward the compression surface.[14] Figure 16 shows the origin to be a large pore at the tensile surface from which twist hackle is emanating, whereas in Figure 16(b) the origin is a porous region in direct contact with the ground surface. Figure 17 is an example of a surface flaw origin resulting from compositional inhomogeneity in 3Y-TZP bend bars. EDAX confirmed the presence of CaO which was responsible for an excessive grain growth, thus weakening the zirconia locally where the stress concentrated.

2.2. *Fractographic Montage of Origins*

With ceramic testing, a probability function such as the two-parameter Weibull distribution is often used to describe the strength data.

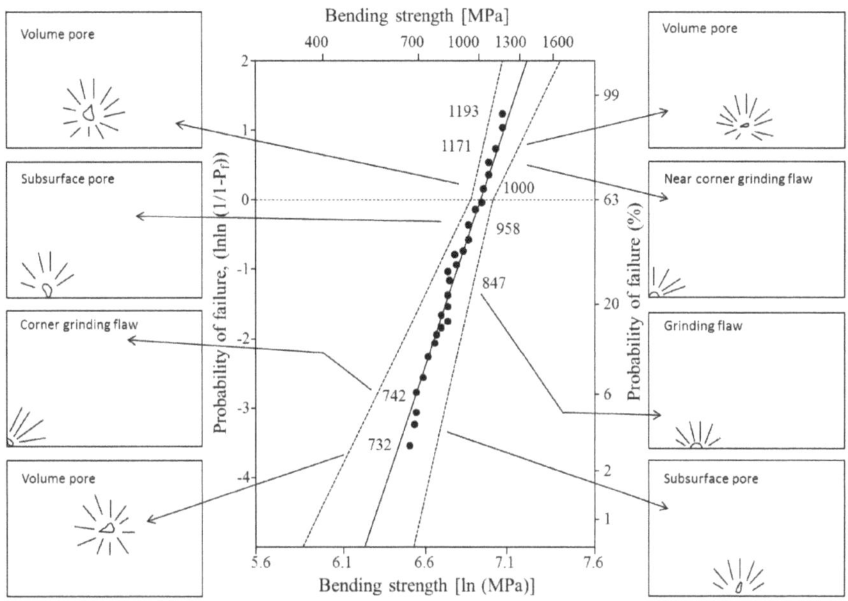

Figure 18. Fractographic montage or labeling of fracture origins on a Weibull plot

A fractographic montage is helpful to better understand the data distribution in correlation with the type of critical flaws as recommended in the ASTM C1322.[1] If no images are shown, the Weibull graph can also be labeled describing the flaw population with letters and/or colors.[13] Figure 18 is a schematic illustration of such a Weibull fractographic montage. The drawings are replaced by SEM or stereomicroscopic images. A minimum of the three weakest and three best specimens should be analyzed using fractography.

3. Quantitative Fractography and Fracture Mechanics

Dental ceramics are brittle materials following the principle of linear elastic fracture mechanics (LEFM). Several fracture toughness tests have been developed and described in the ASTM C1421 standard among which the surface crack in flexure (SCF) test is one[2] which uses fractographic analysis for crack size determination. In this test,

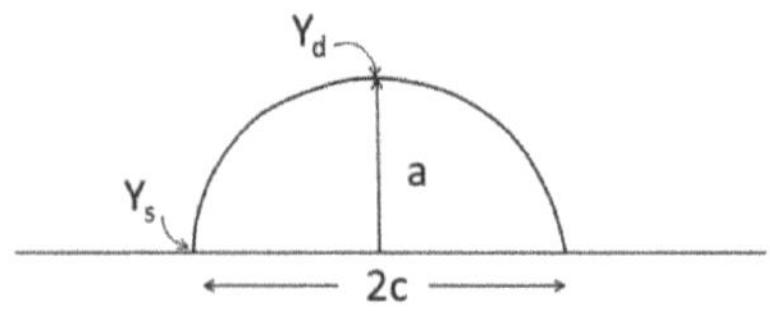

Figure 19. Pre-crack in an SCF broken bend bar. The critical crack depth a and width $2c$ are measured for determination of the maximum Y *stress* intensity shape factor (either Y *depth* or Y *surface*) based on Newman and Raju equations

a small but sharp pre-crack is introduced with a Knoop indenter with a slight tilt of 0.5° (to make the pre-crack easier to discern and measure after fracture), the indentation zone and associated residual stress field is further removed by polishing, and the bend bar is fractured in 4 point bending (σ_f flexural strength). The fracture toughness (K_{Ic}) is calculated using fractographic techniques for the crack size measurement (depth a and width $2c$), and Newman and Raju equations[2,16] for the Y-stress intensity shape factor coefficient for both the deepest point of the pre-crack periphery (Y_d) and the point at the surface (Y_s) (Figure 19), with the maximum Y (Y_d or Y_s) being finally used in the fracture toughness Eq. (1):

$$K_{Ic} = Y \sigma_f \sqrt{a}, \tag{1}$$

where a is the crack depth, σ_f the flexural strength, and Y the stress intensity shape factor (based on Newman and Raju).

This SCF standard has been applied to several dental ceramics including mica glass-ceramic[17] and leucite-based porcelains with varying composition and leucite crystal content.[18,19] The identification of the critical crack boundary by fractographic means is dependent on the microstructure of the ceramic and the final fracture surface roughness. Coarser microstructures increase the difficulty to correctly interpret the crack size as reported for mica glass-ceramic.[17] An example of such crack size identification after SCF testing in liquid nitrogen is shown in Figure 20 for a feldspathic dental porcelain.[18]

Quantitative fractography is also used to obtain fracture toughness estimates from strength-tested specimens by determining the

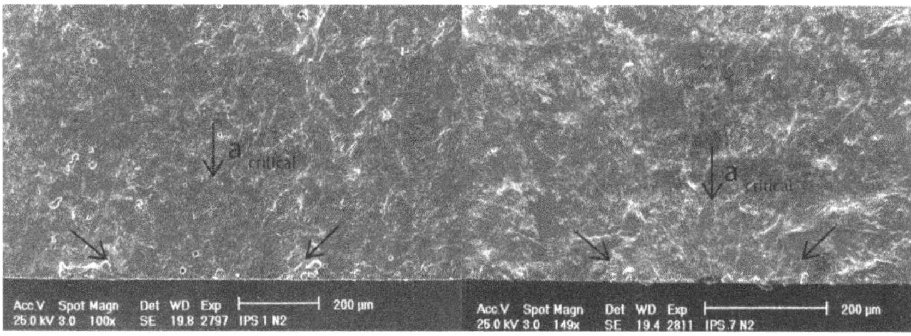

Figure 20. Dental porcelain fracture surfaces in an SCF test.[18] The critical pre-crack size (width and depth) from a Knoop indentation is marked with arrows

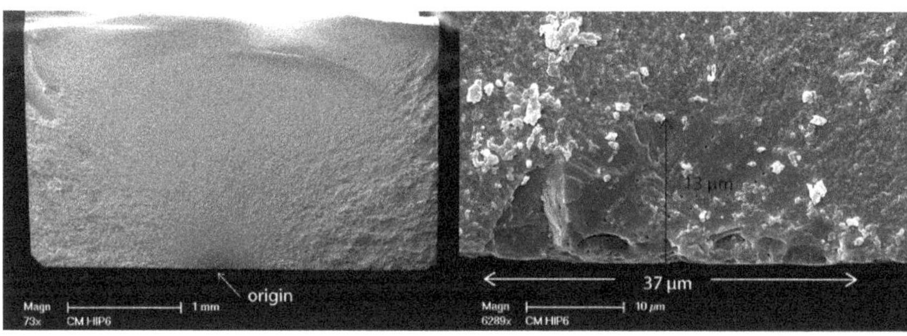

Figure 21. Fracture surface of a 3Y-TZP specimen broken in 4-point bending. The critical flaw (origin) is a localized excessive grain growth flaw of 13 × 37 μm. The flexure strength was 680 MPa

size and location of the critical crack and correlating these flaws with ceramic processing issues. Examples of such application to strength-tested ceramic specimens is provided in Figure 21 on zirconia bend bars in which the critical flaws on the surface responsible for failure is related to excessive grain growth at the surface due to a localized concentration of CaO as a sinter additive.[15] Fracture toughness estimates can be calculated from critical crack size measurements (width and depth). In Figure 21, the flexure strength was 680 MPa. The critical flaw size is 37 μm wide and 13 μm deep. Based on Raju–Newman equations, the Y factor is 1.4 for this specimen, which gives a K_{Ic} estimate of 3.4 MPa√m. This is far lower than classic dense 3Y-TZP which has a fracture toughness around 4.5–5.0 MPa√m. Other work using fracture mechanics relationships and Newman and Raju Υ calculations have been successfully applied to moisture-assisted subcritical crack growth effects on alumina glass-infiltrated ceramic and alumina porcelain.[20]

Fracture toughness estimates were also calculated based on quantitative fractography for other dental ceramics such as lithium disilicate and amorphous glass,[21] and 3Y-TZP[22] using calculations of the Υ factor based on Randall's[23] interpretation of Irwin's work.[24]

Alternatively, the researcher can use approximations of stress intensity shape factors (Υ) as provided in the ASTM-C1322[1] for surface flaws that are semi-circular ($c = a$) or semi-elliptical cracks depending on the c length with respect to a. Figure 22 is adapted from the ASTM C1322,[1] reproducing examples of Υ factor values for small surface crack shapes in flexure test bars. Such rapid

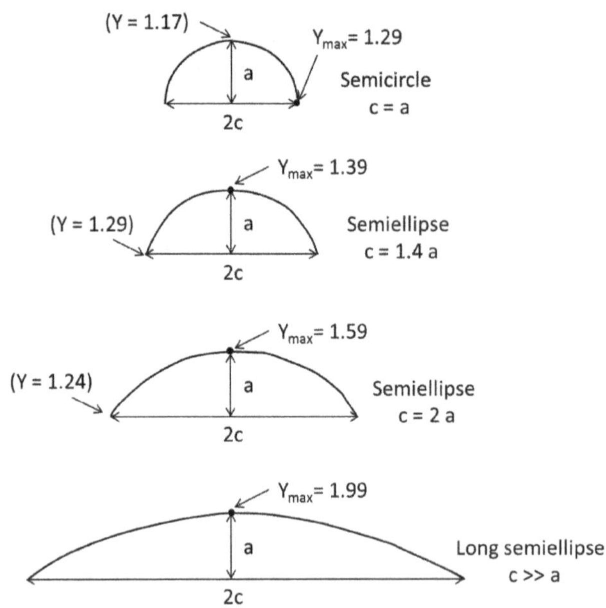

Figure 22. Stress intensity factor Υ for semi-circular or semi-elliptical surface cracks in tension stress fields. Adapted from Ref. [1]

approximations are useful to determine fracture toughness estimates based on crack size measurements and flexural strength values for bend bars or, alternatively, estimate the strength from known K_{Ic} and critical crack size.

4. Clinical Failure Analysis

4.1. *A Systematic Approach*

Dental ceramics have been developed for specific restorative needs such as inlays, onlays, crowns, bridges, implant abutments, and implants. Clinical and mechanical considerations will dictate the choice of the ceramic material to restore or replace a tooth and are part of the daily work in every dental office or medical institution treating patients. Although ceramic restorations in Dentistry overall have a very good long-term outcome, 1–5% may fracture prematurely within the first 5 years of service (Figure 23). These sudden fractures occur without any warning during chewing and are often due to a combination of negatively affecting factors such as ceramic processing flaws in the dental laboratory, grinding damage, design deficiencies, thermal residual stresses in conjunction with

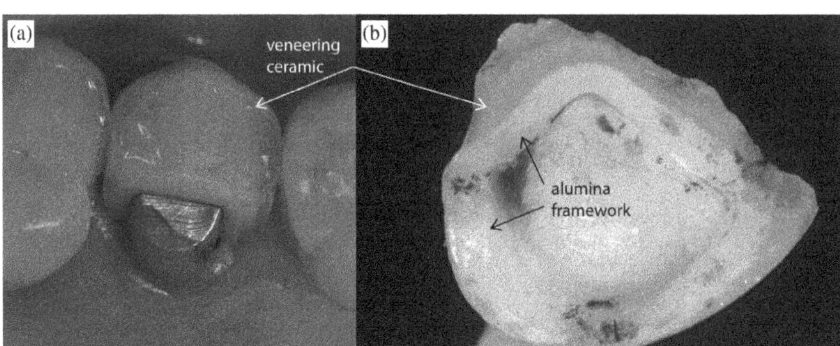

Figure 23. Premolar clinical fracture of a Procera® alumina crown made of an alumina framework layered with a veneering ceramic (Nobel Rondo™). (a) and (b) show the recovered broken part before cleaning on which fractographic analysis will be performed. Adapted from Ref. [25].

mechanical loading, chewing impacts, and localized excessive pressure visible from contact wear. The possibility of recovering a broken part (Figure 22(b)) and analyzing it fractographically helps in understanding the premature failure and forwarding the needed feedback to all the actors involved (dentist, dental laboratory technician, manufacturer, and patient).

Fractography has been applied to assess clinical ceramic broken parts mainly as a descriptive approach[11,25–31] as fracture origins are rarely well-defined flaws as encountered in strength-tested specimens for crack size measurements. Few papers have applied with success fracture mechanic principles based on determination of critical flaw sizes on broken ceramic restorations for stress estimates.[9,10,32–34] Descriptive fractography can be successfully performed, providing that key fractographic features are identified on the ceramic broken surface using a microscope and the methods described earlier.

Before starting with the fractographic analysis, relevant information connected to the failure event and the material need to be collected. Hence, knowledge of the ceramic material, time to failure, circumstances of the fracture event, intraoral location of the broken part, and possibly an intraoral photograph (Figure 23) are very useful in the overall investigation. A *systematic approach* of every failure case is recommended and is described in the following example (Figures 23–25), which has been published in greater detail.[25] The first step is to document the broken part with an overall image under a stereomicroscope (Figures 23 and 24). Areas of interest labeled with numbers (Figure 24) are selected based on the presence of some easy-to-spot surface crack features (compression curl, arrest lines, larger hackle). Lateral illumination will help in making these features sticking out at low magnifications under the stereomicroscope. Gold coating (Figure 24) can enhance some fractographic features such as a compression curl, hackle, and arrest lines, and will provide a good opinion as to the direction of the cracking and aid in simplifying the search for the origin before starting SEM. An overall drawing while viewing under the optical stereomicroscope helps to quickly secure topographic information (Figure 24).

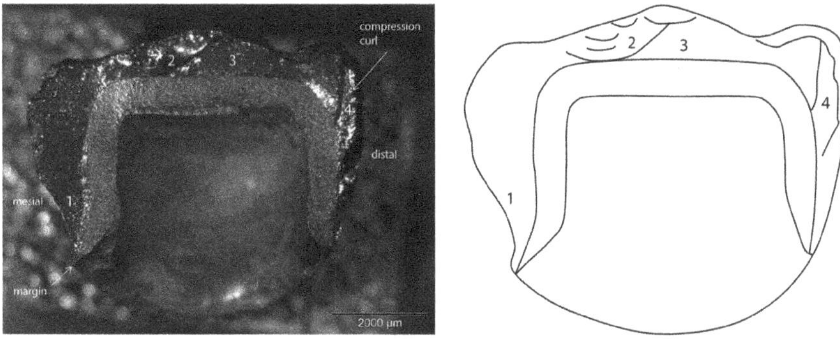

Figure 24. Gold coating and viewing under the stereomicroscope of the fractured part of Figure 23. A quick drawing is performed of the key features seen at low magnification and the zones of interest labeled 1–4 for further analysis under the SEM. Adapted from Ref. [25]

A higher depth of field and power of SEM (Figure 25) are needed to visualize in greater detail smaller crack features such as hackle, wake hackle, and twist hackle. Each zone of interest (1–4) is viewed at higher magnification, and key features indicate the direction of crack propagation (dcp), which is then mapped locally.

In zone 4 of Figure 25(a) is the compression curl which was already identified as such in the stereomicroscope. Several wake hackles (Figure 25(b)) confirm the dcp exiting on that distal crown side. The glassy veneering ceramic of zone 3 (Figure 25(d)) shows again wake hackle, indicating that the crack moved toward the compression curl. Zone 2 (Figure 25(c)) may confuse a beginner fractographer as it shows cracking of the crown from the occluding surface downward to the alumina framework as shown by the multiple arrest lines and wake and twist hackles. However, a big arrest line stops the crack and no further hackles are entering from there inside the alumina framework. This is a secondary event and should not be confused as the fracture origin. Zone 1 (Figure 25(e)) is of key interest. It shows a series of hackles and wake hackles within the veneering ceramic (Figure 25(f)), with the crack path going straight up toward the occlusal side. The origin is to be searched at the

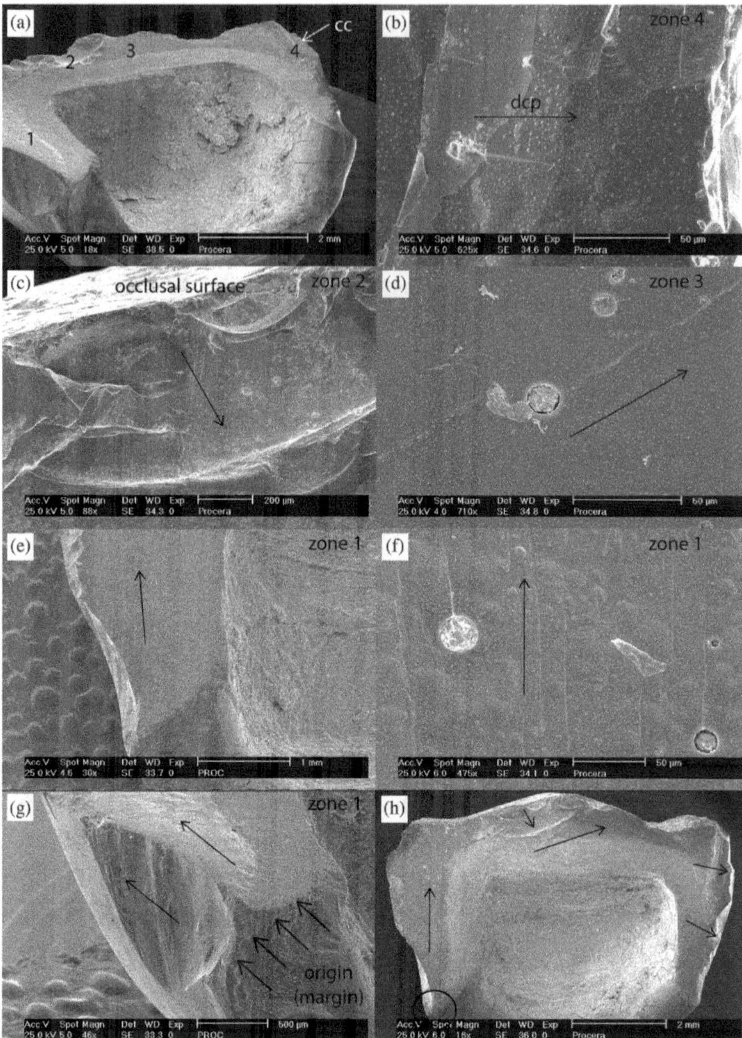

Figure 25. SEM of the broken part following a systematic approach. Zones of interest (1–4) illustrate key features for the dcp. Zone 4: Compression curl (cc) (a) and wake hackle (b). Zone 3 (d): Hackle in the veneering ceramic. Zone 2 (c): Surface crack arrested at the border with the alumina framework. Zone 1: Wake hackle (e, f). Margin ceramic chip and fracture origin (g). (h): Summary of the overall dcp and crack origin (circle) located at the mesial margin

mesial margin in zone 1 (Figure 25(g)). A veneering ceramic chip of approximately 2 × 1 mm is visible containing several arrest lines, hackle, and wake hackles. No clear origin was identified, but the black arrows at the margin indicate the area where the crack started (Figure 25(g)). The overall crack path is marked on the fracture surface of the broken part (Figure 25(h)) as well as the origin site (ellipse) indicating a failure from the mesial margin. This is not surprising as margins in dental restorations are areas subjected to Hoop stress. This mesial margin, possibly weakened by the ceramic chip, was the starting point of the catastrophic fracture which occurred 4 years after intraoral service during a chewing episode.[25] From the margin, the crack propagated upward, toward the occlusal surface, then rotated over the corner of the alumina framework to exit at the distal side of the crown. The cement used was a glass-ionomer cement which has a weak adhesion to tooth substrates (dentin, enamel) and no chemical bond to alumina or metal. Resin-based cements nowadays provide a better adhesion to the tooth substrate and to ceramics. It could have added a few MPas in the fracture strength by bonding the ceramic crown to the tooth substrate, but the problem of clinical failure is far more complex than narrowing it down to a cement issue.

Publications of clinical failures can use fractographic montages[11,31] based on an initial overview and adding detailed views of selected zones of interest which allows to follow the search and identification of key fractographic features.

4.2. *Thin Margin Origins*

Thin ceramic margins are problematic as the machining and laboratory processing of the ceramic may be complex even for high-strength materials such as alumina or zirconia. Cervical margin origins have been identified in 22 fractured alumina crowns recovered for fractographic analysis.[30] Dominant Hoop stresses combined with thin margin design, machining, and complex laboratory handling were responsible for premature fracture. An example of such thin margin finishing is shown in Figure 26 of cervical margin fracture origins.

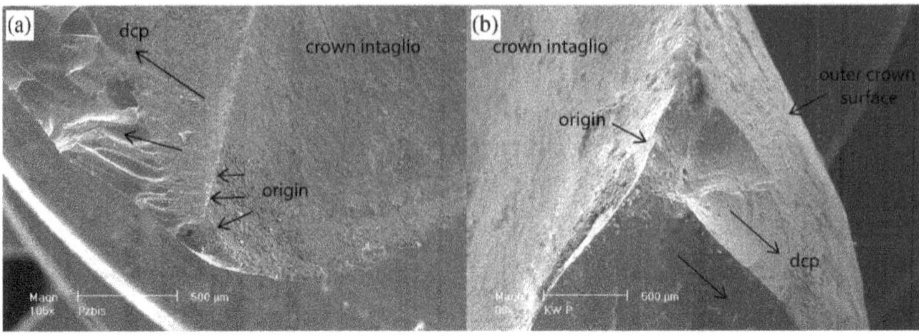

Figure 26. Fracture origins starting at the inner side (intaglio) of the alumina crown framework at the cervical margin

4.3. *Contact Wear, Grinding Damage*

Occlusal contact wear is often connected to the fracture event when a partial chip-type fracture of the veneering ceramic is involved. The veneering ceramics are mainly silica-based with low fracture toughness around 0.7–0.9 MPa√m and fracture strengths around 70–100 MPa. These esthetic but weak ceramics are layered over an existing high-strength framework (alumina, zirconia, metal) for the final crown shape and will undergo cyclic loading with variable loads from the antagonist tooth or restorative material having different hardness and state of surface roughness. It is therefore not surprising to see on the occluding surface, with time, a wear pattern. What is critical is the localized loading magnitude and frequency, the surface roughness state, and surface damage. A rough ceramic surface will lower the fracture strength of the ceramic as well as any grinding damage introduced from adjusting the occlusion. Examples of fracture origins related to contact wear and grinding damage are shown in Figures 27 and 28. The first case (Figure 27) shows a clinical ceramic chip fracture in which contact wear and occlusion played a role.

A silicon impression was taken intraorally of the fractured surface, poured in epoxy resin and gold coated for SEM analysis. This technique is called the replica technique[35] and is helpful in clinical fractures when the broken part cannot be retrieved without damage

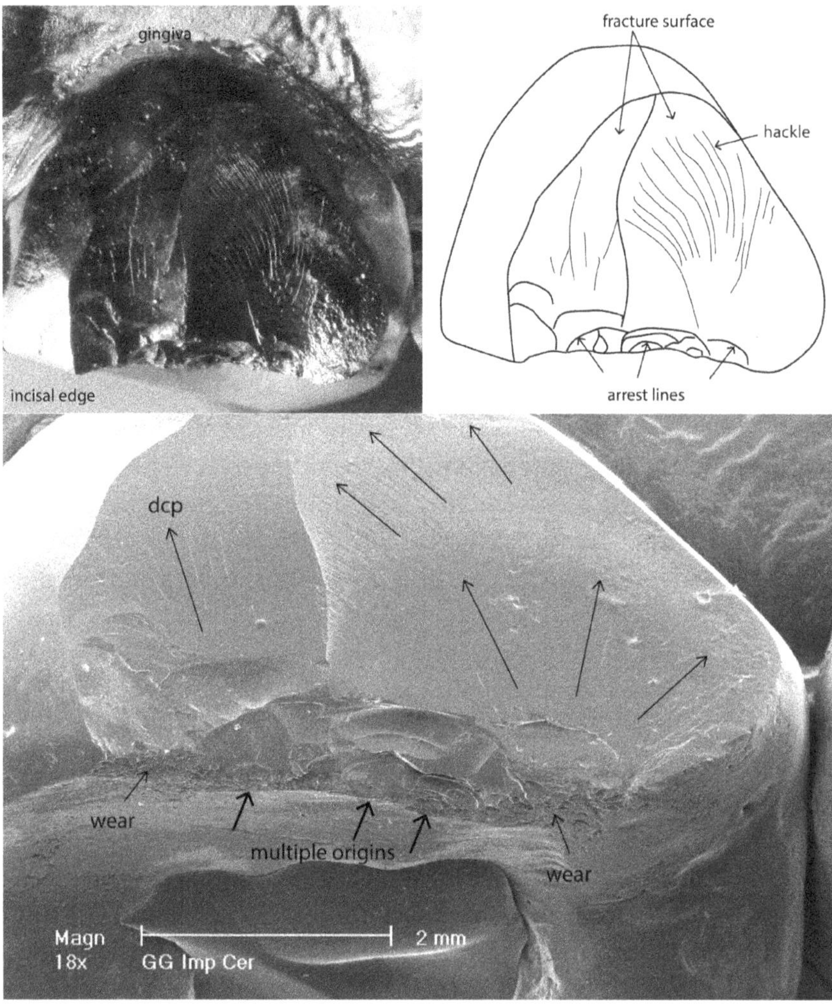

Figure 27. Gold-coated epoxy replica of a veneering ceramic chip of a premolar crown viewed under stereo and SEM. Low magnification under the SEM shows multiple origins at the incisal edge arrested by multiple arrest lines. The fracture propagated toward the gingival margin as seen from hackle, wake hackle, and twist hackle. The presence of incisal wear indicates pressure and friction during chewing and lateral excursions, exceeding the resistance of the weak veneering ceramic

or made available for failure analysis. The reproduction of details is excellent providing that no biofilm is adherent on its surface. On the gold-coated epoxy replica, features such as hackle, wake hackle, twist hackle, and arrest lines can be seen on the fracture surface of the veneering ceramic. A quick drawing helps to capture the surface morphology and characteristic features. Further analysis with the SEM shows a jagged incisal edge with multiple starter cracks (black arrows) followed by arrest lines. The fracture propagated to the gingival side of the crown as seen by the hackle, wake and twist hackles. The incisal ridge shows some wear indicating friction during chewing and lateral excursions, exceeding the resistance of the weak veneering ceramic. This early fracture most probably occurred due to a slightly too long incisal cusp which underwent shearing during lateral chewing movements, resulting in microchipping over time until a bigger fracture chipped off portions of the veneering ceramic. More information regarding this case can be found in the literature.[36]

Figure 28 illustrates more contact wear chip fractures origins (a–d) as well as grinding damage from occlusal adjustment (e,f). Figures (a) and (b) are porcelain fractures in a porcelain-fused-to-metal crown after 1 year, starting at the occlusal contact wear surface and moving downward, toward the gingiva. This case was already seen in Figure 11 for documentation of a compression curl. Figures (c) and (d) show a veneering ceramic chip fracture starting from a localized contact wear zone at the occluding surface. Figures (e) and (f) illustrate a chip fracture of a veneering ceramic in conjunction with diamond grinding damage. Higher magnification of the ground surface shows brittle cracking of the ceramic (f). These cases all illustrate the technical challenges in Dentistry, which are well-distributed occluding contacts on ceramic restorations, recognizing excessive wear, and smoothening by polishing these worn surfaces as well as those adjusted for occlusion purposes with diamond burs. Longitudinal clinical studies are still lacking with regard to the use of fractography when reporting survival and success data, but a recent report has provided some classification suggestions based on fractographic analysis of clinical fractures.[37] Further clinical retrospective evaluation

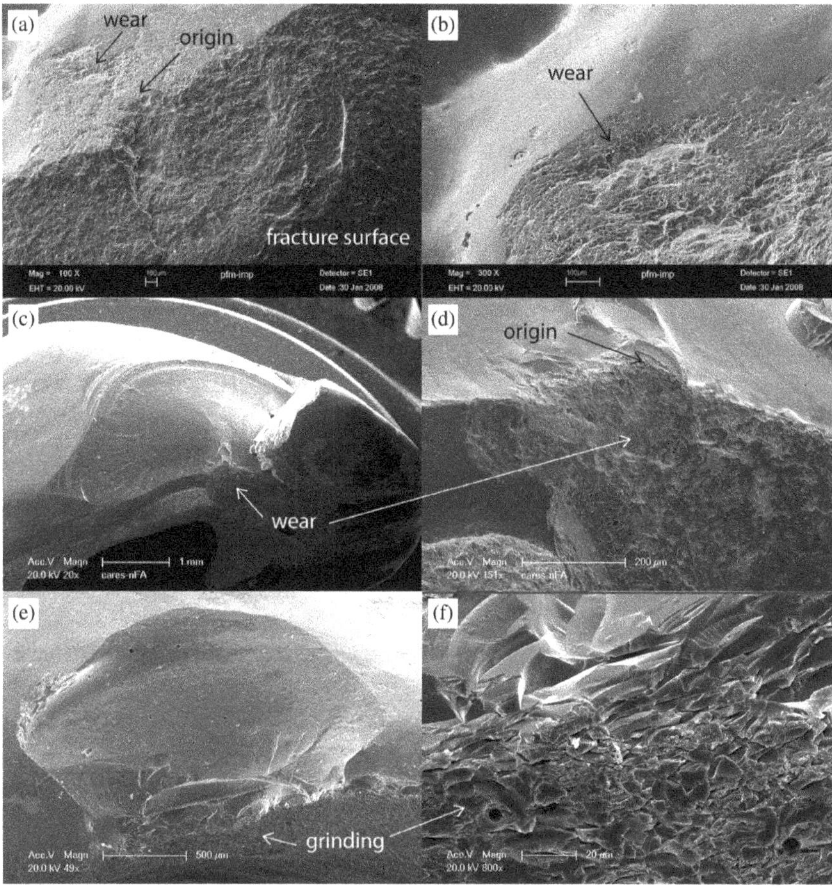

Figure 28. Chip fractures of veneering ceramics. Contact wear origins are illustrated in Figures (a–d). Diamond grinding damage origin associated with brittle fracture failure mode is shown in Figures (e,f)

of chippings of veneering ceramics over zirconia framework have confirmed occlusal contact wear as failure origins.[38]

5. Conclusions

The purpose of this chapter is to familiarize the fractographer with dental ceramic issues regarding fracture analyses. The most powerful tool for clinical failure analysis is a descriptive (qualitative) fractography, consisting of a thorough search on the fracture surface of characteristic crack feature indicators of the overall crack propagation direction and thus pinpointing back to the area of crack origin. A systematic approach should however be applied covering the entire fracture surface with zones of interest for more detailed microscopy including SEM. The hunt for information regarding the circumstances of failure and the processing details in the laboratory remain difficult to get as these may be biased by the issue of free replacement. Design, processing, handling, choice of the ceramic for restorative purposes, biting habits, and the oral environment are parameters to consider when analyzing clinical failures. Quantitative and qualitative fractography should be part of every strength test and follow the guidelines provided in existing standards and books. The knowledge of critical flaw and type of flaw population existing within a tested ceramic is of outmost importance if improvement in the ceramic material and processing are to be expected. There is enough information within the dental literature which can guide the reader for more in-depth applications of fractography to dental ceramics.

Acknowledgments

This work is a result of years of invaluable personal teaching received by Janet and George Quinn with respect to the application of fractography to ceramic fractures of dental restorative materials. Janet was a leader within the dental materials community, working at the American Dental Association — former Paffenbarger Research Center focusing on failure analysis of dental materials. Very sadly, she passed away in 1998.[39] George Quinn, her husband, has worked most of his life for the National Institute of Standards and Technology developing standards related to strength testing, fracture mechanics, and fractography. His NIST recommended practice guide on fractography of ceramics and glasses[5] was the kick off for the dental materials community to get more involved in using fractography on *in vitro* and *in vivo* ceramic dental materials.

References

1. ASTM-C1322-15, Standard Practice for Fractography and Characterization of Fracture Origins in Advanced Ceramics (ASTM International, **2015**).
2. ASTM-C1421-16, Standard Test Methods for Determination of Fracture Toughness of Advanced Ceramics at Ambient Temperature (ASTM International, **2016**).
3. ASTM-C1678-10, Practice for Fractographic Analysis of Fracture Mirror Sizes in Ceramics and Glasses (ASTM International, **2010**).
4. Fréchette, V. D. In: *Advances in Ceramics*, Vol. 28. (Westerville, Ohio: The American Ceramic Society, **1990**).
5. Quinn, G. D. *A NIST Recommended Practice Guide: Fractography of Ceramics and Glasses*. Special Publication 960-16e2. (Washington, D.C.: National Institute of Standards and Technology, **2016**). Available at: http://dx.doi.org/10.6028/NIST.SP.960-16e2: 2016.
6. Hull, D. *Fractography: Observing, Measuring and Interpreting Fracture Surface Topography* (Cambridge University Press: **1999**), 366 (pp.).
7. Freiman, S. W.; Mecholsky, J. J. J. *The Fracture of Brittle Materials: Testing and Analysis*. First Edition. (Hoboken, New Jersey, USA: The American Ceramic Society. Published by John Wiley & Sons, Inc., **2012**).
8. Varner, J., In: *Engineering Materials Handbook, Metals Park, Ohio*, Schneider, S. J. (ed.), Vol. 4 (Ohio: ASM International, **1991**), pp. 635–644.
9. Kelly, J. R.; Giordano, R.; Pober, R.; Cima, M. J. *Int. J. Prosth.* **1990**, *3* (5), 430–440.
10. Thompson, J. Y.; Anusavice, K. J.; Naman, A.; Morris, H. F. *J. Dent. Res.* **1994**, *73* (12), 1824–1832.
11. Quinn, J. B.; Quinn, G. D.; Kelly, J. R.; Scherrer, S. S. *Dent. Mater.* **2005**, *21* (10), 920–929.
12. Quinn, G. D.; Eichler, J.; Eisele, U.; Rodel, J. *J. Am. Ceram. Soc.* **2004**, *87* (3), 513–516.
13. Quinn, G. D.; Hoffman, K.; Quinn, J. B. *Dent. Mater.* **2012**, *28* (5), 502–511.
14. Scherrer, S. S.; Cattani-Lorente, M.; Vittecoq, E.; de Mestral, F.; Griggs, J. A.; Wiskott, H. W. *Dent. Mater.* **2011**, *27* (2), e28–e42.

15. Scherrer, S. S.; Cattani-Lorente, M.; Yoon, S.; Karvonen, L.; Pokrant, S.; Rothbrust, F.; Kuebler, J. *Dent. Mater.* **2013**, *29* (9), e180–e190.
16. Newman, J. C.; Raju, I. S. *Eng. Fract. Mech.* **1981**, *15* (1–2), 185–192.
17. Quinn, J. B.; Lloyd, I. K. *J. Am. Ceram. Soc.* **2000**, *83* (12), 3070–3076.
18. Scherrer, S. S.; Kelly, J. R.; Quinn, G. D.; Xu, K. *Dent. Mater.* **1999**, *15* (5), 342–348.
19. Cesar, P. F.; Yoshimura, H. N.; Miranda, W. G.; Miyazaki, C. L.; Muta, L. M.; Rodrigues, L. E. *J. Biomed. Mater. Res. B* **2006**, *78b* (2), 265–273.
20. Taskonak, B.; Griggs, J. A.; Mecholsky, J. J., Jr.; Yan, J. H. *Dent. Mater.* **2008**, *24* (5), 700–707.
21. Della Bona, A.; Mecholsky, J. J., Jr.; Anusavice, K. J. *Dent. Mater.* **2004**, *20* (10), 956–962.
22. Ramos, C. M.; Cesar, P. F.; Bonfante, E. A.; Rubo, J. H.; Wang, L.; Borges, A. F. S. *J. Mech. Behav. Biomed. Mater.* **2016**, *57*, 215–223.
23. Brown, W. F.; Strawley, J. E. *Plain Strain Crack Toughness Testing of High Strength Metallic Materials* (ASTM STP 410, **1966**), pp. 88–126.
24. Irwin, G. R. *J. Appl. Mech.* **1957**, *24*, 361–364.
25. Scherrer, S. S.; Quinn, G. D.; Quinn, J. B. *Dent. Mater.* **2008**, *24* (8), 1107–1113.
26. Scherrer, S. S.; Quinn, J. B.; Quinn, G. D.; Kelly, J. R. *Int. J. Prosth.* **2006**, *19* (2), 185–192.
27. Lohbauer, U.; Amberger, G.; Quinn, G. D.; Scherrer, S. S. *J. Mech. Behav. Biomed. Mater.* **2010**, *3* (8), 623–629.
28. Lohbauer, U.; Belli, R.; Arnetzl, G.; Scherrer, S. S.; Quinn, G. D. *Case Studies in Engineering Failure Analysis* **2014**, *2*, 100–106.
29. Belli, R.; Scherrer, S. S.; Reich, S.; Petschelt, A.; Lohbauer, U. *Case Studies in Engineering Failure Analysis* **2014**, *2*, 91–99.
30. Oilo, M.; Quinn, G. D. *J. Mech. Behav. Biomed. Mater.* **2016**, *53*, 93–103.
31. Basilio Mde, A.; Delben, J. A.; Cesar, P. F.; Rizkalla, A. S.; Santos Junior, G. C.; Arioli Filho, J. N. *J. Mech. Behav. Biomed. Mater.* **2016**, *60*, 187–194.
32. Taskonak, B.; Mecholsky, J. J., Jr.; Anusavice, K. J. *J. Dent. Res.* **2006**, *85* (3), 277–281.
33. Taskonak, B.; Yan, J.; Mecholsky, J. J., Jr.; Sertgoz, A.; Kocak, A., *Dent. Mater.* **2008**, *24* (8), 1077–1082.

34. Du, Q.; Swain, M. V.; Zhao, K., *Quintessence Int.* **2014**, *45* (5), 369–376.
35. Scherrer, S. S.; Quinn, J. B.; Quinn, G. D.; Wiskott, H. W. *Dent. Mater.* **2007**, *23* (11), 1397–1404.
36. Scherrer, S. S.; Quinn, J. B.; Quinn, G. D. *Key Eng. Mater.* **2009**, *409*, 72–80.
37. Moraguez, O. D.; Wiskott, H. W.; Scherrer, S. S. *Clin. Oral Invest.* **2015**, *19* (9), 2295–2307.
38. Koenig, V.; Vanheusden, A. J.; Le Goff, S. O.; Mainjot, A. K. *J. Dent.* **2013**, *41* (12), 1164–1174.
39. Scherrer, S. S.; Carey, C. *Dent. Mater.* **2009**, *25* (1), 2–3.

Chapter 9

Bioactive Glasses for the Development of Dental Restorative Materials

José Bauer*,§, Ceci Nunes Carvalho†,¶, Edilausson Moreno Carvalho*, and Rodrigo França‡,||

**Discipline of Dental Materials, Federal University of Maranhão (UFMA) Rua dos Portugueses, 1966, 65080-805, São Luís, Brazil*

†Department of Endodontic, Dental School of UNICEUMA — Universidade Ceuma, Rua Josué Montello Nº 1, Renascena II, 65075-120, São Luis, MA, Brazil

‡Dental Biomaterials Research Laboratory, University of Manitoba, 780 Bannatyne Avenue, Winnipeg, Manitoba R3E 0W2, Canada

§bauer@ufma.br
¶ceci.carvalho@ceuma.br
||Rodrigo.Franca@umanitoba.ca

The use of bioactive glasses in developing materials for use in dentistry is rising every day. Numerous researchers have published enlightening articles on the development and characterization of new biomaterials containing bioactive glass. This chapter will discuss the types of bioactive glass and how these materials have been applied to the development of new dental restorative materials.

1. Introduction

The development of bioactive materials in dentistry has been a dominant topic in recent publications in the field of dental materials. At present, there are different groups of researchers in the world in quest of an objective: to include bioactive glasses in restorative materials with the intention of developing "*smart materials*". We searched the PubMed database using the keywords "glass + bioactive + dental + materials". This figure definitely shows an increasing trend toward research related to bioactive materials, indicating that the use of bioactive materials in Dentistry has been a "big" research topic in the past two decades.

Figure 1 shows that in the last 20 years, scientific publications involving bioactive restorative materials have increased considerably. Basically, bioactive particles are included in restorative materials with a view to bringing about benefits such as neutralization of acid pH, bacterial inhibition, action against metalloproteinases enzymes, and, particularly, stimulation of enamel and dentin remineralization.

Today, there are innumerable bioactive glasses available to researchers. The first bioactive glass was invented by Larry Hench at

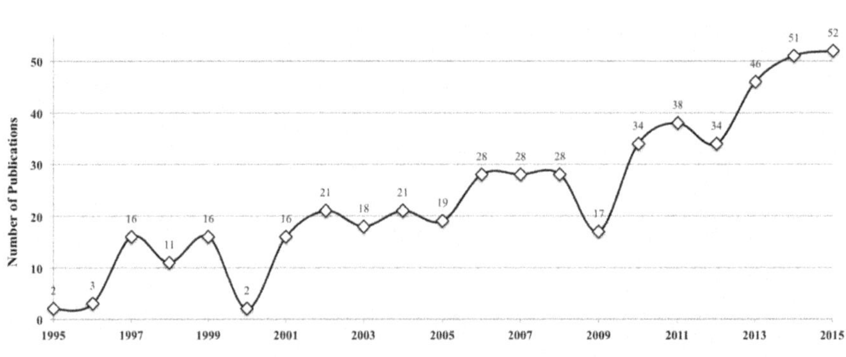

Figure 1. Number of scientific publications involving bioactive restorative materials from 1995 to 2015

the University of Florida in 1969. The main discovery was that a glass with the composition 46.1 mol.% SiO_2, 24.4 mol.% Na_2O, 26.9 mol.% CaO, and 2.6 mol.% P_2O_5, later termed 45S5 and Bioglass, exhibited notable properties of interaction with live tissues. The name "Bioglass" was trademarked by the University of Florida as a name for the original 45S5 composition. It should therefore only be used in reference to the 45S5 composition and not as a general term for bioactive glasses.[1] This glass exhibits the highest bioactivity index and is still considered the gold standard of bioactive materials.

Recently, a new bioactive glass, denominated Biosilicate, was developed by a group of researchers at the University of São Carlos, under the guidance of Prof. Edgar D. Zanotto who worked in collaboration with Prof. Larry L. Hench. The purpose of developing this biosilicate was to find a glass that would have a high bioactivity index, and simultaneously present superior mechanical properties that would favor better obtainment of particles.[2]

Bioactive glasses containing niobium have also drawn attention. Researchers at the Nuclear and Energy Research Institute ("Instituto de Pesquisas Energéticas e Nucleares — IPEN"), under the guidance of Prof. José Roberto Martinelli, have developed a bioactive niobium phosphate glass with high mechanical strength and great chemical stability for use in bone grafting. The precursor of the bioactive glass developed by Martinelli was the vitreous system P_2O_5–PbO–Nb_2O_5–K_2O, also called niobium phosphate, containing lead, developed by Prof. Oswaldo Luiz Alves of the State University of Campinas.[3]

In spite of the large number of bioactive glasses on the market, this chapter will be devoted to these three bioactive glasses only: (i) 45S5, (ii) Biosilicate, and (iii) niobium phosphate.

2. Bioactive Glasses

2.1. *Bioglass (45S5)*

There are diverse glasses and glass-ceramics containing silica in their composition used in biomedical applications. The chemical compositions, morphological characteristics, and mechanical properties of these glasses may be adjusted according to the interest of the research.

The first bioactive glass was developed by Larry Hench, who in 1971, developed an Na_2O–CaO–P_2O_5–SiO_2 system with a high bioactivity index.

The majority of bioactive glasses are silicate based, and to present high bioactivity, the concentrations of SiO_2 must be around 60% in mol, have high relative contents of Na_2O and CaO, and maintain a high CaO/P_2O_5 ratio.

For this material to be bioactive, a chemical action must occur on the material surface after its insertion in the body. A carbonated hydroxyapatite layer is formed on the material surface, which promotes the bond interface with the tissue.[4–9] Three fundamental factors are necessary for a silicate glass to present bioactivity: (1) its composition must contain an SiO_2 content lower than 60% in mol; (2) high relative Na_2O and CaO contents; and (3) a high Ca/P ratio. These factors allow the glass surface to become reactive when in contact with an aqueous medium. The physicochemical mechanisms involved in the formation of the bioactive bond with tissue and the sequence of cellular events are presented in Table 1.

Table 2 lists the stages of reactions on bioactive material surfaces. The mechanisms involved in Stage 1 (ionic exchange) and Stage 2

Table 1. Sequence of interfacial events involved in bond formation between bone tissue and bioactive materials

Stages	Events
1	Bioactive glass in contact with body fluids
2	Formation of SiOH bonds
3	Transformation of SiOH + SiOH → Si–O–Si + H_2O
4	Adsorption of Ca + PO_4 + CO_3
5	Carbonated hydroxyapatite formation
6	Action of macrophages
7	Approximation of mesenchymal cells
8	Differentiation of mesenchymal cells
9	Bone matrix formation
10	Bone matrix crystallization

Table 2. Stage of reactions in bioactive implants

Stages of superficial reactions	**Events**
1	Rapid exchange of Na^+ and K^+ ions with H^+ and H_3O^+ ions of the $Si–O–Na^+ + H^+ + OH^-$ solution → $Si–OH^+ + Na^+$ (solution) + OH^+. This stage is frequently controlled by the process of diffusion.
2	Loss of soluble silica in the form of $Si(OH)_4$ into the solution, resulting in the breakage of the Si–O–Si bonds and formation of Si–OH at the interface of the vitreous solution. This stage is frequently controlled by the interfacial reactions.
3	Condensation and repolymerization of the layer rich in SiO_2 on the surface, depleting alkaline cations and alkaline earth elements.
4	Migration of Ca^{+2} e PO_4^{-3} groups to the surface by means of the layer rich in SiO_2 forming a film rich in $CaO–P_2O_5$ on the surface of the layer rich in SiO_2, followed by the growth of an amorphous film rich in $CaO–P_2O_5$ by incorporating soluble calcium and phosphate from the solution.
5	Crystallization of the amorphous film of $CaO–P_2O_5$ by incorporating OH, CO_3^{-2} anions, or F^- from the solution to form a layer of hydroxyl, carbonate, and fluorapatite.

(silica network dissolution) are described precisely; however, the mechanisms that act in Stage 3 (condensation and repolymerization of silica) are not well known. The superficial reactions involved in Stages 1–4 are being determined for a large number of vitreous compositions.[4–9]

The ratio of carbonated hydroxyapatite formation (Stage 4) and time of onset of crystallization (Stage 5) vary considerably. When the ratio of formation becomes excessively slow, no formation of bond between the implant material and bone tissue occurs, and the material presents no bioactivity.

This entire bioactivity mechanism has led to 45S5 being a success among the bioactive glasses. The 45S5 bioglass has been used in over a million patients to repair bone defects in the jaw and in orthopedics.[1,4] Hench, in 2006,[6] wrote, "After 30 years, as a result of satisfactory contracts and commercial relationships, Bioglasses are sold in 35 countries. A wide variety of other bioactive materials are also now in use worldwide". In the field of Dentistry, in 2009, 40 years after the discovery of 45S5, the one millionth tube of tooth paste containing 45S5 was sold. This material occludes dentinal tubules and remineralizes the surface of teeth, thereby eliminating the cause of dentinal hypersensitivity.[7]

However, the bioactive glass 45S5 has shown disadvantages such as low mechanical strength and low fracture toughness. On the other hand, innumerable researchers have incorporated 45S5 glass into the development of dental restorative materials with excellent results.[10–15]

2.2. *Biosilicate*

Today, we know that other materials may also be bioactive, such as for example, new compositions of glasses, glass ceramics, and the family of calcium phosphate ceramics.[16] Thus, a new bioactive glass, called Biosilicate, was developed. The inventors had in mind the development of a material that would preserve the high bioactivity index shown by bioactive glasses and would simultaneously have superior biomechanical properties. Its composition is very close to that used in 45S5, with a microstructure controlled to prevent crystallization during the production of the glass ceramic. Thus, in 1997, after promising results, a patent was deposited about the obtainment of highly bioactive glass ceramics.[17] An important characteristic of Biosilicate is the possibility of obtaining more regular and less abrasive particles without cutting surfaces, therefore, less aggressive to gingival and mucosal tissues. Some researchers have shown that this material is a high-strength, high-toughness glass-ceramics with bioactivity equivalent to that of the grandfather 45S5 bioactive glass.[18–20]

In a recent review of studies developed with Biosilicate, this product was shown to present a high potential for use in restorative material. The authors described, "Biosilicate has been evaluated in 28 theses and dissertations and in more than 30 scientific papers over the last 20 years. These studies have demonstrated its efficiency for regenerating bone tissue and treating dental hypersensitivity.

Biosilicate presents some important features for bone tissue regeneration: it is highly bioactive, osteoconductive, osteoinductive, non-cytotoxic, non-genotoxic and has antibacterial properties".[2,21–25] On the other hand, few studies in the field of restorative materials have been developed with this bioactive material.

2.3. *Niobium Phosphate Glass*

One of the disadvantages of some bioactive glasses is their poor chemical durability in aqueous media; however, this durability may be modified with the addition of niobium oxide. The addition of niobium (Nb) creates a vitreous structure made up of chains (–O–P–O-Nb–O–P–O–) or in some cases, predominantly bonds of the (–O–Nb–O–Nb–O–) type, making the glass more chemically stable as the niobium oxide content is increased.[26] This modification may contribute to increasing the bioactivity[26–29] and biocompatibility.[28] Small concentrations of Nb_2O_5 added to bioactive glasses may also increase the velocity of binding and formation of bone tissue to glass.[30,31]

This gain in performance may be explained in the following manner: in simulated body fluid (SBF), the Nb–OH functional groups acquire a negative charge and induce apatite formation with the deposition of an amorphous calcium compound. Afterward, an amorphous form of calcium phosphate is transformed into hydroxyapatite.[32] Moreover, niobium pentoxide alone is capable of promoting crystallization and mineralization of the surrounding tissues.[33] As opposed to silica, Nb actively participates in the osseointegration reaction due to its elevated biocompatibility.[34] The incorporation of Nb pentoxide (Nb_2O_5) may also increase the radiopacity and hardness of experimental adhesive materials.[35,36]

In spite of the 45S5 bioglasses having elevated bioactivity, its use is restricted to applications in which high mechanical strength is not required.

Whereas, a niobium phosphate glass has demonstrated high mechanical strength, high chemical stability, biocompatibility, bioactivity, and its flexural strength values were higher than those of 45S5 glass[37] and close to those of Biosilicate.[38]

This study gave origin to a patent under the title "Bioactive niobium phosphate glasses for osseointegrated applications" (WO 2004026781 A1) deposited in 2003. Because of these promising results, researches have been developed with niobium phosphate with the purpose of developing intelligent restorative materials in diverse fields of Dentistry.[39–41]

3. Restorative Materials Containing Bioactive Glasses

Initially, bioactive glasses in Dentistry were mainly used for coating titanium implants[42] or for the treatment of dentin hypersensitivity.[7]

Bioactive particles have been incorporated into glass ionomer cements, composites and, ultimately, in adhesive systems. Therefore, we are going to discuss each of these materials separately.

3.1. *Glass Ionomer Cements*

Glass ionomer cements are exceptional restorative materials, mainly used in primary teeth. The antimicrobial properties of glass ionomer cements are directly related to the quantity of fluoride released by these materials.[43] The fluoride ion (F^-) is capable of diminishing demineralization and increasing remineralization of a carious tissue, and in low concentration, modifying the metabolism of the bacteria that cause caries. F^- may also interfere in the adhesion of the biofilm pellicle to the tooth and inhibition of microbial growth.[43,44]

In spite of all these positive characteristics, this material also has clinical and mechanical limitations, such as unfavorable esthetics due to is low translucence, sensitivity of manipulation technique, sensitivity to water during setting, short working time, low fracture strength, low resistance to hardness and wear, and low bond strength.[44–48]

To improve these limitations of conventional glass ionomer cement, resin monomers were added to its composition. Thereby, in addition to fluoroaluminosilicate glass, there is also bisphenol glycidyl methacrylate (BisGMA), triethylene glycol dimethacrylate (TEGDMA), urethane dimethacrylate (UDMA), and 2-hydroxy ethyl methacrylate, (HEMA) in the composition of the powder, thus giving rise to the resin-modified glass ionomer cements (RMGICs). In spite of the addition of these resin monomers to the conventional glass ionomer cements having improved the clinical and mechanical properties of these materials, the RMGICs do not present bioactivity as yet.[44,46,49,50] The powder composition of the glass ionomer cement was designed so that the glass can react with the weak acid, polycarboxylic acid, and even if it contains both calcium and phosphate, it does not show any bioactivity.[51]

On the other hand, the incorporation of 45S5 into glass ionomer cements may favor the formation of an Si-rich layer capable of stimulating the deposition of carbonated hydroxyapatite [$Ca_{10}(PO_4)_6(OH)_2$], which is responsible for the induction of osseointegration and remineralization of the hard tissues of teeth.

One study evaluated the release of Si, Ca, and P ions from conventional glass ionomer cement and resin-modified glass ionomer cement doped with 45S5 (10 and 30 wt.%). The authors demonstrated that the addition of 45S5 to these materials provided the precipitation of Ca-P on the surface, capable of mineralizing human dentin *in vitro*. This modification may also provide the materials with antimicrobial properties.[52] These same authors evaluated the mechanical strength (compressive strength, modulus, and Vickers hardness) of glass ionomers doped with 45S5 (10% and 30%). Their results demonstrated that the addition of 45S5 particles to the GICs decreased the compressive strength and modulus of elasticity. This suggests that the 45S5 particles might be only loosely attached to the GIC matrix. Thus, 45S5 particles probably acted as fillers that had not been adhered into the matrix of GIC leading to decreased mechanical properties. This could also be seen with resin-modified GICs, especially when a higher weight fraction (30%) of 45S5 particles was used. Another explanation is that 45S5 is less reactive for poly acrylic acid, and therefore less surface reaction of BAG occurs. The addition of 45S5 to GIC may increase the microhardness of the material surface after 180 days of storage in water due to the deposition of Si- and Ca-based precipitates. The increase in microhardness may also be linked to the Ca^{2+} released from the bioactive glass to form carboxylate salt leading to an increase in the degree of polymerization in the silicate network.[53]

However, innumerable studies have shown that the incorporation of bioactive glasses could reduce the mechanical properties of GICs.[51,54,55] But, their clinical use ought to be restricted to applications where their bioactivity can be beneficial, such as root surface fillings and liners in dentistry, and where high compressive strength is not necessarily needed.[54]

The addition of bioactive glasses to GIC may not compromise the mechanical performance of the material, but provide a bioactive potential. Matsuya *et al.*[53] evaluated the bioactivity of the new GIC in the SBF and found no apatite formation on the surface of the newly set cement at least within 4 weeks. This may perhaps have been due to the presence of polyacrylic acid that inhibited the apatite formation, and concluded it might be difficult to obtain a bioactive glass ionomer cement. These results indicated that polyacrylic acid suppresses the apatite forming ability of bioactive glass.[56]

Choi *et al.*[57] found that an addition of sol–gel derived glass with a bioactive composition ($70SiO_2{\cdot}25CaO{\cdot}5P_2O_5$) added to the commercial GIC did not significantly alter the diametral tensile strength and induced the precipitation of an apatite bone-mineral phase on the surface after immersion in a SBF, showing *in vitro* bone bioactivity.

With the purpose of evaluating the impact on the mechanical properties of demineralized dentin in contact with modified-GIC+45S5, Khoroushi *et al.*[58] demonstrated that resin-modified glass ionomer (RMGI) containing bioactive could compensate for this loss of strength of demineralized dentin. They found the mean FS of demineralized dentin increased by almost 20% after contact of modified-GIC with 45S5.

These characteristics make it possible to use GICs with the addition of bioactive glass on carious dentin, or with partial removal of the carious tissue, which would make it possible for dentin remineralization to occur. These results are very encouraging for the use of this potential combination for the mineralization of dentin capping.[59]

A large step forward in recent studies published was the obtainment of nanoparticles of bioactive glasses for overcoming the problem of the reduction in mechanical properties of GIC when bioactive glass was added. In 2016, Valenezhad *et al.*[44] showed that the addition of 10% of bioactive glass nanoparticles was an optimal concentration for cell adherence and acceptable mechanical properties.

Encouraging results were also found with the addition of Biosilicate to two modified GICs. The addition of 2% biosilicate did not harm the compressive strength of the materials tested, and increased the bond strength to dentin.[60] However, ion release and bioactive compound formation tests with this mixture need to be evaluated.

Another interesting point of view adopted recently was the development of bioactive glasses containing fluoride. This may lead to the development of a material with the capacity for increasing bone mass and mineral density, improving the resistance of the apatite structure to acid attack, and better antibacterial properties. This new bioactive material is an interesting candidates for various clinical applications, such as dentinal tubule occlusion in the treatment of dentin hypersensitivity.[61] In SBF, this new bioactive glass can form fluorapatite, which is more acid resistant than carbonated hydroxyapatite.[62]

In the meantime, there are no published studies with the inclusion of NbG glass in modified GIC; however, there are some studies in progress. The preliminary results have indicated that the inclusion of NbG glass did not reduce the flexural strength of two modified-GICs, when added in the concentrations of 5%, 10%, and 20% by weight (Table 3).

Table 3. Results of the flexural strength (MPa) test of RMGICs with the addition of niobium phosphate (NbG) bioactive glass in different concentrations*

Materials	Control	5%	10%	20%
Vitro Fil LC	28.41 ± 7.95	33.06 ± 8.4	25.70 ± 4.4	29.16 ± 7.82
Resiglass	45.67 ± 9.31	46.77 ± 9.95	46.73 ± 9.95	52.49 ± 8.98

Note: *Unpublished data.

Table 4. pH values of two RMGI with 20% NbG over 7 days*

Mixture	pH	24 h	48 h	72 h	96 h	120 h	144 h	168 h
Resiglass	pH 7	5.2	6.0	6.7	6.7	6.7	6.7	6.8
	pH 4	4.8	5.0	4.9	5.0	4.7	4.8	4.8
Vitro Fil LC	pH 7	6.0	6.9	7.4	7.5	7.4	7.4	7.3
	pH 4	5.7	5.9	6.0	6.1	5.8	5.9	5.9

Note: *Unpublished data.

This result may be related to the greater chemical stability of the NbG glass that would work as filler, as opposed to 45S5 glass that undergoes solubility, exposing the material to degradation. The pH monitoring data over the course of 7 days in two conditions of pH (4 and 7) with 20% NbG are described in Table 4.

These data demonstrated that the NbG glass in the concentration of 20% tended to neutralize the acid pH in the medium and of the GIC. The increase in the initial pH is important to inhibit bacterial growth and paralyze the demineralization process. Another important finding obtained with the inclusion of NbG particles in modified GIC was the possibility of deposition of precipitates responsible for bioactivity (Figure 2).

3.2. *Composites*

Some studies have been published, with the inclusion of bioactive glasses in composites, and some fields of Dentistry, such as restorative dentistry, Orthodontics and Endodontics. These researches have reported success with the inclusion of bioactive glasses in resin composites, orthodontic bracket bonding materials and endodontic filling materials.

The bioactive glass incorporated into an endodontic sealer contributed to an increase in ion release, promoting an alkaline pH in the medium.[63]

Although the antimicrobial effect of bioactive glasses has not yet been completely understood, it may be related to the elevation of pH in aqueous suspensions. It has been reported the bioactive glass

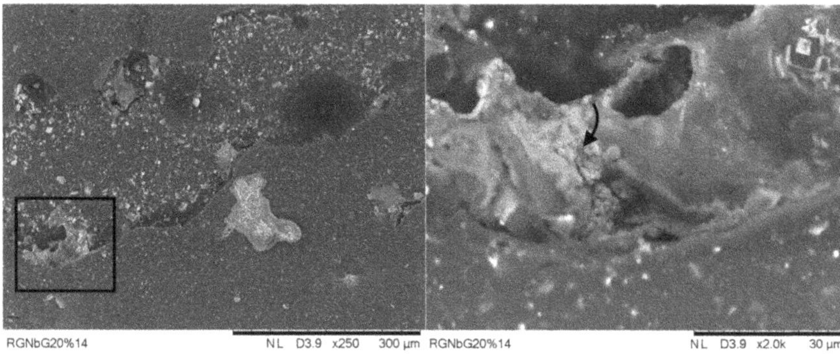

Figure 2. Precipitation (black arrow) in a sample of RMGI (Resiglass) with 20% NbG after 14 days immersion in a phosphate-buffered saline solution. (Unpublished data — Further analysis is required to determine the composition of precipitates)

S53P4 had a greater antiseptic effect than that observed for calcium hydroxide, and apparently this effects would not be related to pH only.[64,65]

Another important finding was that the addition of 45S5 particles to resin cements for endodontic filling made this material a powerful inhibitor of MMP and collagen degradation.[66] The reduction of MMPs has been shown to have a positive effect on bone formation.[67]

On the market, it is possible to find an endodontic filling material called BC Sealer (calcium silicates, monobasic calcium phosphate, zirconium oxide, tantalum oxide), which the manufacturer suggests has bioactivity, anti-inflammatory, and anti-bacterial capacity, without post-operative complications. Zhang *et al.*[68] demonstrated that this material has a high pH, close to 12, and that this contributed to the elimination of bacteria such as *Enterococcus faecalis*.

In the same study, the authors demonstrated that the small particle size and hydrophilic nature of the BC Sealer allows it to flow into all aspects of the canal anatomy, and this favors a high bond strength to root dentin.[69] Shokouhinejad *et al.*[70] compared the bond strength of the EndoSequence cement, BC Sealer, and AH Plus either in the presence or absence of a *smear layer*. In conclusion, the bond strength of this new bioceramic cement was equal to that of AH Plus with or without the *smear layer*. This good performance of bond strength to root dentin of bioactive cements may also be linked to the formation and deposition of by-products at the cement/dentin interface.

The BC Sealer cement shows high calcium ion release.[71] However, this does not mean that this material presents the capacity for bioactivity, in spite of the presence of precipitates (Figure 3) on the root dentin surface, which suggested a possible bioactivity. Readouts made by X-ray diffraction (XRD) did not confirm the presence of hydroxyapatite (Unpublished data).

Bioactive glasses have also been used in an attempt to develop a bioactive gutta-percha capable of filling the root canal system in a humid environment, without the use of any filling cement.[72] New composites containing phosphated glasses, capable of releasing ions to form a precipitate and promote sealing have been evaluated.[10,12,72,73] These experimental materials showed desirable properties for an endodontic filling material, such as alkaline capacity, adhesion to root dentin,[12,72] radiopacity, and bioactivity.[10,73] A group of researchers have developed a commercial product (BioGuta) with the addition of 45S5 glass to the polymer matrix of gutta-percha that showed promising results as a single root canal filling material. This material (under investigation) made the resulting composite materials bioactive and improved their immediate sealing ability.

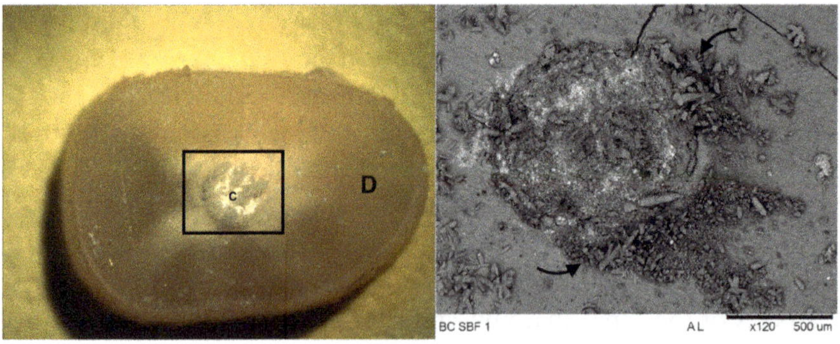

Figure 3. Precipitation in root dentin surface (black arrows) stimulated by BC sealer. (C — Cement BC sealer. D — Root dentin)

Recently, Carvalho *et al.*[39,40] developed and patented a gutta-percha with a high concentration of NbG glass. Preliminary results showed that this material is self-adhesive, bioactive, has antimicrobial properties, and has a bond strength similar to that obtained with the well-established filling cement AH Plus.

In an small scale, studies have also been conducted in the field of Orthodontics for the development of materials containing bioactive particles used for bracket bonding. Up to now, there are only three studies that have evaluated the inclusion of bioactive glasses in bonding materials.[74–76]

The function of this incorporation of bioactive glasses is to prevent bacterial colonization around brackets. The presence of bacteria around brackets may lead to demineralization of the enamel surface and formation of incipient caries, denominated white spot (WSL). The high prevalence of WSL still causes concern as they could lead to carious lesions and esthetic alterations that would compromise the orthodontic treatment. According to Tufekci *et al.*[77] the prevalence of WSL during orthodontic treatment (nearly 50% of patients after 12 months) is due to many factors: (1) fixed orthodontic appliances make oral hygiene more difficult;[78] (2) increase bacterial flora around the bracket;[79] and (3) reduce the pH at the enamel interface, resulting in mineral loss.[80]

As has been described in different points of this chapter, the incorporation of bioactive glasses may solve this problem, due to their bactericidal and pH neutralizing action. Brown *et al.*[74] suggested that the incorporation of 45S5 glass into bracket bonding materials could lead to the development of smart materials that provide a reservoir of ions crucial to remineralization or to protect enamel against demineralization. In same way, another study showed that smart materials had the best preventive effect against WSL formation and helped to reduce superficial enamel softening surrounding orthodontic brackets when compared with a conventional resin adhesive.[75] Altmann *et al.*[76] developed a material for bracket bonding, containing an antibacterial monomer (1,3,5-tri acryloyl hexahydro-1,3,5-triazine) and bioactive glass (phosphate invert glass/niobium pentoxide). The authors found very promising results, such as a significant reduction in bacterial growth, deposition of phosphate content, high degree of conversion, and acceptable bond strength values. These authors have evaluated these materials in both *in situ* and *in vivo* studies.

Bioactive fillers have also been added to resin composites with the purpose of reducing biofilm aggregation on the restorative material surface, and thereby reducing leakage at the restoration interface. Thus, the researchers have attempted to reduce the high clinical failure rate of resin-composite restorations in posterior teeth. Exploration into bioactive filler potential for use in resin-based dental restorative composites has only very recently begun.[81] It is of the utmost importance for the restorative material to inhibit bacterial growth, and if it is not capable of preventing this growth, it should be capable of providing ions so that remineralization of the demineralized dental substrate may occur. Xu *et al.*[82] showed that a plaque pH of 6.0–5.5 is potentially cariogenic, and pH of 5.5–4 is cariogenic or of danger to cavity formation. So, it is desirable for Ca/PO_4 composite to be "smart", to increase the release of caries-inhibiting ions at a lower pH, when the Ca and PO_4 ions are most needed.

On the other hand, the addition of bioactive glass to the composite must not compromise its mechanical properties and clinical performance. An excellent performance as regards the properties was obtained with the incorporation of 5, 10, and 15 (wt.%) of bioactive glass (45S5) into resin composite. Resins containing bioactive glass (BAG composite) showed comparable or better properties than commercial resins (Heliomolar, Filtek Z250 and Filtek Supreme Plus) that were attributed to: (1) a higher filler content; and (2) a microstructure morphology with better promotion of the toughening mechanisms of crack deflection and bridging.[81] The same group of researchers succeeded in proving that a resin composite containing 15 (wt.%) of bioactive glass inhibited biofilm formation and penetration into marginal gaps of restorations.[83,84] Some studies have successfully added bioactive glasses to composites containing silver (Ag) to combine regenerative and antibacterial properties in one and the same material.[85,86]

3.3. *Adhesive Systems*

Adhesive systems must penetrate into the entire demineralized collagen network, so that after polymerization, the collagen fibers will be protected against degradation caused by the MMPs.[87,88]

However, different studies have shown that adhesive systems contain hydrophilic monomers that may be cleaved by the action of H_2O, leaving the collagen fibers unprotected.[89–91] Some studies have demonstrated that the interface with dentin produced by the conventional adhesives deteriorates within a short period.[35,88,92,93] This behavior may compromise the clinical performance of the material and favor the appearance of secondary caries, marginal staining, and sensitivity.[93,94]

Various alternatives have been observed for improving the behavior of the bond interface.[95] Application of chlorhexidine solutions in different concentrations,[96] multiple layers of adhesives,[97,98] electrical currents,[99] appliances that improve the infiltration of adhesives into the collagen layer,[100] longer time of application/agitation, and longer light activation time[98,101] are changes in the application protocol which lead to an increase in the number of steps, and consequently in clinical time.

Some authors have suggested the addition of inorganic particles to the resin matrix to improve the mechanical behavior of the material.[93,102] Particles differing in nature have been used colloidal silica,[102] zirconium,[103] Ytterbium trifluoride,[104] and barium borosilicate.[93] On the other hand, the addition of inorganic particles to the resin matrix must not function only as a reinforcement to improve the mechanical properties. An alternative found in the literature was the incorporation of particles to inhibit the action of MMPs and bacteria, and to stimulate remineralization of the collagen matrix.[105]

At present, growing interest in new restorative materials has been observed, associated with bioactive glasses (45S5) that induce remineralization of the bond interface by means of phosphate and calcium ion release,[15,88,106–113] favoring the elevation of pH at the interface, acting as an antimicrobial agent,[112,114–116] and inhibiting MMPs.[105]

In the field of development of bioactive adhesive systems, a group led by Salvatore Sauro has obtained excellent results with the addition of bioglass (45S5). Their studies have pointed toward a bioactive adhesive system that remineralizes the collagen fibers, recovers the mechanical properties of dentin, stabilizes the bond strength values, and reduces nanoleakage.[107]

The incorporation of bioactive particles into dental adhesives can also act as a filler to improve the mechanical properties of the material. Some manufactures have reinforced adhesives systems by adding fillers as a component.[117] This material could therefore act as a stress absorbing layer, because of its lower elastic modulus, by allowing deflection between composite/dentine and improving marginal seal.[118] Furthermore, adhesives with fillers may have radiopacity, and prevent clinicians from being misled into interpreting adhesive radiotransparency as gap formation or recurrent caries at the restoration margin.[119]

On the other hand, there is no etch-and-rinse and self-etch adhesive capable of completely replacing water in the extrafibrillar and intrafibrillar collagen compartments with resin monomers.[120,121] The objective of adding bioactive particles is to stimulate remineralization in areas where the collagen is unprotected and to compensate degradation of the polymer matrix.

Taubock *et al.*[112] incorporated 20 wt.% of ultrafine particles (SiO_2–Na_2O–CaO–P_2O_5–Bi_2O_3) into the Bis-GMA/TEGDMA matrix. A material with bioactive properties and capacity to raise the pH in aqueous suspensions, as a result of the release of alkali ions, mainly Na^+, and the incorporation of protons (H^+) into the corroding material, gave these particles their anti-microbial activity.[122,123] This author added Bi_2O_3 with the purpose of making the adhesive system radiopaque.

Recently, a study demonstrated that the incorporation of niobium phosphate glass (40 wt.%) alone was capable of providing the adhesive system with radiopacity (Figure 4). The addition of this bioactive glass also provided an increase in the degree of conversion, hardness, and stabilized the bond strength after 6 months of storage in water.[41]

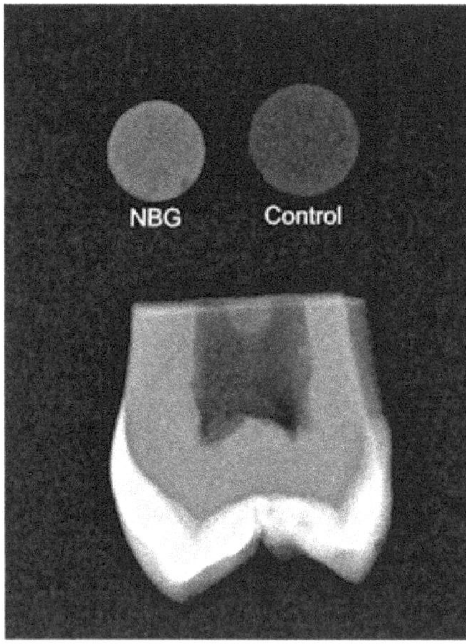

Figure 4. Radiopacity of human tooth and two adhesive systems: control (no addition of glass particles) and an experimental adhesive containing 40% NbG

Along the same lines, the addition of the same NbG glass did not change the degree of conversion, increased the hardness, and provided the commercial adhesive systems (Prime Bond, Dentsply) with radiopacity, but it was not capable of preventing the reduction in bond strength after 6 months of storage. However, it was possible to observe particles of NbG glass obliterating the entrance of dentinal tubules and within the adhesive layer (Figure 5) (Unpublished data).

The use of an adhesive system doped with bioactive glasses would be of greater use in deep cavities and/or under carious tissue. Up to now, new studies have been found in the literature with bioactive adhesive systems under carious dentin.

A bioactive glass impregnated in carious dentin could interrupt the process of demineralization,[124] bacterial growth,[125] and the enzymatic action of metalloproteinases.[11,50,106,126–128] The application of bioactive glass in caries-affected dentin creates a smear layer rich in minerals,[129] which could remineralize dentin and recover the

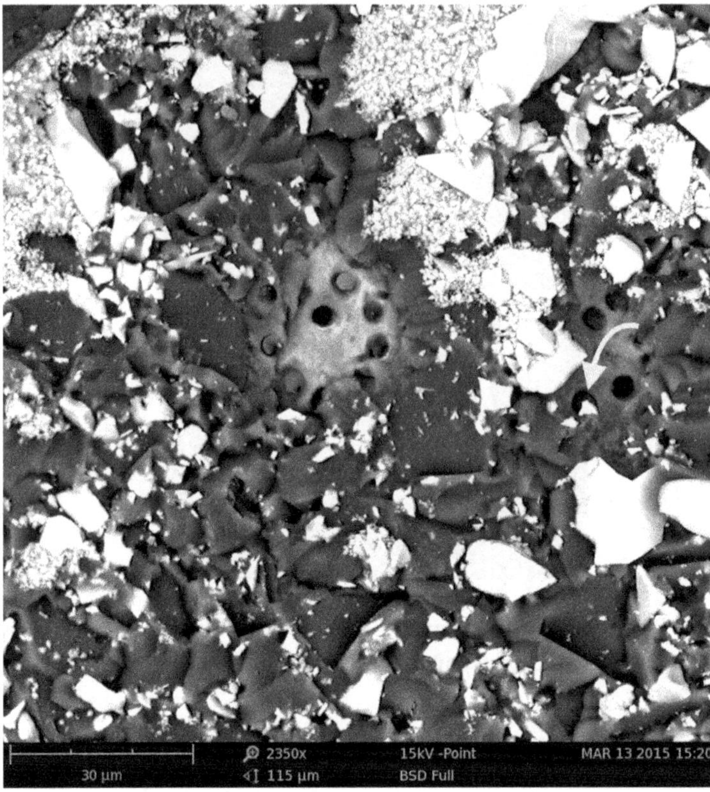

Figure 5. Presence of NbG particles at the entrance of the dentinal tubules (white arrow) and within the adhesive layer

mechanical properties of this tissue. Moreover, the presence of bioactive glass microparticles acts as a link for binding with functional monomers (MDP) of adhesive materials.[50,130]

Studies in progress have presented interesting results, showing that the bioactive NbG glass was capable of increasing the bond strength values only to dentin from which carious tissue had been completely removed. Airborne particle abrasion with microparticles of NbG in deep dentin may have sealed the entrance to the dentinal tubules (Figure 6), making it difficult for the passage of water to occur or serving as a link with the restorative material, and thus increasing the bond strength values. Other studies with a "bioactive adhesive" and bioactive glass need be conducted to evaluate their

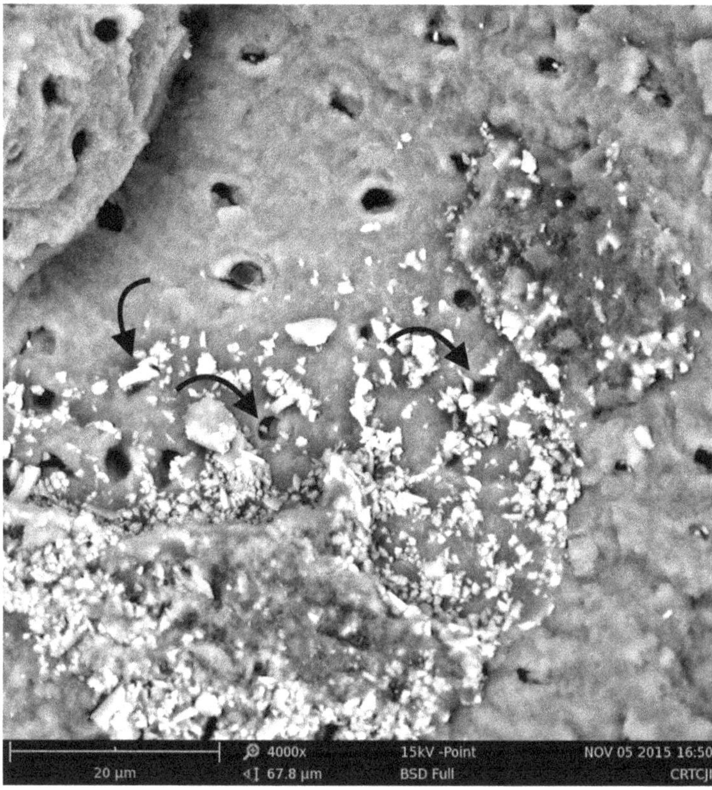

Figure 6. NbG microparticles in dentinal tubules (white arrows) after airborne particle abrasion with bioactive glass

ability to remineralize hybrid layers or affected dentin and to restore the mechanical properties of structures. At this time, many researchers are looking for adhesive materials capable of remineralizing hybrid layers and completely restoring the mechanical properties of mineral-depleted dental collagen structures within resin-bonded interfaces through biomimetic apatite formation.[131]

4. Conclusions and Outlook

The first bioactive glass formulations were developed over 40 years ago. However, some mechanisms by which these materials interact with body tissues remain not fully elucidated. The use of bioactive particles in dentistry generated a lot of research that enabled the development of biomaterials with the most varied applications. Although various formulations of bioactive glasses have been reported in the literature, this chapter has focused on only three of them, as well as their inclusion in restorative materials commonly used.

However, most of the literature on the application of bioactive glass in restorative materials consists of laboratory research. Given the promising results found in this work, further studies are necessary in order to prove the clinical application for these biomaterials.

Acknowledgments

The authors are grateful to Foundation for the Support of Scientific and Technological Research of Maranhão (FAPEMA–BEPP 6527/ 2014).

References

1. Jones, J. R. *Acta Biomater.* **2013**, *9*, 4457.
2. Siqueira, R. L.; Zanotto, E. D. *Quim. Nova* **2011**, *34*, 1231.
3. Aranha, N. *Vidros Niobofosfatos: Preparação, caracterização e propriedades* (PhD Dissertation, **1994**).
4. Hench, L. L. *J. Am. Ceram. Soc.* **1991**, *74*, 1487.
5. Hench, L. L.; Jones, J. R.; Sepulveda, P. In: *Futures Strategies for Tissue and Organ Replacement*, Polak, J. M.; Hench, L. R.; Kemp, P., eds. (London: Imperial College Press, **2002**), p. 3.
6. Hench, L. L. *J. Mater. Sci. Mater. Med.* **2006**, *17*, 967.
7. Hench, L. L. *New J. Glass Ceram.* **2013**, *3*, 67.
8. Cao, W.; Hench, L. L. *Ceram. Inter.* **1996**, *22*, 493.
9. Ogino, M.; Hench, L. L. *J. Non-Cryst. Solids* **1980**, *38*, 673.
10. Mohn, D.; Bruhin, C.; Luechinger, N. A.; Stark, W. J.; Imfeld, T.; Zehnder, M. *Int. Endod. J.* **2010**, *43*, 1037.
11. Osorio, R.; Yamauti, M.; Sauro, S.; Watson, T. F.; Toledano, M. *J. Endod.* **2012**, *38*, 1227.
12. Marending, M.; Bubenhofer, S. B.; Sener, B.; De-Deus, G. *Int. Endod. J.* **2013**, *46*, 317.

13. Tauböck, T. T.; Zehnder, M.; Schweizer, T.; Stark, W. J.; Attin, T.; Mohn, D. *Dent. Mater.* **2014**, *30*, 868.
14. Sauro, S.; Vijay, S.; Deb, S. *Eur. Polym. J.* **2012**, *48*, 1466.
15. Sauro, S.; Osorio, R.; Osorio, E.; Watson, T. F.; Toledano, M. *J. Biomater. Sci. Polym. Ed.* **2012**, *24*, 940.
16. Kokubo, T. ed., *Bioceramics and their Clinical Applications* (Boca Raton: CRC Press, **2008**).
17. Hench, L. L.; La, T. G.; Filho, O. P.; Zanotto, E. U. S. Patent WO/1997/041079, **1997**.
18. Peitl, O.; La Torre, G.; Hench, L. L. *J. Bio. Mater. Res.* **1996**, *30*, 509.
19. Peitl, O.; Zanotto, E. D.; Hench, L. L. *J. Non-Cryst. Solids* **2001**, *292*, 115.
20. Peitl, O.; Zanotto, E. D.; Serbena, F. C.; Hench, L. L. *Acta Biomater.* **2012**, *8*, 321.
21. Moura, J.; Teixeira, L.N.; Ravagnani, C.; Peitl, O.; Zanotto, E. D.; Beloti, M. M.; Panzeri, H.; Rosa, A. L.; de Oliveira, P. T. *J. Biomed. Mater. Res. A* **2007**, *82*, 545.
22. Tirapelli, C.; Panzeri, H.; Soares, R. G.; Peitl, O.; Zanotto, E. D. *Braz. Oral Res.* **2010**, *24*, 381.
23. Martins, C. H.; Carvalho, T. C.; Souza, M. G.; Ravagnani, C.; Peitl, O.; Zanotto, E. D.; Panzeri, H.; Casemiro, L. A. *J. Mater. Sci. Mater. Med.* **2011**, *22*, 1439.
24. Pintado-Palomino, K.; Peitl, O.; Zanotto, E. D.; Tirapelli, C. *J. Dent.* **2015**, *43*, 1099.
25. Crovace, M. C.; Souza, M. T.; Chinaglia, C. R.; Peitl, O.; Zanotto, E. D. *J. Non-Cryst. Solid.* **2015**, *432*, 90.
26. Carbonari, M. J. *Desenvolvimento de vidros niobofosfato bioativos* (PhD Dissertation, **2003**).
27. Sene, F. F.; Martinelli, J. R.; Gomes, L. *J. Non-Cryst. Solid.* **2004**, *348*, 63.
28. Denry, I. L.; Holloway, J. A.; Nakkula, R. J.; Walters, J. D. *J. Biomed. Mater. Res. B. Appl. Biomater.* **2005**, *75*, 18.
29. Bertolini, M. J.; Zaghete, M. A.; Gimenes, R.; Padovani, G. C. *Dent. Mater.* **2008**, *24*, 124.

30. Plenk, H.; Pfluger Jr., G.; Bohler, N.; Gottsauner-Wolf, F.; Schider, S. In: *Biomaterials and Biomechanics*, Ducheyne, P.; Van der Perre, G.; Aubert, A. E., eds. (Amsterdam: Elsevier, **1984**), p.61.
31. Stefanovich, Y. S.; Sigaev, V. N. *Glass Phys. Chem.* **1995**, *21*, 253.
32. Kokubo, T.; Kim, H. M.; Kawashita, M. *Biomater.* **2003**, *24*, 2161.
33. Karlinsey, R. L.; Hara, T. A.; Yi, K.; Duhn, C. W. *Biomed. Mater.* **2006**, *1*, 16.
34. Velten, D.; Eisenbarth, E.; Schanne, N.; Breme, J. *J. Mater. Sci. Mater. Med.* **2004**, *15*, 457.
35. Leitune, V. C.; Collares, F. M.; Takimi, A.; Lima, G. B.; Petzhold, C. L.; Bergmann, C. P. *J. Dent.* **2013**, *41*, 106.
36. Leitune, V. C.; Takimi, A.; Collares, F. M.; Santos, P. D.; Provenzi, C.; Bergmann, C. P. *Int. Endod. J.* **2013**, *46*, 205.
37. Hench, L. L.; Wilson, J. In: *An Introduction to Bioceramics*, Hench, L. L.; Wilson, J., eds. (London: World Scientific Publishing, **1993**), p. 1.
38. Peitl, O. *Vitro-cerâmica bioativa de alto desempenho mecânico* (PhD Dissertation, **1995**).
39. Carvalho, C. N.; Wang, Z.; Shen, Y.; Gavini, G.; Martinelli, J. R.; Manso, A.; Haapasalo, M. *Int. Endod J.* **2016**, *49*, 1048.
40. Carvalho, C. N.; Freire, L. G.; de Carvalho, A. P. L.; Duarte, M. A. H.; Bauer, J.; Gavini, G. *Braz. Dent. J.* **2016**, *27*, 325.
41. Bauer, J.; Carvalho, E. M.; Carvalho, C. N.; Meier, M. M.; de Souza, J. P.; de Carvalho, R. M.; Loguercio, A. D. *Int. J. Adhes. Adhes.* **2016**, *69*, 110.
42. Thomas, M. V.; Puleo, D. A.; Al-Sabbagh, M. *J. Long Term Eff. Med. Implants.* **2005**, *15*, 585.
43. Neelakantan, P.; John, S.; Anand, S.; Sureshbabu, N.; Subbarao, C. *Oper. Dent.* **2011**, *36*, 80.
44. Valanezhad, A.; Odatsu, T.; Udoh, K.; Shiraishi, T.; Sawase, T.; Watanabe, I. *J. Mater. Sci. Mater. Med.* **2016**, *27*, 3.
45. Lohbauer, U. *Materials* **2009**, *3*, 76.
46. Silva, R. M.; Santos, P. H. N.; Souza, L. B.; Dumont, V. C.; Soares, J. A.; Santos, M. H. *Mater. Res. Bull.* **2013**, *48*, 118.
47. Fleming, G. J.; Marquis, P. M.; Shortall, A. C. *Dent. Mater.* **1999**, *15*, 87.

48. Aratani, M.; Pereira, A. C.; Correr-Sobrinho, L.; Sinhoreti, M. A.; Consani, S. *J. Appl. Oral Sci.* **2005**, *13*, 356.
49. Xie, D.; Chung, I. D.; Wu, W.; Mays, J. *Dent. Mater.* **2004**, *20*, 470.
50. Sauro, S.; Watson, T. F.; Thompson, I.; Toledano, M.; Nucci, C.; Banerjee, A. *Eur. J. Oral Sci.* **2012**, *120*, 168.
51. Ana, I. D.; Matsuya, S.; Ohta, M.; Ishikawa, K. *Biomaterials* **2003**, *24*, 3061.
52. Yli-Urpo, H.; Vallittu, P. K.; Närhi, T. O.; Forsback, A. P.; Väkiparta, M. *J. Biomater. Appl.* **2004**, *19*, 5.
53. Matsuya, S.; Matsuya, Y.; Ohta, M. *Dent. Mater. J.* **1999**, *18*, 155.
54. Yli-Urpo, H.; Lassila, L. V.; Närhi, T.; Vallittu, P. K.; *Dent. Mater.* **2005**, *21*, 201.
55. Mousavinasab, S. M.; Khoroushi, M.; Keshani, F.; Hashemi, S. *J. Contemp. Dent. Pract.* **2011**, *12*, 41.
56. Kamitakahara, M.; Kawashita, M.; Kokubo, T.; Nakamura, T. *Biomaterials* **2001**, *22*, 3191.
57. Choi, J. Y.; Lee, H. H.; Kim, H. W. *J. Mater. Sci. Mater. Med.* **2008**, *19*, 3287.
58. Khoroushi, M.; Mousavinasab, S. M.; Keshani, F.; Hashemi, S.; *Oper. Dent.* 2013, *38*, E1.
59. Xie, D.; Zhao, J.; Weng, Y.; Park, J. G.; Jiang, H.; Platt, J. A. *Eur. J. Oral Sci.* **2008**, *116*, 479.
60. Osorio, E.; Fagundes, T.; Navarro, M. F.; Zanotto, E. D.; Peitl, O.; Osorio, R.; Toledano-Osorio, M.; Toledano, M. *J. Adhes. Sci. Technol.* **2015**, 29.
61. Shah, F. A. *Mater. Sci. Eng. C Mater. Biol. Appl.* **2016**, *58*, 1279.
62. Brauer, D. S.; Karpukhina, N.; O'Donnell, M. D.; Law, R. V.; Hill, R. G. *Acta Biomater.* **2010**, *6*, 3275.
63. Krithikadatta, J.; Indira, R.; Dorothykalyani, A. L. *J. Endod.* **2007**, *33*, 1473.
64. Stoor, P.; Söderling, E.; Salonen, J. I. *Acta Odontol. Scand.* **1998**, *56*, 161.
65. Zehnder, M.; Söderling, E.; Salonen, J.; Waltimo, T. *J. Endod.* **2004**, *30*, 220.
66. Osorio, R.; Yamauti, M.; Sauro, S.; Watson, T. F.; Toledano, M. *J. Endod.* **2012**, *38*, 1227.

67. Braux, J.; Velard, F.; Guillaume, C.; Bouthors, S.; Jallot, E.; Nedelec, J. M.; Laurent-Maquin, D.; Laquerrière, P. *Acta Biomater.* **2011**, *7*, 2593.
68. Zhang, H.; Shen, Y.; Ruse, N. D.; Haapasalo, M. *J. Endod.* **2009**, *35*, 1051.
69. Nagas, E.; Uyanik, M. O.; Eymirli, A.; Cehreli, Z. C.; Vallittu, P. K.; Lassila, L. V.; Durmaz, V. *J. Endod.* **2012**, *38*, 240.
70. Shokouhinejad, N.; Gorjestani, H.; Nasseh, A. A.; Hoseini, A.; Mohammadi, M.; Shamshiri, A. R. *Aust. Endod. J.* **2013**, *39*, 102.
71. Borges, R. P.; Sousa-Neto, M. D.; Versiani, M. A.; Rached-Júnior, F. A.; de-Deus, G.; Miranda, C. E. S.; Pécora, J. D. *Int. Endod. J.* **2012**, *45*, 419.
72. Alani, A.; Knowles, J. C.; Chrzanowski, W.; Ng, Y. L.; Gulabivala, K. *Dent. Mater.* **2009**, *25*, 400.
73. Mohn, D.; Zehnder, M.; Imfeld, T.; Stark, W. J. *Int. Endod. J.* **2010**, *43*, 210.
74. Brown, M. L.; Davis, H. B.; Tufekci, E.; Crowe, J. J.; Covell, D. A.; Mitchell, J. C. *Angle Orthod.* **2011**, *81*, 1014.
75. Manfred, L.; Covell, D. A.; Crowe, J. J.; Tufekci, E.; Mitchell, J. C. *Angle Orthod.* **2013**, *83*, 97.
76. Altmann, A. S.; Collares, F. M.; Leitune, V. C.; Arthur, R. A.; Takimi, A. S.; Samuel, S. M. *Clin. Oral Investig.* **2017**, *21*, 93.
77. Tufekci, E.; Dixon, J. S.; Gunsolley, J. C.; Lindauer, S. J.; *Angle Orthod.* **2011**, *81*, 206.
78. Gomes, S. C.; Varela, C. C.; da Veiga, S. L.; Rösing, C. K.; Oppermann, R. V. *Eur. J. Orthod.* **2007**, *29*, 477.
79. Lundström F.; Krasse, B. *Eur. J. Orthod.* **1987**, *9*, 117.
80. Featherstone, J. D. *J. Am. Dent. Assoc.* **2000**, *131*, 887.
81. Khvostenko, D.; Mitchell, J. C.; Hilton, T. J.; Ferracane, J. L.; Kruzic, J. J. *Dent. Mater.* **2013**, *29*, 1139.
82. Xu, H. H.; Weir, M. D.; Sun, L. *Dent. Mater.* **2009**, *25*, 535.
83. Hyun, H. K.; Salehi, S.; Ferracane, J. L. *Dent. Mater.* **2015**, *31*, 1599.
84. Khvostenko, D.; Hilton, T. J.; Ferracane, J. L.; Mitchell, J. C.; Kruzic, J. J. *Dent. Mater.* **2016**, *32*, 73.
85. Chatzistavrou, X.; Fenno, J. C.; Faulk, D.; Badylak, S.; Kasuga, T.; Boccaccini, A. R.; Papagerakis, P. *Acta Biomater.* **2014**, *10*, 3723.

86. Chatzistavrou, X.; Velamakanni, S.; DiRenzo, K.; Lefkelidou, A.; Fenno, J. C.; Kasuga, T.; Boccaccini, A. R.; Papagerakis, P. *Mater. Sci. Eng. C Mater. Biol. Appl.* **2015**, *52*, 267.
87. De Munck, J.; Van Landuyt, K.; Peumans, M.; Poitevin, A.; Lambrechts, P.; Braem, M.; Van Meerbeek, B. *J. Dent. Res.* **2005**, *84*, 118.
88. Hashimoto, M.; Nagano, F.; Endo, K.; Ohno, H. *Jpn. Dent. Sci. Rev.* **2011**, *47*, 5.
89. Yiu, C. K. Y.; King, N. M.; Pashley, D. H.; Suh, B. I.; Carvalho, R. M.; Carrilho, M. R. O. *Biomaterials* **2004**, *25*, 5789.
90. Malacarne, J.; Carvalho, R. M.; De goes, M. F.; Svizero, N.; Pashley, D. H.; Tay, F. R.; Yiu, C. K.; Carrilho, M. R. *Dent. Mater.* **2006**, *22*, 973.
91. Manso, A. P.; Bedran-Russo, A. K.; Suh, B.; Pashley, D. H.; Carvalho, R. M. *Dent. Mater.* **2009**, *25*, 744.
92. Peumans, M.; Kanumilli, P.; De Munck, J.; Van Landuyt, K.; Lambrechts, P.; Van Meerbeek, B. *Dent. Mater.* **2005**, *21*, 864.
93. Martins, G. C., Meier, M. M., Louguercio, A. D., Reis, A., Gomes, J. C., Gomes, O. M. M. *J. Adhes. Dent.* **2014**, *16*, 107.
94. Van Meerbeeck, B.; De Munk, J.; Yoshida, Y.; Inoue, S.; Vargas, M.; Vijay, P.; Van Landuyt, K.; Lambrechts, P.; Vanherie, G. *Oper. Dent.* **2003**, *28*, 215.
95. Reis, A.; Carrilho, M.; Breschi, L.; Louguercio, A. D. *Oper. Dent.* **2013**, *38*, E1.
96. Carrilho, M. R. O.; Tay, F. R.; Pashley, D. H.; Tjäderhane, J.; Carvalho, R. M. *Dent. Mater.* **2005**, *21*, 232.
97. D'Arcangelo, C.; Vanini, L.; Prosperi, G. D.; Bussolo, G. D.; Angelis, F. D. *J. Adhes. Dent.* **2009**, *11*, 109.
98. Ito, S.; Tay, F. R.; Hashimoto, M.; Yoshiyama, M.; Saito, T.; Brackett, W. W.; Waller, J. L.; Pashley, D. H. *J. Adhes. Dent.* **2005**, *7*, 133.
99. Pasquantonio, G.; Tay, F. R.; Mazzoni, A.; Suppa, P.; Ruggeri Jr A.; Falconi, M. *Dent. Mater.* **2007**, *23*, 513.
100. Mena-Serrano, A.; Garcia, E. J.; Louguercio, A. D.; Reis, A. *Clin. Oral Invest.* **2014**, *18*, 729.
101. Cadenaro, M.; Breschi, L.; Rueggeberg, F. A.; Agee, K.; Di Lenarda, R.; Carrilho, M.; Tay, F. R.; Pashley, D. H. *Dent. Mater.* **2009**, *25*, 39.

102. Conde, M. C., Zanchi, C. H., Rodrigues, J. R. S. A.; Carreno, N. L.; Ogliari, F. A.; Piva, E. *J. Dent.* **2009**, *37*, 331.
103. Lohbauer, U.; Wagner, A.; Belli, R.; Stoetzel, C.; Hilpert, A.; Kurland, H. D.; Grabow, J.; Muller, F. A. *Acta Biomater.* **2010**, *6*, 4539.
104. Collares, F. M.; Klein, M.; Santos, P. D.; Portella, F. F.; Oligari, F.; Leitune, V. C.; Samuel, S. M. *J. Appl. Oral Sci.* **2013**, *21*, 533.
105. Osorio, R.; Osorio, E.; Medina-Castillo, A. L.; Toledano, M. *J. Dent. Res.* **2014**, *93*, 1258.
106. Peters, M. C.; Bresciani, E.; Barata, T.; Fagundes, T. C.; Navarro, R. L.; Navarro, M. F.; Dickens, S. H. *J. Dent. Res.* **2010**, *89*, 286.
107. Sauro, S.; Osorio, R.; Watson, T. F.; Toledano, M. *J. Mater. Sci. Mater. Med.* **2012**, *23*, 1521.
108. Hashimoto, M.; Lijima, M.; Nagano, F.; Ohno, H.; Endo, K. *J. Biomed. Mat. Res. B Appl. Biomater.* **2010**, *94*, 127.
109. Profeta, A. C.; Mannocci, F.; Foxton, R. M.; Thompson, I.; Watson, T. F.; Sauro, S. *Eur. J. Oral Sci.* **2012**, *120*, 353.
110. Kim, Y. K.; Gu, L. S.; Bryan, T. E.; Kim, J. R.; Chen, L.; Liu, Y.; Yoon, J. C.; Breschi, L.; Pashley, D. H.; Tay, F. R. *Biomaterials* **2010**, *31*, 6618.
111. Ryou, H.; Niu, L. N.; Dai, L.; Pucci, C. R.; Arola, D. D.; Pashley, D. H.; Tay, F. R. *J. Dent. Res.* **2011**, *90*, 1122.
112. Taubock, T. T.; Zehnder, M.; Schweizer, T.; Stark, W. J.; Attin, T.; Mohn, D. *Dent. Mater.* **2014**, *30*, 868.
113. Hashimoto, M.; Nakamura, K.; Kaga, M.; Yawaka, Y. *Dent. Mater.* **2008**, *24*, 457.
114. Gubler, M.; Brunner, T. J.; Zehnder, M.; Waltimo, T.; Sener, B.; Stark, W. J. *Int. Endod. J.* **2008**, *41*, 670.
115. Ten Cate, J. M. *J. Dent. Res.* **2012**, *91*, 813.
116. Melo, M. A. S., Guedes, S. F. F., Xu, H. H. K., Rodrigues, L. K. A. *Trends Biotechnol.* **2014**, *31*, 459.
117. Van Landuyt, K. L.; Snauwaert, J.; De Munck, J.; Peumans, M.; Yoshida, Y.; Poitevin, A.; Coutinho, E.; Suzuki, K.; Lambrecths, P.; Van Meerbeek, B. *Biomaterials* **2007**, *28*, 3757.
118. Montes, M. A.; De Goes, M. F.; Da Cunha, M. R.; Soares, A. B. *J. Dent.* **2001**, *29*, 435.

119. Opdam, N. J.; Roeters, F. J.; Verdonschot, E. H. *J. Dent.* **1997**, *25*, 391.
120. Tay, F. R.; Pashley, D. H. *J. Dent. Res.* **2009**, *88*, 719.
121. Brackett, M. G.; Li, N.; Brackett, W. W.; Sword, R. J.; Qi, Y. P.; Niu, L. N.; Pucci, C. R.; Dib, A.; Pashley, D. H.; Tay, F. R. *J. Dent.* **2011**, *39*, 238.
122. Allan, I.; Newman, H.; Wilson, M. *Biomaterials* **2001**, *22*, 1683.
123. Sepulveda, P.; Jones, J. R.; Hench, L. L. *J. Biomed. Mater. Res.* **2002**, *61*, 301.
124. Banerjee, A. *Br. Dent. J.* **2013**, *214*, 107.
125. Waltimo, T.; Brunner, T. J.; Vollenweider, M.; Stark, W. J.; Zehnder, M. *J. Dent. Res.* **2007**, *86*, 754.
126. Sauro, S.; Watson, T. F.; Thompson, I.; Banerjee, A. *J. Dent.* **2012**, *40*, 896.
127. Sauro, S.; Watson, T. F.; Thompson, I. *J. Dent.* **2010**, *38*, 411.
128. Wang, Z.; Jiang, T.; Sauro, S.; Wang, Y.; Thompson, I.; Watson, T. F.; Sa, Y.; Xing, W.; Shen, Y.; Haapsalo, M. *J. Dent.* **2011**, 39, 746.
129. Bakry, A. S.; Takahashi, H.; Otsuki, M.; Tagami, J. *Dent. Mater.* **2013**, *29*, 357.
130. Carvalho, E. M.; Lima, D. M.; Carvalho, C. N.; Loguercio, A. D.; Martinelli, J. R.; Bauer, J. *J. Prosthodont. Res.* **2015**, *59*, 129.
131. Sauro, S.; Pashley, D. H. *Int. J. Adhes. Adhes.* **2016**, *69*, 39.

Chapter 10

Dental Adhesives

Marcelo Giannini*,‡, Patrícia Makishi*,§,
Ronaldo Hirata†,¶, and Carolina Bosso André*,‖

*Department of Restorative Dentistry,
Piracicaba Dental School, State University
of Campinas-SP, Brazil
†Department of Biomaterials and Biomimetics,
New York University, College of Dentistry
New York, USA

‡giannini@fop.unicamp.br
§pmakishi@hotmail.com
¶rh1694@nyu.edu
‖carolina.bosso@gmail.com

Adhesive dentistry is among the fastest growing fields in dental science. The treatment methods are a continuous learning process for practitioners and require adaptation to new technologies, materials, clinical techniques, and research findings. A realistic prediction about the success of a dental restoration requires a deep understanding of the bonding mechanism, including mechanical, chemical, and biological viewpoints, as well as the consideration of the risks and contributing factors that may affect the durability of dental restorations. *In vitro* bonding evaluations as marginal adaptation, bond strength, and interaction of the bond with the tooth substrate are well recognized as comparative tools of the restorative materials bonding performance *in vivo*.

1. Introduction

1.1. *Mineralized Dental Tissues*

Human teeth contain two mineralized tissues called enamel and dentin. Enamel is the hardest tissue of the human body and is composed of minerals, which make up 96% of its composition.[1] The remainder of its composition is water and some proteins, such as amelogenins and enamelins. The main mineral component is the hydroxyapatite, which is formed by calcium phosphate crystals. The enamel has high Young's modulus (approximately 83 GPa) and high tensile strength (approximately 42 MPa) because of its high mineralization level. However, when enamel is stressed transversally to its prismatic orientation, the strength is significantly weaker (approximately 11 MPa).[2,3] Enamel rod or prims are the basic units of dental enamel (Figure 1), which is formed by ameloblast cells during the early stage of enamel formation.[1]

The amelo–dentinal junction is the interfacial area between enamel and underlying dentin (Figure 2) which has biomechanical

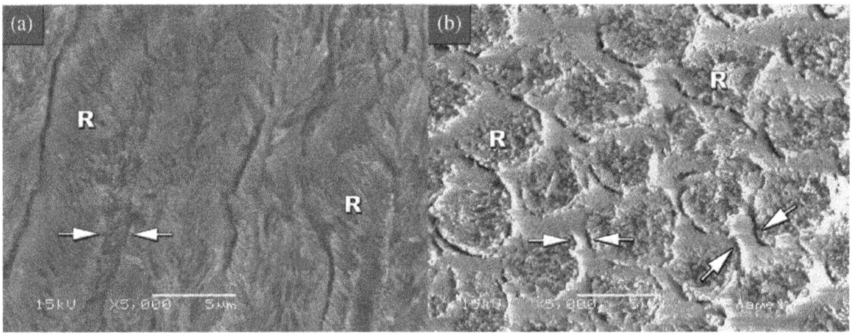

Figure 1. SEM images showing the human dental enamel (R: rods; Arrows: interrod area) from a transversal cut (a) and from a longitudinal cut (b) (5,000× magnification)

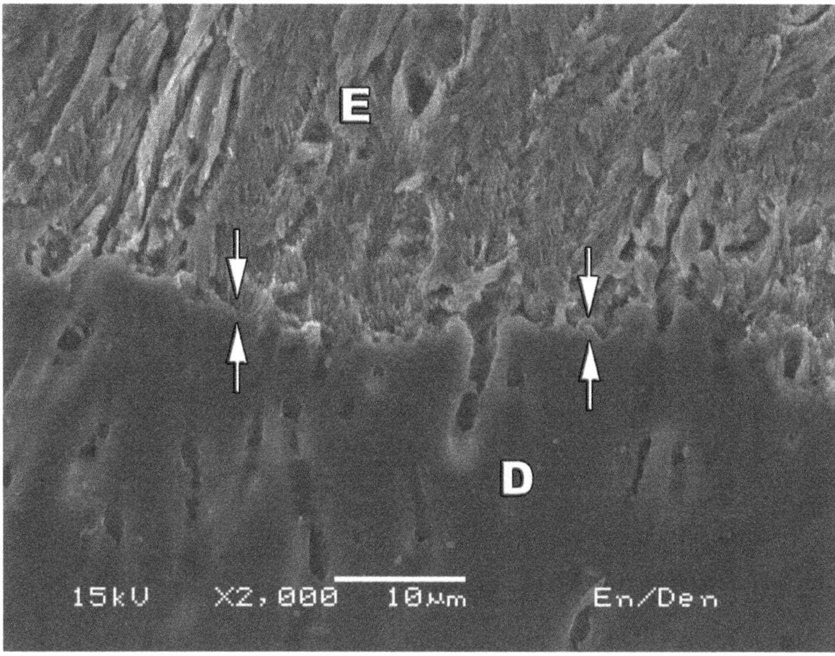

Figure 2. SEM image showing the amelo-dentinal junction (between arrows), that is the interfacial region between the dentin (D) and enamel (E) (2,000× magnification)

properties that avoid catastrophic tooth fractures from the cracks formed in outer enamel.[3,4] Unlike enamel, the dentin is a complex dental tissue in terms of morphology, composition, and physiology. The composition depends on the analysis location, and the main components are minerals (70–45% by weight), organic content (33–18%), and water (22–12%). The inorganic phase is basically hydroxyapatite, which is deposited around collagen fibrils during the dentinogenesis. Besides collagen, other organic components are present, such as glycoproteins and proteoglycans. The dentin structural units are the dentinal tubules and intertubular and peritubular (or intratubular) dentin (Figure 3).[1]

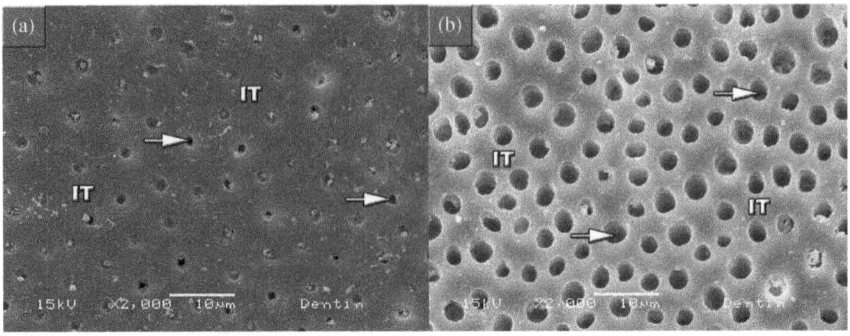

Figure 3. SEM images showing the structural units of dentin (Arrow: dentinal tubule, IT: Intertubular dentin and Intratubular dentin: whitish aspect around the tubules) for occlusal superficial dentin close to enamel (a) and deep dentin close to pulp chamber (b) (2,000× magnification)

1.2. *Historic of Bonding Agents*

The improvement of bonding agents had run parallel with the morphological and physiological mineralized hard dental tissues studies. Adhesion to enamel began with Buonocore *et al.*, 1955, in which the phosphoric acid altered, morphologically and chemically, the enamel surface.[5] For dentin, the starting point was when Nakabayashi *et al.*, 1982, infiltrated adhesive monomers into conditioned dentin, which has been called as hybrid layer or resin–dentin interdiffusion zone.[6] The first dentin bonding agents contained glycerophosphoric acid dimethacrylate,[7,8] *n*-phenylglycine glycidyl methacrylate (NPG-GMA),[9] polyurethane resin[10] orcyanoacrylate.[11]

The second generation of adhesives contained halophosphorous esters of unfilled resins such as Bis-GMA, and poor clinical results were obtained with these adhesives.[12,13] At the beginning of the 1990s, some commercial dental adhesive brands became available for use with composite resin in direct restorations. This third generation introduced the concept of a "primer" for dentin bonding and was combined with etched enamel with phosphoric acid. Primers were hydrophilic solutions of organic or mineral acids that were able to modify or partially remove the smear layer, allowing the monomer resins to penetrate into dentinal tubules resulting in resin tags formation. Also, these adhesives were able to chemically bond with calcium from hydroxyapatite; however, the early microleakage in dentin margins of composite restorations was not completely avoided.[14,15]

The application of phosphoric acid to etch the dentin was suggested by Fusayama *et al.*, 1979,[16] but was clinically accepted only during the nineties. The "total-etch" (enamel and dentin etching) or the etch-and-rinse adhesives combined with wet-bonding technique have been used until now (Figures 4 and 5). Hydrophilic monomers infiltrate into the wet demineralized dentin forming the hybrid layer or resin–dentin interdiffusion zone.[17] The first acidic hydrophilic monomer used in a commercial self-etching adhesive was the phenyl-P. This category of bonding agent was also introduced during the 1990s.[18,19] Many acidic resin monomers for self-etching systems have been developed; however, the methacryloyloxi-decyl-dihydrogen-phosphate (10-MDP) functional monomer seems to be the most effective in bonding resin-based materials to dentin.[20,21]

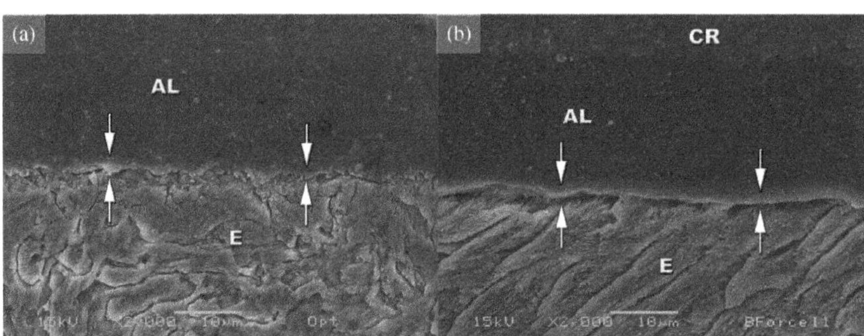

Figure 4. SEM images showing the resin–enamel interfaces with etch-and-rinse (a) and self-etching adhesive systems (b). Arrows show the enamel–adhesive interfaces (E: enamel; AL: adhesive layer; CR: composite resin) (2,000× magnification)

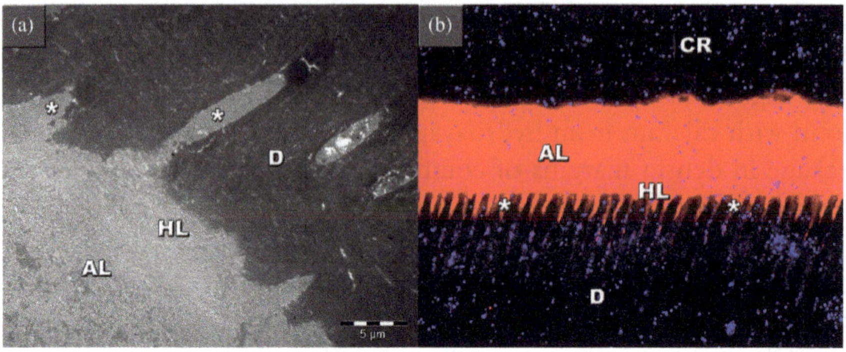

Figure 5. TEM image (a) showing the resin–dentin interface of an etch-and-rinse adhesive. The hybrid layer (HL) corresponds to the infiltration of adhesive resin monomers into dentin with exposed collagen by acid etching (1,100× magnification) (Vermelho PM and Giannini M, 2011). Confocal laser microscopy image (b) showing the resin–dentin interface of an etch-and-rinse adhesive. The rhodamine dye (red) was incorporated to the bonding agent (25× objective lens). (*: resin tags; AL: adhesive layer; D: dentin; CR: composite resin)

2. General Composition

Contemporary bonding agents contain resin monomers (hydrophobic and hydrophilic ones), organic solvents (such as acetone, alcohol, and/or water), chemical initiator system, inhibitor, fillers (such as colloidal silica, pyrogenic silica, and silicate glasses), and other compounds (such as copolymers, desensitizing agents, sources of fluoride, and antibacterial agents). Alcohol and acetone are monomers solvents, indispensable for a good penetration of the monomers, while water is important for the hydrolysis of functional monomers and to re-expand the collapsed collagen network for the etched dentin technique. The fillers increase the polymer's intrinsic strength and also promote fluoride release depending on its composition. Initiators are responsible for polymerizing the monomers, while inhibitors increase the shelf life of the adhesive systems.[22]

Regarding hydrophilic resin monomers, they can be wetting agents, responsible for penetrating into etched tooth surface and bond to calcium from hydroxyapatite and to collagen fibrils, which are called adhesion-promoting functional monomers. The wetting agents have small molecular dimensions and in uncured state they are present as a fluid resin that is solvable in water, alcohol, and/or acetone. The most popular wetting agent is the 2-hydroxyethyl methacrylate (HEMA).[22]

2.1. *Functional Adhesive Monomers*

Functional monomers are acidic, have hydrophilic properties, and can bond to calcium of the hydroxyapatite via chelate or ionic bond. Their etching aggressiveness depends on the acidity of adhesive monomeric composition. In general, dihydrogen acids are more acidic that monohydrogenic ones because dihydrogen acids form more protons following the dissociation reaction. Sulfonic acid, phosphate, phosphonate, and carboxyl groups have been used in commercial products. They act as wetting agents, demineralize the dentin surface by causing proton release from functional groups, and function as adhesion promoters by chemical reaction.[22–24]

NPG-GMA and N-tolylglycine glycidyl methacrylate (NTG-GMA) have also been used as adhesion promoting monomers and are co-initiators as is dimethylaminoethyl methacrylate (DMAEMA).[23,25] The 4-methacryloyloxyethyl trimellitate anhydride (4-META) and 4-methacryloyloxyethyl trimellitic acid (4-MET) present two carboxylic groups which are responsible for the demineralizing properties and enhancing the wetting. These functional monomers are indicated for adhesion to enamel, dentin, amalgam, metals alloys, or gold. The 4-META functional monomer is an organic acid anhydride derived from carboxylic acid and is able to chelate to calcium from hydroxyapatite. The salicylic group of N-methacryloyl-5-aminosalicylic acid (5-NMSA) also chelates with calcium.[20,22,27,28]

The dihydrogenphosphate group of 10-MDP dissolves partially the smear layer and etches the dentin surface, reacting chemically with calcium from hydroxyapatite of enamel or dentin and forming calcium salt. Studies have shown that 10-MDP forms stronger and more stable ionic bonds with calcium than with other functional monomers.[20,22,28] 10-MDP has also been shown to bond alloy metals, composites, and zirconia ceramics, and for this reason is used in the new multimodes and single-step adhesives.

Other functional monomers such as 11-methacryloyloxy-1,10-undecanedicarboxylic acid (MAC-10), 4-acryloyloxyethyl trimellitate anhydride (4-AETA), Di-HEMA-phosphate, and HEMA-phosphate are the main ingredients of some commercial adhesives. The amide monomers bonds to collagen via a hydrogen bridge bond between the carboxyl and amide groups of the monomer with the carboxyl groups of collagen.[24,29]

The methacryloyloxy dodecylpyridinium bromide (MDPB) is a hydrophobic monomer compound with antibacterial agent (dodecylpyridinium bromide).[30,31] The hydrophilicity of the spacer group of functional monomers determine their hydrophilic behavior and susceptibility to hydrolysis in aqueous solutions by water uptake. The ester group of acrylates, phosphate, and carboxyl groups used in functional monomers can hydrolyze in water.[22]

The main less-hydrophilic adhesive resin monomers are the UDMA, Bis-GMA, TEG-DMA, other dimethacrylates, and monomers. They are responsible for the formation of a densely cross-linked polymer film following the polymerization reaction. They also keep the surface hydrophobic against water uptake.[32,33]

3. Adhesive Systems

3.1. *Etch-and-Rinse Adhesive Systems*

This category of adhesives involves a previous etching with phosphoric acid, rinsing with water, and applying the adhesive on a wet demineralized dentin. Etch-and-rinse adhesives can be used following two or three steps; the first step being the acid etching for both types of these adhesives. After etching for 15 s, the dentin is rinsed with water to remove the acid gel and the mineral dissolved. The demineralized dentin must be wet, and water occupies the spaces of the removed mineral by the acid etching step.[34,35]

The acid etching removes the smear layer and smear plugs, demineralizing the dentin 5–10 μm in depth. In this demineralized area, the resin monomers are able to infiltrate forming the "hybrid layer" or "resin–dentin interdiffusion zone",[6] which represents the replacement of mineral with adhesive resin monomers (Figure 6). When a three-step etch-and-rinse adhesive is used, an adhesive solution known as primer is applied before hydrophobic bonding resin (third step), while for two-step etch-and-rinse adhesives, a single combined solution of hydrophilic and hydrophobic monomers is used. The primer is a solution containing basically HEMA and a solvent such as water or ethanol. The bonding resin is less hydrophilic and contains Bis-GMA, TEG-DMA, UDMA, other hydrophobic resins, and other components. The two-step etch-and-rinse adhesives are often used in Restorative Dentistry and represent a combination of primer and bonding resin in a single but complex mixture.[17,21]

If the demineralized dentin is poorly infiltrated with resin monomer or if it slowly hydrolyses and leaches resin monomers from the hybrid layer due to poor polymerization, the intrinsic matrix metaloproteinases (MMP) activity of dentin matrix can be expressed, leading to an attack on the denuded collagen. This behavior could weaken the hybrid layer, accelerating the loss of resin and collagen degradation. Studies have demonstrated that the hydrophilic characteristic of the adhesive monomers could compromise the long-term bonding effectiveness and that insufficient resin infiltration or an incompletely

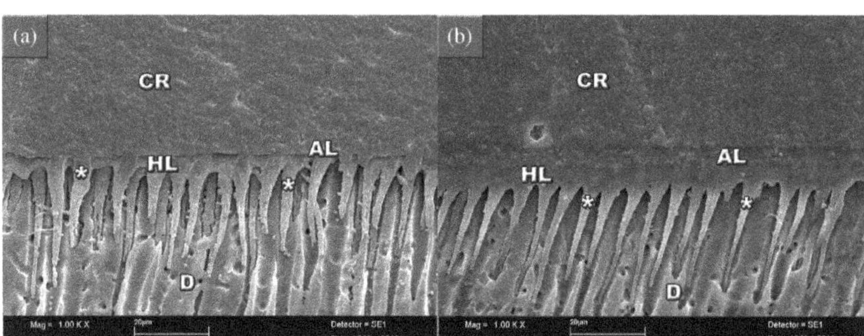

Figure 6. SEM images showing the resin–dentin interfaces with two-steps (a) and three-steps (b) etch-and-rinse adhesives (HL: hybrid layer; *; resin tags: D: dentin; AL: adhesive layer; CR: composite resin) (1,000× magnification) (Carvalho *et al.*, 2013)

cured hydrophilic monomer could remain at the bottom of the hybrid layer, leading to leakage. Consequently, both factors may expose the collagen matrix, which may be degraded by proteolytic enzymes.[36–38]

In an attempt to enhance the mechanical properties and reduce biodegradation rates, studies have focused on the incorporation of MMP inhibitors in the bonding procedure, such as chlorhexidine, galardin, and flavonols.[39,40] Studies have reported the use of chlorhexidine, which exhibits an inhibitory effect against MMPs and cysteine cathepsins (another class of collagenolytic enzymes).[41,42] However, controversial results regarding the pre-treatment of dentin with chlorhexidine before bonding have been reported. While some studies have shown long-term preservation of integrity of the hybrid layers and bonding efficacy, other studies indicated no detrimental effect on the bond strength or the sealing ability.[37,43–46]

Another approach would be to inactivate the endogenous MMPs via biomodification of the dentin matrix with collagen cross-linkers. Glutaraldehyde has been used as a cross-linking agent for years.[31,38] Other cross-linkers agents, such as proanthocyanidin extract and carbodiimide have been used to inactivate the proteolytic activity of MMPs and increase the bond strength of adhesives to dentin.[47–49]

3.2. *Self-Etching Adhesive Systems*

The main characteristic of self-etching systems is the use of non-rinse acidic monomers, i.e. no phosphoric acid etching and water rinsing steps are required. The acidic monomers are present on formulation, which are responsible for micromechanical and chemical bonding. These two bonding mechanism have provided good results in the laboratory and the clinic, especially for the self-etching primers. The three-steps etch-and-rinse adhesives have also been described as effective bonding agents when compared to self-etching primers.[21,50,51]

The self-etching primers are applied in two steps: primer and bonding. The acidic primers are aqueous solution containing organic solvents, wetting agent (such as HEMA), and a functional monomer with carboxyl or phosphate groups. The fluid bonding resin is less hydrophilic and is mixed with primer to reduce the hydrophilicity of the resin monomers, which are in contact with dentin, giving a more hydrophobic outer surface to bond with the restorative composite.[22]

The all-in-one or single-step self-etching adhesives are the most simplified bonding agents. They are a complex aqueous solution containing hydrophilic and hydrophobic resin monomers, organic solvents, initiators, and other components, depending on the commercial product. Studies have indicated that this category of self-etching system, as well as two-steps etch-and-rinse adhesives produced less durable composite restorations, according to clinical and laboratory investigations.[21,50,51]

Based on the acidic aggressiveness of self-etching adhesives, they are classified as "mild" (pH around 2) and "strong" (pH < 1). For mild pH self-etching adhesives, the collagen fibrils are only partially exposed, with residual hydroxyapatite still attached to the collagen fibrils and available for chemical interaction with functional monomers (Figure 7). For strong self-etching adhesive solutions, the dentin etching is similar to the effects found with 37% phosphoric acid etching.[21,23]

In order to reduce the hydrophilicity and increase the bonding durability, some single-step self-etching adhesives are free of HEMA

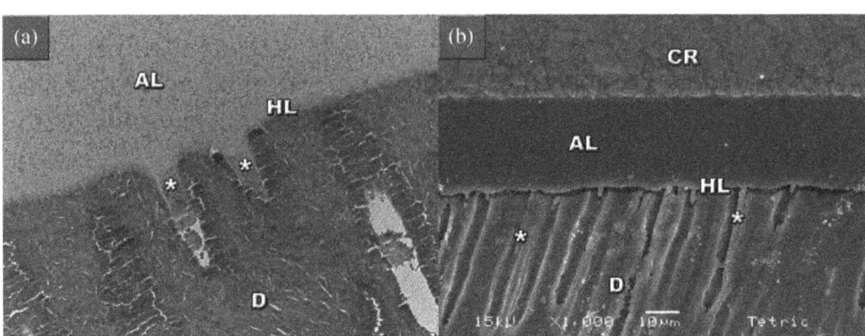

Figure 7. TEM image showing the resin–dentin interface with two-step self-etching adhesive (a) (3,000× magnification) (Vermelho PM, master thesis — 2011). SEM image showing the resin–dentin interfaces with single-step self-etching adhesive (b) (HL: hybrid layer; *: resin tags; D: dentin; AL: adhesive layer; CR: composite resin) (1,000× magnification)

monomer. These HEMA-free self-etching adhesives also contain a functional monomer, such as carboxylic acid monomers, which also play the role of wetting agents.[52–54] However, some concerns have been raised for the clinical use of simplified all-in-one adhesives, because the degree of conversion seems to be low when compared to two-step self-etching and etch-and-rinse adhesives. The low conversion rate can compromise the mechanical strength and form an adhesive film that behaves as a semi-permeable membrane, with high permeability through polymerized adhesive layer.[55–59]

4. Advances and Future Perspectives in Adhesive Dentistry

A trend in adhesive dentistry is to provide simple and time-effective chairside solutions. One of these examples is the multimode adhesives, or so-called universal adhesives. The multimode adhesives contain 10-MDP and are self-etch adhesives designed using the same concept as that used for all-in-one adhesives; however, they incorporate the versatility of being adaptable to different clinical situations such as the use on enamel, dentin, alloy, ceramic, or composite substrates. A long-term investigation indicated that current universal adhesives may perform equally well on an etched enamel substrate as a conventional adhesive system, without leakage; however, they may have a bonding performance that is equal to or inferior than a conventional self-etching adhesive when using dentin as a substrate, with similar degradation patterns at the tooth–dentin interface.[60] In addition, this new category of adhesive system exhibited good long-term bonding performance to sandblasted indirect resin composite. However, the use of separate bottles of silane and bonding resin resulted in superior bond strength for etched-glass-based ceramic.[61] Thus, it can be speculated that the bonding performance of universal adhesives are manufacturer- and substrate-specific.

Another issue that should be addressed is that the bond formation between the resin composite and tooth structure can be challenging because two different interfaces must be considered: that between the dentin/enamel substrate and adhesive system, and that between the adhesive system and resin composite. Polymerization shrinkage of methacrylate-based resin composites during curing may result in contraction stress and a loss of marginal adaptation, which may lead to early failures. Current resin composite technology is focused on the polymeric matrix, developing systems with reduced polymerization shrinkage stress to reduce the contraction stress during the polymerization.[62] For posterior restorations, a new category of resin composites have been examined to reduce the polymerization shrinkage and stress with a single increment, known as bulk-fill. Due to the differences in filler loading and resin matrix characteristics of this new category of resin composites, the mechanical properties can be expected to be material dependent. Studies have demonstrated that bulk-fill composites have higher volumetric shrinkage than conventional composites, even when their polymerization shrinkage values are lower.[63] However, in a Class I cavity, less volumetric polymerization contraction than that in a conventional composite was observed when a bonding agent was applied.[64] Therefore, it can be assumed that current adhesives and resin composites play a major role in the long-term success of restorations and that their mechanical and chemical properties should be considered as a combined set.[65,66]

The ultimate goal in dental materials science is the development of self-adhesive restorative materials, without the need for an adhesive to bond to the tooth substrate. Ideally, these materials should also provide aesthetic characteristics, with great functionality and durable bonding at affordable costs. Attempts have been made regarding the development of self-adhesive resin composites with the incorporation of functional monomers that serve as adhesion promoters to hydroxyapatite[67]; however, the separate use of adhesive and resin composite components still results in superior bonding performance.[68] Once the limitations related to the mechanical and chemical properties of these restorative materials are properly addressed, it will be possible to have even simpler and faster procedures with durable bonding in the future.

Restorative techniques and dental materials have evolved significantly over the years, expanding our clinical options. It appears reasonable to assume that much of this evolution was based on *in vitro* and *in vivo* evaluation tests. Although the current evaluation methods provide good information on the biomechanical properties of restorative materials, it is of crucial importance for researchers to investigate the materials from different aspects, developing even more sophisticated yet clinically relevant methods to evaluate the performance of restorative materials.

The introduction of digital technologies is reshaping the model for research and clinical care in three dimensions. One example is the use of optical coherence tomography (OCT) to follow-up on adhesive restorations over time and to non-invasively predict the bond durability.[69] This field is a very revolutionary and exciting field for diagnostic and treatment in Dentistry. Within the range of non-invasive imaging techniques, OCT has been reported to be a promising high-resolution biomedical optical method to examine the microstructural details of hard and soft oral tissues over a small distance. This technology implements high-resolution, volumetric, and cross-sectional tomographic imaging of the internal microstructure of materials and biological tissues on the micron-scale based on depth-resolved optical reflectivity.[70] This technique has been applied in Dentistry to characterize caries,[71] assess gaps between the resin–tooth interface in two-dimensional (2D) and three-dimensional (3D) images,[68,69] and evaluate voids and internal defects in restorations.[72] More recently, studies have investigated the association between real-time OCT findings related to the marginal adaptation of restorative materials and the bond strength,[69] gap formation and the bond strength,[73] and the effect of marginal sealing ability on demineralization progress.[74] It has thus been possible to better understand and mimic the degradation process *in vitro* using different factors in the same sample, which is clearly clinical relevant. Chairside diagnosis will also open new horizons into non-invasive procedures, and OCT can be a helpful tool in the selection of the most appropriate treatments and preventive measures. It is assumed that Dentistry will continue to advance and that new, better, smarter technologies will continue to emerge and affect both research and clinical practice.

Acknowledgments

This book chapter was partially supported by the São Paulo Research Foundation (FAPESP #2013/22823-9 and #2009/51674-6), the Coordination for the Improvement of Higher Education Personnel (CAPES #1777-2014 and #1778-2014) and The National Council for Scientific and Technological Development (CNPq #307217-2014-0). The authors are grateful to Dr. Adriana Oliveira Carvalho and Dr. Paulo Moreira Vermelho for providing SEM and TEM images.

References

1. Nanci, A. *Ten Cate's Oral Histology — Development, Structure, and Function*, 8th Edn. (Amsterdam: Elsevier, **2013**).
2. Staines, M.; Robinson, W. H.; Hood, J. A. A. *J. Mater. Sci.* **1981**, *16*, 2551.
3. Giannini, M.; Soares, C. J.; de Carvalho, R. M. *Dent. Mater.* **2004**, *20*, 322.
4. Imbeni, V.; Kruzic, J. J.; Marshall, G. W.; Marshall, S. J.; Ritchie, R. O. *Nat. Mater.* **2005**, *4*, 229.
5. Buonocore, M. G. *J. Dent. Res.* **1955**, *34*, 849.
6. Nakabayashi, N.; Kojima, K.; Masuhara, E. *J. Biomed. Mater. Res.* **1982**, *16*, 265.
7. Kramer, I. R. H.; McLean, J. W. *Br. Dent. J.* **1952**, *93*, 150.
8. Buonocore, M.; Wileman, W.; Brudevold, F. *J. Dent. Res.* **1956**, *35*, 846.
9. Bowen, R. L. *J. Dent. Res.* **1965**, *44*, 895.
10. Lee, H. L.; Cupples, A. L.; Schubert, R. J.; Swartz, M. L. *J. Dent. Res.* **1971**, *50*, 125.
11. Causton, B. E.; Johnson, N. W. *J. Dent. Res.* **1981**, *60*, 1315.
12. Ziemiecki, T. L.; Dennison, J. B.; Charbeneau, G. T. *Oper. Dent.* **1987**, *12*, 27.
13. Tyas, M. J. *Aust. Dent. J.* **1991**, *36*, 298.
14. Duke, E. S.; Robbins, J. W.; Snyder, D. S. *Quintessence Int.* **1991**, *22*, 889.

15. Prati, C.; Nucci, C.; Montanari, G. *J. Prosthet. Dent.* **1991**, *65*, 401.
16. Fusayama, T.; Nakamura, M.; Kurosaki, N.; Iwaku, M. *J. Dent. Res.* **1979**, *58*, 1364.
17. Swift, E. J. Jr.; Perdigão, J.; Heymann, H. O. *Quintessence Int.* **1995**, *26*, 95.
18. Wang, T.; Nikaido, T.; Nakabayashi, N. *Dent. Mater.* **1991**, *7*, 59.
19. Watanabe, I.; Nakabayashi, N.; Pashley, D. H. *J. Dent. Res.* **1994**, *73*, 1212.
20. Yoshida, Y.; Nagakane, K.; Fukuda, R.; Nakayama, Y.; Okazaki, M.; Shintani, H.; Inoue, S.; Tagawa, Y.; Suzuki, K.; De Munck, J.; Van Meerbeek, B. *J. Dent. Res.* **2004**, *83*, 454.
21. De Munck, J.; Van Landuyt, K.; Peumans, M.; Poitevin, A.; Lambrechts, P.; Braem M.;Van Meerbeek B. *J. Dent. Res.* **2005**, *84*, 118.
22. Van Landuyt, K. L.; Snauwaert, J.; De Munck, J.; Peumans, M.; Yoshida, Y.; Poitevin, A.; Coutinho, E.; Suzuki, K.; Lambrechts, P.; Van Meerbeek, B. *Biomaterials* **2007**, *28*, 3757.
23. Tay, F. R.; Pashley, D. H. *Dent. Mater.* **2001**, *17*, 296.
24. Moszner, N.; Salz, U.; Zimmermann, J. *Dent. Mater.* **2005**, *21*, 895.
25. Bowen, R. L.; Bennett, P. S.; Groh, R. J.; Farahani, M.; Eichmiller, F. C. J. *Dent. Res.* **1996**, *75*, 606.
26. Nakabayashi, N. *Oper. Dent.* **1992**, *5*, 125.
27. Chang, J. C.; Hurst, T. L.; Hart, D. A.; Estey, A. W. *J. Prosthet. Dent.* **2002**, *87*, 216.
28. Hanabusa, M.; Yoshihara, K.; Yoshida, Y.; Okihara, T.; Yamamoto, T.; Momoi, Y.;Van Meerbeek, B. *Eur. J. Oral Sci.* **2016**, *124*, 204.
29. Nishiyama, N.; Suzuki, K.; Asakura, T.; Komatsu, K.; Nemoto, K. *J. Dent. Res.* **2001**, *80*, 855.
30. Imazato, S.; Russell, R. R.; McCabe, J. F. *J. Dent.* **1995**, *23*, 177.
31. André, C. B.; Gomes, B. P.; Duque, T. M.; Stipp, R. N.; Chan, D. C.; Ambrosano, G. M.; Giannini, M. *J. Dent.* **2015**, *43*, 466.
32. Asmussen, E.; Peutzfeldt, A. *Dent. Mater.* **1998**, *14*, 51.
33. Sideridou, I.; Tserki, V.; Papanastasiou, G. *Biomaterials* **2002**, *23*, 1819.
34. Bertolotti, R. L. *J. Esthet. Dent.* **1991**, *3*, 1.
35. Kanca, J. 3rd. *Quintessence Int.* **1992**, *23*, 625.
36. van Strijp, A. J.; Jansen, D. C.; DeGroot, J.; ten Cate, J.; Everts, V. *Caries Res.* **2003**, *37*, 58.

37. Pashley, D. H.; Tay, F. R.; Yiu, C.; Hashimoto, M.; Breschi, L.; Carvalho, R. M.; Ito, S. *J. Dent. Res.* **2004**, *83*, 216.
38. Pashley, D. H.; Tay, F. R.; Breschi, L.; Tjaderhane, L.; Carvalho, R. M.; Carrilho, M.; Tezvergil-Mutluay, A. *Dent. Mater.* **2011**, *27*, 1.
39. Islam, S.; Hiraishi, N.; Nassar, M.; Yiu, C.; Otsuki, M.; Tagami, J. *J. Dent.* **2012**, *40*, 1052.
40. Perdigao, J.; Reis, A.; Loguercio, A. D. *J. Esthet. Restor. Dent.* **2013**, *25*, 219.
41. Tersariol, I. L.; Geraldeli S.; Minciotti, C. L.; Nascimento, F. D.; Paakkonen, V.; Martins, M. T.; Carrilho, M. R.; Pashley, D. H.; Tay, F. R.; Salo, T.; Tjaderhane, L. *J. Endod.* **2010**, *36*, 475.
42. Tjaderhane, L.; Nascimento, F. D.; Breschi, L.; Mazzoni, A.; Tersariol, I. L.; Geraldeli, S.; Tezvergil-Mutluay, A.; Carrilho, M. R.; Carvalho, R. M.; Tay, F. R.; Pashley, D. H. *Dent. Mater.* **2013**, *29*, 116.
43. Gurgan, S.; Bolay, S.; Kiremitci, A. J. *Oral Rehabil.* **1999**, *26*, 836.
44. de Castro, F. L.; de Andrade, M. F.; Duarte Junior, S. L.; Vaz, L. G.; Ahid, F. J. *J. Adhes. Dent.* **2003**, *5*, 129.
45. Turkun, M.; Turkun, L. S.; Kalender, A. *Quintessence Int.* **2004**, *35*, 469.
46. Carrilho, M. R.; Geraldeli, S.; Tay, F.; de Goes, M. F.; Carvalho, R. M.; Tjaderhane, L.; Reis, A. F.; Hebling, J.; Mazzoni, A.; Breschi, L.; Pashley, D. *J. Dent. Res.* **2007**, *86*, 529.
47. Bedran-Russo, A. K.; Pereira, P. N.; Duarte, W. R.; Drummond, J. L.; Yamauchi, M. *J. Biomed. Mater. Res. B. Appl. Biomater.* **2007**, *80*, 268.
48. dos Santos, P. H.; Karol, S.; Bedran-Russo, A. K. *J. Biomech.* **2011**, *44*, 1691.
49. Zhang, Z.; Beitzel, D.; Maid, H.; Mutluay, M.; Tezvergil-Mutluay, A.; Tay, F. R.; Pashley, D. H.; Arola *D. Dent. Mater.* **2016**, *32*, 211.
50. Reis, A. F.; Arrais, C. A.; Novaes, P. D.; Carvalho, R. M.; De Goes, M. F.; Giannini, M. *J. Biomed. Mater. Res. B Appl. Biomater.* **2004**, *71*, 90.
51. Reis, A. F.; Giannini, M.; Pereira, P. N. *Dent. Mater.* **2007**, *23*, 1164.
52. Cantanhede de Sa, R. B.; Carvalho, A. O.; Puppin-Rontani, R. M.; Ambrosano, G. M. B.; Nikaido, T.; Tagami, J.; Giannini, M. *J. Adhes. Dent.* **2012**, *14*, 543.
53. Mahdan, M. H. A.; Nakajima, M.; Foxton, R. M.; Tagami, J. *J. Dent.* **2013**, *41*, 861.

54. Van Landuyt, K. L.; De Munck, J.; Ermis, R. B.; Peumans, M.; Van Meerbeek, B. *Clin. Oral Investig.* **2014**, *18*, 1045.
55. Ferracane, J. L.; Greener, E. H. *J. Biomed. Mater. Res.* **1986**, *20*, 121.
56. Tay, F. R.; Pashley, D. H.; Suh, B. I.; Carvalho, R. M.; Itthagarun, A. *J. Dent.* **2002**, *30*, 371.
57. Bae, J. H.; Cho, B. H.; Kim, J. S.; Kim, M. S.; Lee, I. B.; Son, H. H.; Um, C. M.; Kim, C. K.; Kim, O. Y. *J. Biomed. Mater. Res. B Appl. Biomater.* **2005**, *74*, 822.
58. Cadenaro, M.; Antoniolli, F.; Sauro, S.; Tay, F. R.; Di Lenarda, R.; Prati, C.; Biasotto, M.; Contardo, L.; Breschi, L. *Eur. J. Oral Sci.* **2005**, *113*, 525.
59. Nunes, T. G.; Garcia, F. C.; Osorio, R.; Carvalho, R.; Toledano, M. *Dent. Mater.* **2006**, *22*, 963.
60. Makishi, P.; André, C. B.; Ayres, A.; Martins, A. L.; Giannini M. *Oper. Dent.* **2015**, *41*, 305.
61. Makishi, P.; Andre, C. B.; Lyra, e Silva, J. P.; Bacelar-Sa, R.; Correr-Sobrinho, L.; Giannini, M. *Oper. Dent.* **2016**, *41*, 541.
62. Ferracane, J. L. *Dent. Mater.* **2011**, *27*, 29.
63. Fronza, B. M.; Rueggeberg, F. A.; Braga, R. R.; Mogilevych, B.; Soares, L. E.; Martin, A. A.; Ambrosano, G.; Giannini, M. *Dent. Mater.* **2015**, *31*, 1542.
64. Kim, R. J.; Kim, Y. J.; Choi, N. S.; Lee, I. B. *J. Dent.* **2015**, *43*, 430.
65. Garcia, D.; Yaman, P.; Dennison, J.; Neiva, G. *Oper. Dent.* **2014**, *39*, 441.
66. Hirata, R.; Clozza, E.; Giannini, M.; Farrokhmanesh, E.; Janal, M.; Toyar, N.; Bonfante, E. A.; Coelho, P. G. *J. Biomed. Mater. Res. B Appl. Biomater.* **2015**, *103*, 798.
67. Juloski, J.; Goracci, C.; Rengo, C.; Giovannetti, A.; Vichi, A.; Vulicevic, Z. R.; Ferrari, M. *Am. J. Dent.* **2012**, *25*, 239.
68. Makishi, P.; Pacheco, R. R.; Sadr, A.; Shimada, Y.; Sumi, Y.; Tagami, J.; Giannini, M. *Microsc. Microanal.* **2015**, *21*, 1523.
69. Makishi, P.; Thitthaweerat, S.; Sadr, A.; Shimada, Y.; Martins, A. L.; Tagami, J.; Giannini, M. *Dent. Mater.* **2015**, *31*, 190.
70. Huang, D.; Swanson, E. A.; Lin, C. P.; Schuman, J. S.; Stinson, W. G.; Chang, W.; Hee, M. R.; Flotte, T.; Gregory, K.; Puliafito, C. A.; Fujimoto, J. G. *Science* **1991**, *254*, 1178.

71. Nakagawa, H.; Sadr, A.; Shimada, Y.; Tagami, J.; Sumi, Y. *J. Dent.* **2013**, *41*, 80.
72. Nazari, A.; Sadr, A.; Saghiri, M. A.; Campillo-Funollet, M.; Hamba, H.; Shimada, Y.; Tagami, J.; Sumi, Y. *Dent. Mater.* **2013**, *29*, 278.
73. Bakhsh, T. A.; Sadr, A.; Shimada, Y.; Mandurah, M. M.; Hariri, I.; Alsayed, E. Z.; Tagami, J.; Sumi, Y. *J. Dent.* **2013**, *41*, 60.
74. Turkistani, A.; Nakashima, S.; Shimada, Y.; Tagami, J.; Sadr, A. *J. Dent. Res.* **2015**, *94*, 1070.

Chapter 11

Dental Composites — Chemistry and Composition

Carmem S. Pfeifer

Department of Restorative Dentistry, Oregon Health and Science University, 2730 SW Moody Ave., Portland, OR, 97201, USA

pfeiferc@ohsu.edu

Dental composites have significantly evolved since their introduction on the market in the early 1960s. Most of the innovations have focused on the inorganic phase, with the basic chemistry for the organic phase still based on methacrylate polymerizations. The reason for that is the very robust polymerization mechanism, which progresses at faster rates at room temperature, and also the convenience of on demand cure via photoinitiation. The materials are relatively stable and present acceptable mechanical properties. However, the average lifetime of restorations is still only about 10 years in service, with replacements being costly both financially and in terms of tooth structure. The main causes for replacement are secondary caries and fracture. This chapter examines the progress made so far in updating the organic matrix of commercially available systems, as well as perspectives for future developments. Strategies to reduce interfacial and bulk stress development, water sorption and solubility, and overall degradation by hydrolysis and esterase attack are reviewed. Basic concepts in polymerization mechanisms are also summarized.

1. Introduction

Dental composites have become the most popular choice for direct esthetic restorations and are ubiquitously used in dental offices across the globe. Their basic composition consists of an inorganic phase (mostly glass fillers) and an organic matrix. Most of the developments that translated into commercial products since the introduction of the first iteration of direct restorative composites have involved the filler phase. The organic matrix remains mostly based on methacrylate chemistry, since BisGMA was patented by Rafael Bowen in the late 1950s. Even though new monomers have been introduced in the market, more notably in the last 15 years, the basic polymerizable functionality still relies on methacrylates, for a number of different reasons. The main advantage of this chemistry is the fast polymerization rate under mild conditions, usually at room temperature and using photoinitiation. This allows dentists to polymerize the materials on demand, and allows for pigmentation and other types of characterization, making it an excellent choice for highly esthetic restorations. However, in the current state, composite restorations only last an average of 10 years in service, with the main reason for failure being secondary decay, post-operative sensitivity, and fracture.[1] Secondary decay is usually brought about by failure of the adhesive interface. This can be caused by polymerization stress generation that leads to separation of the material from the substrate, in a phenomenon analogous to the delamination due to stress generation in the coatings industry.[2–4] In addition, the adhesive and composite materials are prone to degradation by hydrolysis or enzymatic action via the ester bonds present in the methacrylate.[5,6] This leads not only to the breakdown of the material over time but also acts as the source for potentially toxic leachates.

In spite of the many efforts to replace or aggressively modify methacrylate monomers, very few examples have come to commercial fruition. One notable example is the use of epoxide ring-opening polymerization, which aimed at reducing the inherent stress generation, due to the lower molar shrinkage coefficient of those materials compared to methacrylates. Other efforts have focused on producing more hydrophobic materials to reduce water/salivary degradation, or higher molecular weight monomers to reduce polymerization shrinkage. These examples of novel monomers will be discussed in this chapter, along with an overview of methacrylate polymerization.

2. Current Materials: Methacrylate Chemistry

Methacrylate monomers have the general chemical structure represented in Figure 1. They polymerize via a free-radical mechanism, through chain-growth reactions. Monofunctional methacrylates were the first monomers to be used to produce restorative composites.[7] Due to their high shrinkage values, as well as all the issues involved with linear polymers (high water sorption and solubility, for example), these monomers tended to produce materials with very poor clinical performance.[8–10] Those primitive compositions also used large quartz particles as fillers, leading to unacceptable clinical wear.[11,12] In addition, in those early days, no adhesive was used prior to the application of the composite, which all combined, ultimately gave dental composites a bad reputation. In the late 1950s, Rafael Bowen synthesized the monomer that is still being used today as the main component for many commercial formulations: bisphenol A diglycidyl ether dimethacrylate, widely known as BisGMA (Figure 1). This molecule has a few desirable features: (1) It presents two methacrylate functionalities, one on each end of the molecule, and therefore, is capable of forming a cross-linked network; (2) it has a very stiff backbone, responsible for forming rigid cross-links; (3) it presents two hydroxyl groups, capable of strong secondary intermolecular interactions (these two items combined confer good mechanical properties to the monomer); (4) it presents a relatively high molecular weight (512 g/mol), and therefore, a lot less shrinkage than the first monomethacrylates used.

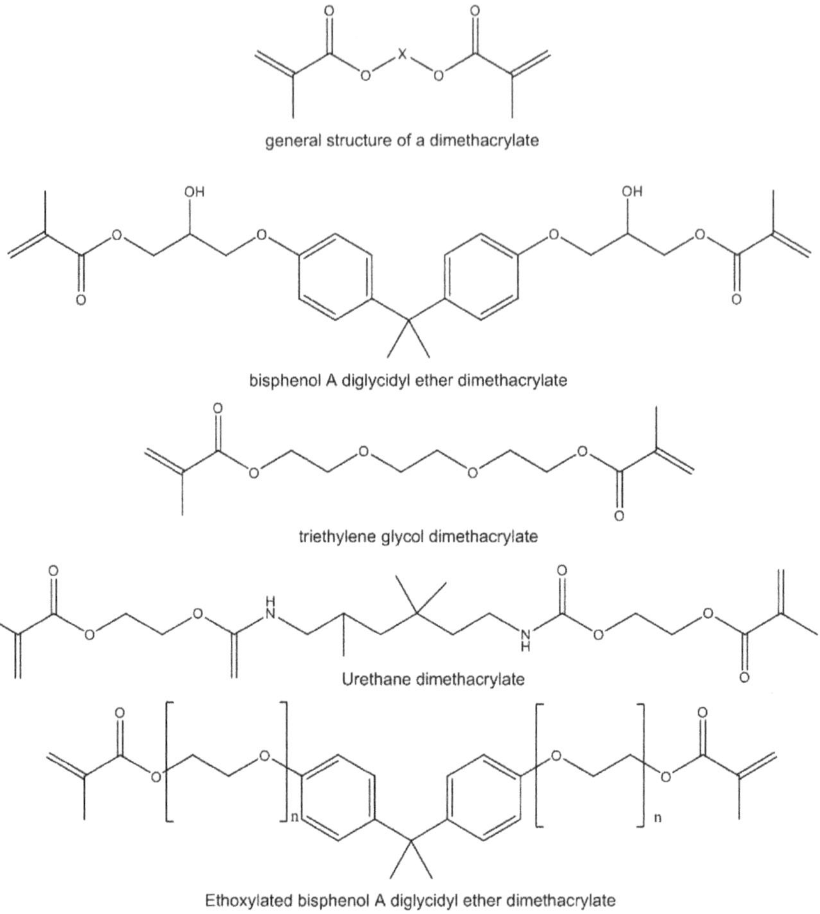

Figure 1. General structure of dimethacrylate monomers and common examples of dimethacrylates used in dental composites

The disadvantage with BisGMA is that the same hydroxyl groups that promote toughening of the network also cause this monomer to present high viscosity, which prohibits the addition of adequate amounts of filler particles — those present as a powder, and are responsible for about 60% of the volume of the material and most of the mechanical properties. For that reason, a low viscosity, di-functional diluent is usually employed. Triethylene glycol dimethacrylate (TEGDMA) is the most common (Figure 1), but its lower molecular weight (286 g/mol) significantly increases the shrinkage of the final material.[13] Therefore, in more modern commercial materials, TEGDMA has been totally or partially replaced by other diluent monomers, such as urethane dimethacrylate and ethoxylate bisphenol A dimethacrylate (UDMA and BisEMA, respectively), which present higher molecular weights (470 and 540 g/mol, respectively — Figure 1). The addition of diluents also has an implication on reaction kinetics, as will be explored in the following sections.

The combination of these high molecular weight di-methacrylate monomers significantly reduced the polymerization shrinkage and improved the mechanical properties compared to the primitive mono-methacrylate versions.

In addition, the use of modern adhesives prior to composite placement, especially with the advent of dentin bonding, has greatly improved interfacial stability. However, the polymerization shrinkage for a typical methacrylate-based composite is still around 4%.[14] Although that does not seem like a significant amount, the fact that the polymerization of these materials takes place confined by the adhesion to the cavity preparation walls leads to the development of interfacial stresses during polymerization, which can lead to the debonding of the restoration and formation of interfacial gaps. In theory, the presence of such gaps may facilitate the colonization of cariogenic bacteria, and it has been proposed that this is the mechanism for the development of secondary decay.[15–17] It has been demonstrated that *S. mutans* can indeed colonize the bottom of such gaps.[18] However, with the current clinical evidence, researchers have still not been able to establish a definitive correlation between stress generation and secondary decay. In fact, many of the low-shrinkage/low-stress materials that present improved performance *in vitro* have failed to show improved performance clinically.[19,20] This is due to the complex, multifactorial nature of dental caries development. Nevertheless, a lot of effort has been placed in developing low-shrinkage/low-stress materials, starting in the 1990s and persisting until today. Those will be addressed in the subsequent sections.

Another facet of methacrylates is the presence of ester bonds in the network. Those bonds have been shown to be labile in aqueous environment and through the action of esterases present in saliva and dentinal tissue.[21–24] A number of studies have demonstrated that methacrylate monomers are prone to degradation by cholinesterase, leading to the formation of products such methacrylic acid, triethylene glycol methacrylate (TEGMA), and bis-hydroxy-propoxy-phenyl-propane (Bis-HPPP), all markers of resin-matrix breakdown, and all of those with potential cytotoxicity effects.[22–24] This effect has been demonstrated to be time- and enzyme-concentration dependent.[22,25–26] However, some controversy still exists as to whether the enzymes present in saliva or dentinal tissues have enough specificity to degrade methacrylate esters, as well as whether the esters are accessible to these enzymes, particularly in the bulk of the material. In any event, it is undeniable that water molecules are definitely small enough and non-specific enough to attack those ester bonds, and simple hydrolysis by water molecules indeed results in the same degradation products. Apart from the potential biocompatibility concerns, the water uptake and degradation of the organic matrix also contributes to the breakdown of the material itself, facilitating crack propagation, especially under fatigue, and ultimately bulk fracture.[27–29] In addition, when used in the more hydrophilic compositions of dental adhesives, the breakdown of esters in methacrylates can be potentiated.[30] Several authors have demonstrated an effect known as “water treeing”, which consists of water seeping through the adhesive layer over time, causing degradation on the margins of the restorations.[31] This has motivated some companies to introduce compositions that are more hydrophobic and/or with alternative chemistries, to improve the resistance to water and enzymatic degradation. In 2012, the National Institute of Dental and Craniofacial Research in the United States has spearheaded an initiative to develop new dental composite monomers departing from methacrylate chemistry (http://grants.nih.gov/grants/guide/rfa-files/RFA-DE-13-001.html). The main goal of this initiative was to double the service life of dental composites. Those new proposed chemistries, along with others available in the literature, will be discussed later in this chapter.

2.1. *Polymerization Kinetics of Cross-Linked Methacrylated Networks*

2.1.1. *Influence of Monomer Choice*

The free-radical, chain growth polymerization reaction of methacrylates can be divided in three non-consecutive phases: initiation, propagation, and termination. Methacrylates are relatively stable in ambient conditions, and therefore, for the reaction to commence, some form of activation needs to take place to generate enough radicals to overcome the energy of activation of methacrylate conversion. This activation can be achieved via thermal, redox, or photochemical mechanisms, or a combination of those, provided that the correct pairing of appropriate initiators and energy source is employed. The concentration of vinyl double bonds can be followed in real time using an infrared spectrometer, and the degree of conversion of monomer to polymer can be calculated.[32,33] Once the first radical is generated, it can attack the first vinyl double bond, and start propagation. At this stage, the reaction is chemically controlled, as the molecular weight of the polymerizing species has not yet increased to the point of significantly increasing viscosity, and molecular mobility remains high. Therefore, the only limiting factor is the availability of initiators/source of energy and monomers. At this stage, propagation and termination reactions occur concomitantly and at similar rates. As the reaction progresses, viscosity starts to increase, and the reaction becomes diffusion-controlled, hindering the mobility of larger molecules and by consequence, termination by bi-molecular interaction. This leads to a significant decrease in the rate of termination. At the same time, small molecule monomers are still relatively free to move, so the rate of propagation increases in relation to termination, leading to auto-acceleration of the reaction (Tromsdorff effect), up until the point when the maximum rate of polymerization is recorded. This effect can be observed in the reaction kinetics curve depicting rate of polymerization as a function of degree of conversion (Figure 2). The gelation of the forming network is an important landmark because it influences the limiting conversion achieved by a monomer system, as well as polymerization stress

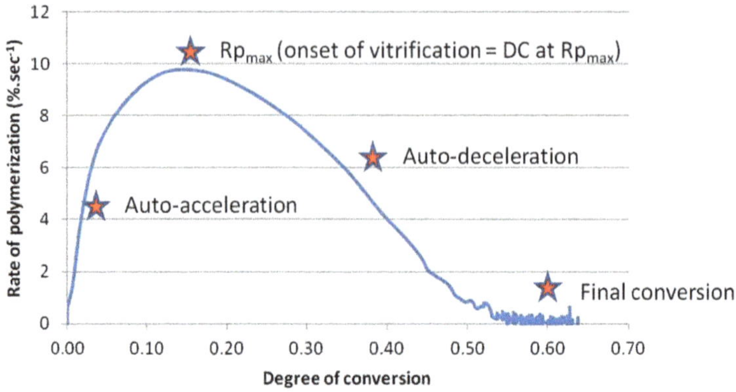

Figure 2. Polymerization kinetics of a dimethacrylate monomers. The graph depicts the rate of polymerization as a function of degree of double bond conversion. Important landmarks are highlighted

relaxation opportunities (Figure 3). The exact gel point is very difficult to determine solely from the reaction kinetics curve, so other tools, such as an oscillating rheometer coupled with an infra-red spectrometer, are often used to determine the conversion at the onset of gelation.[34] As the reaction further progresses, the decrease in mobility affects even small molecule movement, and therefore the rate of propagation also starts to decrease, in a phenomenon known as auto-deceleration, observed after the maximum rate of polymerization is recorded (Figure 2). That point marks the onset of vitrification of the network.[34]

2.1.2. *Implications on Polymerization Stress Development*

At the bottom of the auto-deceleration slope, the network is completely vitrified, and any further conversion results in significant stress build up (Figure 3). This is explained by the fact that the limited amount of conversion that takes place in this phase is a result of the reaction of either trapped monomers or of increased cross-linking. The additional conversion leads to shrinkage, which develops within a non-compliant network, which cannot deform to accommodate the additional dimensional changes.[34] It has long been accepted that any mechanism that can delay the onset of gelation and vitrification as a

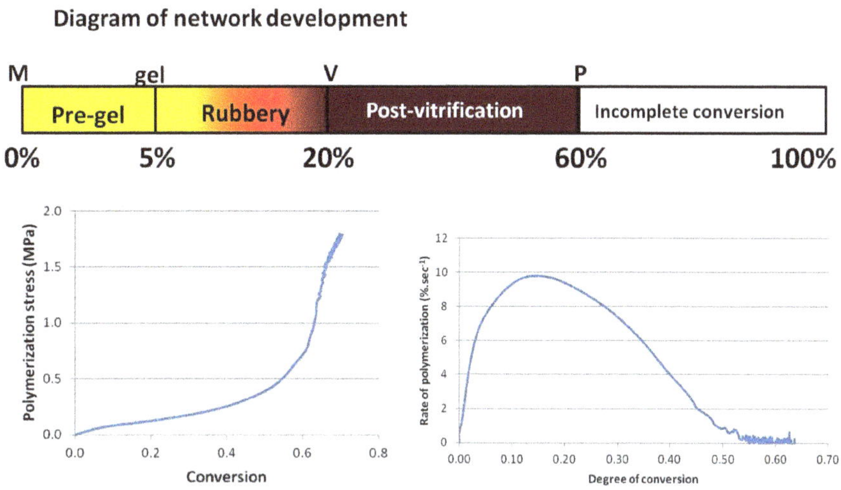

Figure 3. Diagram showing a schematic representation of the different phases of a methacrylate polymerization reaction. The system presents a lot of mobility in the monomeric state (M), until the onset of the gel phase. As the polymerization progresses, it becomes diffusion-controlled, and autoacceleration is a result of decreased rate of termination. The onset of vitrification (V) correlates with the maximum rate of polymerization (the peak of the rate of polymerization versus degree of conversion curve), where the rate of propagation also becomes diffusion-controlled. The reaction decelerates from that point into the vitrified stage, and results in incomplete conversion. The polymerization stress as a function of conversion (left graph) highlights the fact that most of the stress development takes place after the network is vitrified, when small increments in conversion result in significant increases in stress

function of conversion (not time) has a significant impact on polymerization stress development, as stresses can be more easily relaxed in the pre-gel and pre-vitrification stages.[35,36] Those strategies will be explored in the subsequent sections.

In the specific case of photopolymerizations, the rate of polymerization (R_p) can be related to the irradiance (I_a) on the light source by the following equation:

$$R_p = k_p[M]\left(\frac{\varphi I_a}{k_t}\right)^{1/2}$$

where k_p is the rate of propagation, k_t is the rate of termination, φ is the quantum yield of initiation (the number of propagating chains per photon absorbed), and [M] is the monomer concentration at any given time.

The important conclusion from this equation is that the rate of polymerization is dependent on the square root of the irradiance.[34] This means that, for an appreciable reduction in rate of polymerization to take place, the irradiance of the light needs to drop by a factor of 2 orders of magnitude. Many photoactivation protocols proposed in the early 2000s have relied on this principle in an attempt to delay gelation and consequently reduce polymerization stress.[37,38] However, the irradiances proposed were still too high compared to the conventional protocols, and ultimately, the instances where stress reduction was indeed observed could be related to decreased overall degrees of conversion, rather than appreciable changes in reaction kinetics.[39] The development of tools that allowed the measurement of stress simultaneously with conversion in real-time have made possible the demonstration that the final stress development achieved with the photoactivation methods generally known as "soft-start" was actually comparable to continuous methods.[39]

3. Low-Shrinkage and Low Stress Monomer Systems

3.1. *Low-Shrinkage Monomers*

With the aim of reducing shrinkage and ultimately reducing bulk and interfacial stress, researchers and manufacturers have focused on synthesizing new monomers with either higher molecular weight or with intrinsically lower molar shrinkage coefficient. The molar shrinkage coefficient can be calculated with the following equation:

$$VS = [C = C] \times DC \times \kappa,$$

where $[C = C]_0$ is the initial carbon–carbon double-bond concentration (in mol/mL); DC is the fractional degree of conversion, and κ is the molar shrinkage coefficient for methacrylates (20.4 mL/mol).[40]

The coefficient defines the amount of volume loss taking place from the reaction of each polymerizable functionality.

From this equation, it becomes clear that higher molecular weight monomers lead to less shrinkage for the same amount of conversion. This can be easily visualized in Figure 4.

A few examples of monomers with higher molecular weights have made it into commercial products, with notable examples being the dimer acid dimethacrylate (800 g/mol, used in N'Durance®, Septodont-Confidental) and the DX-511, originally a patent from Dupont (895 g/mol, used in Kalore, GC). These monomers' molecular structures are shown in Figure 4. The shrinkage of these commercial materials has been compared to conventional methacrylates, and it has been shown that they indeed produce values 10–30% lower than the controls.[41,42] The resulting stress, however, follows a different ranking, as it depends not only on the nominal shrinkage, but also on the final conversion and stiffness of the resulting network.[41]

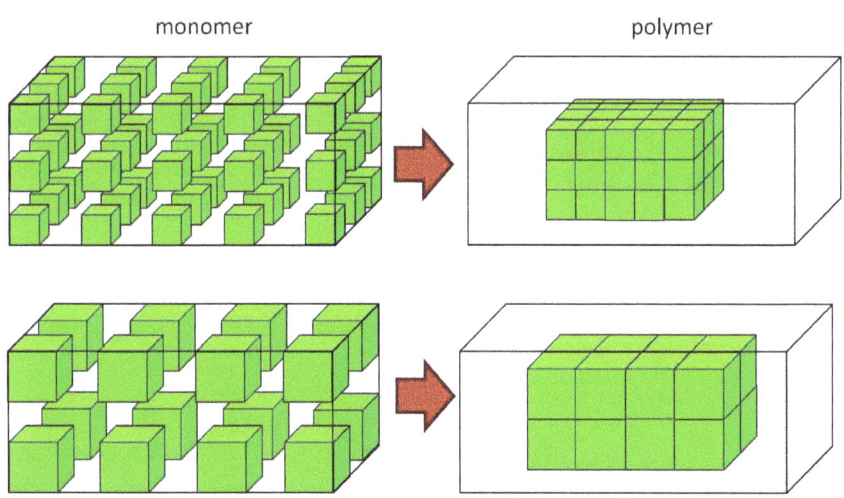

Figure 4. The effect of monomer size on overall polymerization shrinkage is shown in this diagram. The situation depicted on the top shows low molecular weight monomers resulting in greater overall volumetric shrinkage than the polymerization depicted on the bottom. Courtesy of Dr. Josete Meira

Also from the theoretical shrinkage equation, one can predict that some monomers with intrinsically lower molar shrinkage coefficients also lead to less shrinkage. That is the case of ring-opening monomers, such as SOC's and epoxides,[43–45] for which a few examples are shown in Figures 5 and 6. In the case of epoxides, the opening of the ring results in a much lower molar shrinkage coefficient.[46] In other words, even though it is a ring-opening polymerization, there is still net shrinkage, albeit smaller than for methacrylates.

For SOCs monomers, there is actually net expansion of the network. In the case of the only commercial example using epoxide chemistry (Filtek Silorane or Filtek P90, 3M-ESPE), *in vitro* studies have shown that the shrinkage and stress values are indeed lower than for conventional methacrylates (including examples from the same manufacturer), with comparable mechanical properties.[41]

SOCs monomers have also shown great promise, with significantly reduced shrinkage values, on the order of 30% lower than

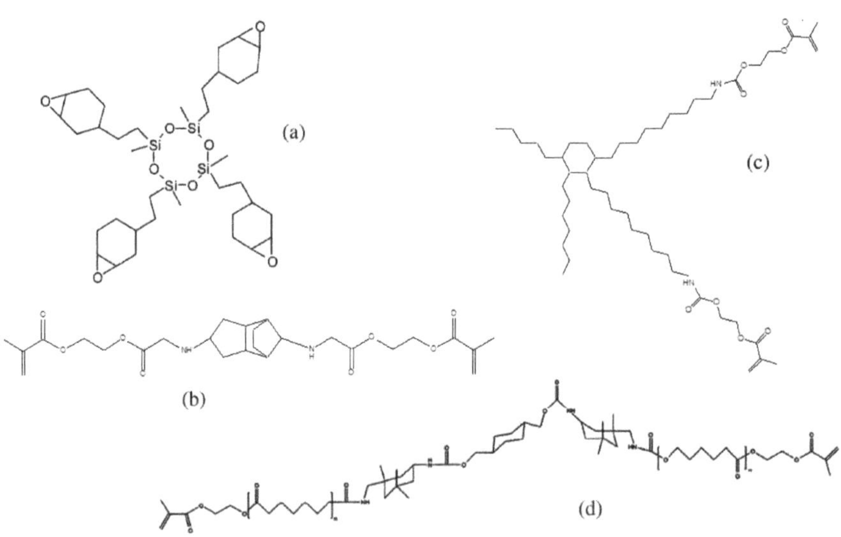

Figure 5. Molecular structure of alternative monomers currently used in commercial products. (a) Oxirane (Filtek LS, 3M-ESPE); (b) TCD-urethane (Venus Diamond, Heraeus Kulzer); (c) Dimeracid cimethacrylate (N'Durance, ConfiDental-Septodont); and (d) DuPont DX-511 (Kalore, GC America)

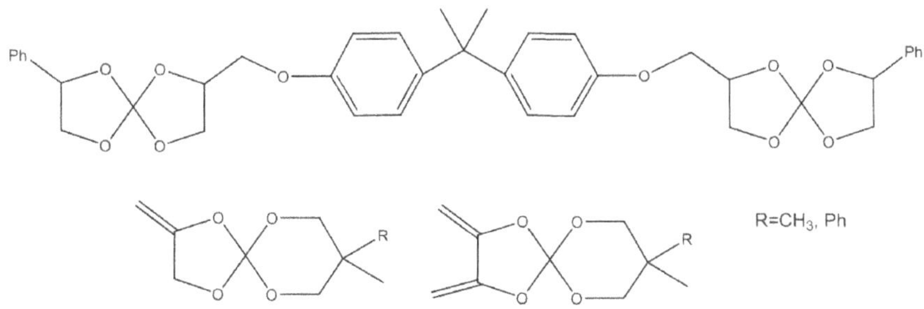

Figure 6. Molecular structure of a few examples of monomers based on spiro-orthocarbonate chemistry[43,44]

methacrylate controls.[44,45] There are not commercial examples for dental products using this chemistry, which can be at least in part attributed to the fact that ring-opening polymerizations do not progress through a free-radical mechanism, but rely on cationic polymerizations, which are far more sensitive to the conditions in the environment, such as moisture.[47] As already mentioned, in clinical testing of the commercially available products, the high molecular weight as well as the ring-opening monomer-based materials were not statistically different from conventional methacrylates in terms of restoration longevity or margin quality.[19,48–50]

3.2. *Thiol-Ene/Thiol-Methacrylate Systems*

Shrinkage reduction has been proposed as a viable strategy to reduce stress at the bonded interface, with some commercial success as already pointed out. Other strategies have focused on reducing stress *per se*, mainly resorting to modifications on the vinyl polymerization reaction directly. One such approach is the use of chain-transfer reactions, which are capable of delaying the point in conversion when gelation and vitrification take place, as is the case with thiol-ene systems, which polymerize through step-growth reactions.[51] These materials present a variety of features that makes them attractive for dental material applications. The chain-transfer reactions of thiol to ene affords delayed network formation, and that, allied to the fact that thiol-ene reactions show much lower molar shrinkage (since the carbon–carbon double bond in this case is only monofunctional), results in stress reduction compared to methacrylate polymerizations.[52,53] Moreover, these are virtually insensitive to oxygen inhibition.[54,55] The major drawback is that the presence of flexible sulfur bonds in the polymer backbone decreases Tg and jeopardizes mechanical properties in general.[54]

In contrast with chain-growth polymerizations, in step-growth reactions the molecular weight of the forming chains does not rise significantly until much later in conversion (Figure 7). In cross-linked networks, this means that the limitation to molecular diffusion and stiffness build up only occurs at the later stages in conversion,[34] which in practice means that the overall stress build up is significantly reduced.[56] For typical thiol-ene systems, the stoichiometric ratio of thiol to ene is kept at 1:1, and the ene monomer structure is carefully selected so that it will not preferentially undergo homopolymerization

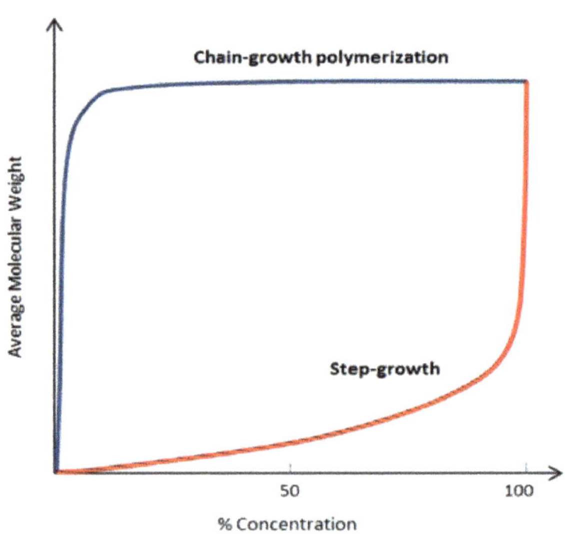

Figure 7. Schematic representation of the molecular weight evolution in chain-growth polymerizations compared with step-growth polymerizations. From: http://polymerdatabase.com/polymer%20chemistry/Chain%20versus%20Step%20Growth.html

through chain growth.[57] With the aim of delaying gelation and reducing stress while still maintaining good mechanical properties, ternary thiol-ene/methacrylates compositions have been proposed.[58,59] In this case, there is competition between chain and step growth mechanisms as the methacrylate can undergo both homopolymerization and chain transfer with the thiol, in addition to the thiol-ene reaction,[60,61] which disturbs the stoichiometric balance and may result in incomplete consumption of the thiol[62] and/or ene.[63] For a series of thiol-ene/methacrylate systems, it has been demonstrated that the ene consumption is delayed until the methacrylate-thiol reaction is largely complete.[64] In turn, methacrylate conversion still progresses at a slower rate, indicating that the chain transfer reactions to thiol are determinant in delaying gelation.

Interestingly, the stress reduction obtained in the ternary system is also achieved with thiol-methacrylates.[65] In those instances, thiols are capable of reducing the kinetic chain length by introducing chain-breaking events.[66] Chain transfer is a chain-breaking mechanism in which the new radical formed through the transfer is considered to be a new initiation site.[34] The addition of chain-transfer agents (thiols being very efficient in this role) in amounts as low as 0.1 wt.% significantly reduces the rate of polymerization and the radical chain length.[66,67] As the thiol concentration increases, the reaction with the methacrylate monomer becomes a more important factor in network development.[62,63] Previously reported data shows, for thiol-methacrylate systems with high thiol concentrations, that the transfer rate constant (k_{tr}) is significantly higher than the propagation rate constant (k_p).[62] This was accompanied by a delay in the auto-acceleration, which in turn was optimized for methacrylate functional groups molar fractions of 60% and 80%.[62] The mechanism through which methacrylate gelation is delayed by chain-transfer to thiol has also been described in studies on thiol-acrylate systems intended for surface functionalization.[68–70] In these cases, amine catalysts were efficiently applied to avoid polymerization through addition to the vinyl, which leads to the advantageous predominance of chain-transfer from carbon-thiol radicals. However, this can also be achieved without resorting to the addition of catalysts by tailoring the reactivity, functionality, and concentration of both the thiol and the acrylate/methacrylate, opening a new avenue to gelation control.

The modification of the kinetic profiles is expected to affect network characteristics and mechanical properties. Thiol monomers added to a methacrylate network will also very likely produce lower Tg values due to the flexibility of the thio-ether bonds incorporated in the polymer backbone through chain-transfer reactions to the methacrylate, but with the benefit of producing more homogeneous networks. By decreasing the breadth of tan delta relative to the cure temperature (meaning narrower Tgs), higher conversion is achieved before gelation, giving opportunity for viscous flow to accommodate the stress generation, which has been demonstrated in ternary thiol-ene/acrylate systems.[54,71] Moreover, because of the chain transfer itself, higher conversion and shorter chains are likely to result[34] and, especially for multifunctional thiols, this is expected to contribute to a tighter network and improved mechanical properties.[64] In the same fashion, backbone structure features, like the presence of cyclic substitutions, may reinforce the resulting polymer network and enhance overall mechanical properties.[54,71]

Specifically for use as dental materials, thiol-ene networks have been investigated in conjunction with methacrylates in ternary systems, to ensure the formation of strong networks.[53,58] The reduction in polymerization stress in those ternary systems reaches 55%, with similar or only modestly diminished mechanical properties.[53] High Tg materials have been designed, resorting to the use of functionalities such as norbornenes,[53] and/or to the synthesis of prepolymerized oligomers.[72,73] The materials can be photoactivated, as already mentioned, but there are concerns with the long-term stability and shelf-life of these materials in base-containing formulations, such as is the case in camphorquinone-amine-initiated composites.[74] The malodor concern is mitigated by the use of high molecular weight thiol species and disappears with polymerization. Even if they are not currently used in commercial formulations, thiol-based materials provide a very versatile platform for stress reduction and water-stable materials, as will be explored further in this chapter.

4. Characterization of Gelation Profiles in Cross-Linked Networks

Rheometry has been classically used to follow mechanical property development during polymerization, and it provides useful information on the gelation behavior.[75] The gel point is defined as the stage of network formation in which one single macromolecule is formed, and that spans the entire sample.[76] There are several experimental routes to determine the onset of gelation. In practice, the rheometer subjects the material to a sinusoidal shear force, at a given strain rate and frequency, and measures the generated stress. From the stress–strain curve, the complex modulus (G^*) is calculated (as the slope of that curve over time). Through a Fourier transform applied to G^*, the elastic and viscous components (storage and loss moduli, G' and G'', respectively) can be determined. When the material is in the unpolymerized state, the viscous component predominates, and the magnitude of G^* was shown to be dependent on the applied frequency.[77] As the material polymerizes and transitions from a viscous liquid (pre-gel) to a visco-elastic solid (post-gel), two phenomena can be observed. First, the magnitude of modulus is no longer frequency-dependent. That way, in multi-frequency experiments, the Winter–Chambon criterion defines the gel point as the stage in conversion where the measured modulus is the same regardless of the frequency applied to the material (Figure 8(a)). Second, the elastic component becomes predominant in the complex modulus determination. Another parameter to determine the onset of gelation then derives: that is the point in conversion where a cross-over between loss and storage moduli development curves is observed (Figure 8(b)).

The practical determination of the cross-over point, however, is somewhat complicated in methacrylates not only because polymerizations are very fast but also because the increase in modulus for some materials exceeds 5 orders of magnitude at full conversion,[78] close to the range limit the rheological apparatus can accommodate. As a consequence, the measurement is conducted with partial cures, generally keeping polymerization rate very slow. For photoactivated systems, it develops that the irradiance used for the testing is much lower than

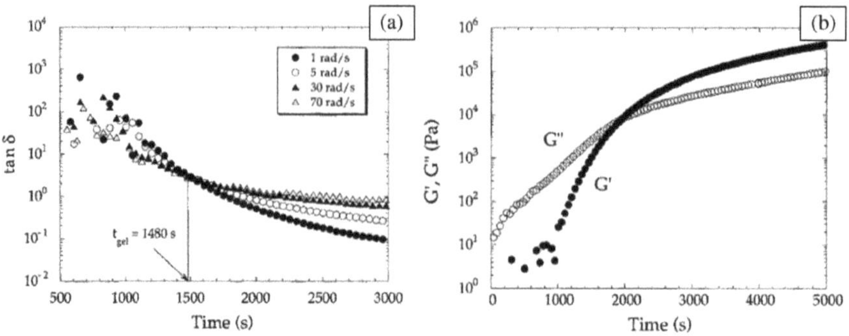

Figure 8. (a) Loss tangent, tan δ, of a trifunctional thiol system plotted as a function of UV exposure time for different frequencies (as labeled in the figure). The intersection of tan δ at a single point ($t = 1{,}480$ s) determines the gel point. (b) Evolution of the elastic (G') and viscous (G'') moduli as a function of exposure time for a trifunctional thiol system. The frequency of oscillation is 10 rad/s. G'' is initially larger than G', but as the photo-cross-linking progresses, G' supercedes G''. From Chiou *et al.*, 1996, Macromolecules

what is practically employed. More meaningful data can be obtained through the simultaneous measurement of modulus and conversion, as shown in the literature.[65,79]

5. Covalent Adaptable Networks

As explained for thiol-ene and thiol-methacrylate networks, the presence of thiols during network formation leads to gelation at much higher conversions compared to traditional chain-growth polymerizations, which ultimately leads to increased conversion and reduced stress. While these polymerizations are advantageous from those standpoints, drawbacks include thiol malodor and the relatively low Tg achieved. Importantly, as with most cross-linked networks used in materials for structural applications, thiol-enes and thio-methacrylates are thermosets, which means once the polymerization reaction is complete, the networks are not amenable to any further rearrangement. More recently, networks capable of undergoing stress relaxation via photo-induced bond rearrangement, also known as "covalent adaptable networks", have been proposed.[80] By definition, these networks contain some type of reversible covalent bond or cross-link that enables the cross-linked structure to respond chemically to an applied stimulus, via breakage and reformation of such bonds.[80] The adaptability of the network can occur via different pathways, including reversible addition and condensation and reversible bond exchange processes.[81] In the bond exchange type, as the reaction progresses and as the external stimulus is applied, the bond density is maintained without chemical degradation, nor compromise to physical properties.[81] These networks find applications as self-healing materials, as well as in high stress/strain situations, such as for restorative dental materials.

Of particular interest for use as dental materials is the addition fragmentation chain-transfer through allyl sulfide functionalities, as proposed recently.[82] As shown in Figure 9, the concentration of radicals and double bonds available to react is kept throughout the reaction, which effectively leads to stress relaxation without impairing

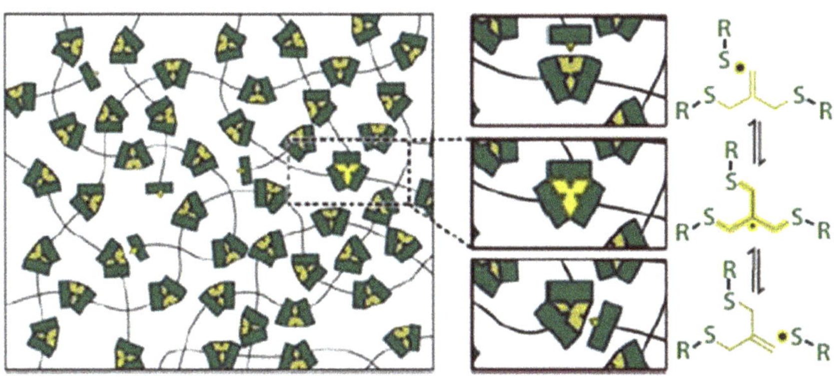

Figure 9. Covalent adaptable network structure based on crosslink units with allyl sulfide groups capable of radical addition-fragmentation to relieve stress during the polymerization. The presence of additional thiol terminated polymer chains allows for the reversible random replacement of existing carbon–sulfur linkages leading to the dissipation of stress throughout the cross-linked polymer network. From http://sigmaaldrich.com/technical-documents/articles/materal-matters/the-progress-in-development.printerview.html (Stansbury and Bowman, *Material Matters* **2010**, *5.3*, 73)

final network properties.[82] When incorporated into thiol/methacrylate networks, this was shown to reduce final stress by as much as 75%, with stress relaxation behavior being denoted by decreased values from a maximum.[82,83] Those systems presented final glass transition temperature above ambient temperature, albeit slightly below that of the unmodified methacrylate network.[82] To alleviate the potential for decreased mechanical properties expected in thiol-containing networks, subsequent studies have used norbornene-functionalized monomers, which were able to keep the stress reduction and alleviate the concern of reduced Tg.[83] Several structure–property relationship studies conducted for applications in different fields have demonstrated the ability of these networks to allow maximum stress relaxation without prejudice to mechanical properties.[83] A variation of this technology is currently being used in one commercial material (Filtek Bulk Fill Posterior, 3M ESPE).

There are other commercial materials based on stress-relaxing monomers, such as what is claimed by DENTSPLY-Caulk, but the formulation is proprietary.[84]

6. Oligomeric Additives

Pre-polymerized compounds have been used in dental composite materials for quite some time, with notable examples in microfilled materials, in which pre-polymerized composite particles are added back into the unpolymerized matrix. In that case, this allows for the incorporation of relatively large amounts of micrometer-sized silica particles, as well as reduces the polymerization shrinkage, via the reduction on the concentration of monomers available to react in the material as being used by the dentist.[85] More recently, the use of loosely cross-linked polymerized particles has been proposed and, given the nanometer size scale of such particles, the term nanogel was coined. Nanogels have been proposed for use in industrial coatings to reduce shrinkage and stress, as well as nanocarriers for drug delivery.[86–88] Recently, they have been proposed for dental applications. To that end, the nanogels are synthesized in solution using a relatively low concentration of cross-linker monomers and chain-transfer agents, to control molecular weight and form networks that can be dispersed into a secondary monomer matrix.[89,90] The addition of the pre-polymerized particle leads to a reduction in shrinkage, and corresponding reduction in stress in resins and highly filled systems, with no prejudice to mechanical properties.[89,90] The nanogel network can be tailored to encompass a wide range of glass transition temperatures via, for example, varying the degree of branching,[91] as well as can be used as a very versatile platform for tethering different functionalities, such as methacrylates (for co-polymerization with the secondary network) and thiols (for further stress reduction via chain-transfer reactions).[92]

Another example of pre-polymerized compounds are thiourethane oligomers.[93–96] The main advantages of thiourethane networks are the sharp glass transition temperature, which denotes a very homogeneous network, and the toughness reported for some formulations.[97–99] Thiourethane networks can also be applied as pre-polymerized additives.[93–96] In these cases, oligomeric particles with molecular weights around 5 kDa are synthesized in solution using multifunctional thiols and isocyanates, in such a way that pendant thiol moieties are left for subsequent reactions and functionalization.[95] The pendant thiol concentration and the ultimate glass transition temperature of the oligomers can be tailored by judicious selection of the starting thiol and isocyanate materials. It has been demonstrated that the addition of thiourethane oligomers to dimethacrylate networks is able to increase the toughness and fracture toughness by at least two-fold,[96] which has been attributed to the introduction of thiocarbamate bonds.[97] In fact, thiol-isocyanate networks have been previously employed in applications where high impact resistance is desirable.[98,99] In addition, the presence of pendant thiol functionalities renders them capable of chain-transfer reactions with the surrounding methacrylate matrix. In addition to the intrinsic reduction in shrinkage achieved with the addition of pre-polymerized particles (as is the case with the aforementioned nanogels), those chain-transfer reactions are able to delay gelation and vitrification.[93] Both these factors contribute to reductions in polymerization stress of up to 60% observed with these materials,[96] as seen in Figure 10.

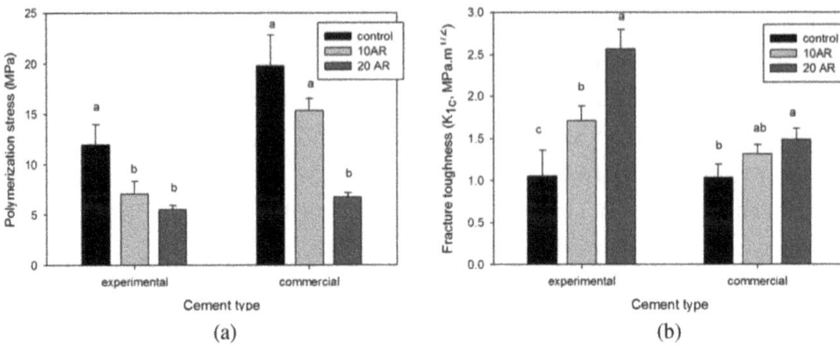

Figure 10. (a) Polymerization stress and (b) Fracture toughness values for the 25wt% filler BisGMA/UDMA/TEGDMA cement and for the commercial cement (RelyX Ultimate) with 0 (control), 10% and 20 wt% of thiourethane oligomer added. Adapted from Ref. [95]

7. Monomers with Increased Hydrophobicity

Dental restorations reside in a relatively harsh environment, where variations in pH, biofilm development, and the presence of moisture and organic solvents are a constant challenge. For that reason, the use of hydrophobic compositions has been proposed as a way to reduce the effects of water aging. Fluorine chemistry has been proposed, with several monomers being synthesized with potential dental applications.[100] Fluorine-derivatives of BisGMA have been shown to produce much lower water sorption and increase the contact angle of resin composites, but with somewhat reduced mechanical properties for some examples.[100] Potential miscibility issues with other co-monomers partly explains the reduced properties, and the addition of moderate amounts of solvents (aldehydes and ketones) has been successful in overcoming the issue.[101,102] More recent work on this chemistry has shown improved mechanical properties in relation to a BisGMA control using monomers derived from urethanes.[103–105] In addition, a few examples of monofunctional fluorinated methacrylates have been proposed for use as adhesive monomers.[106,107] In this case, the rationale is to decrease water percolation through the adhesive barrier, a phenomenon demonstrated with dentin adhesives ("water-treeing"[31]).

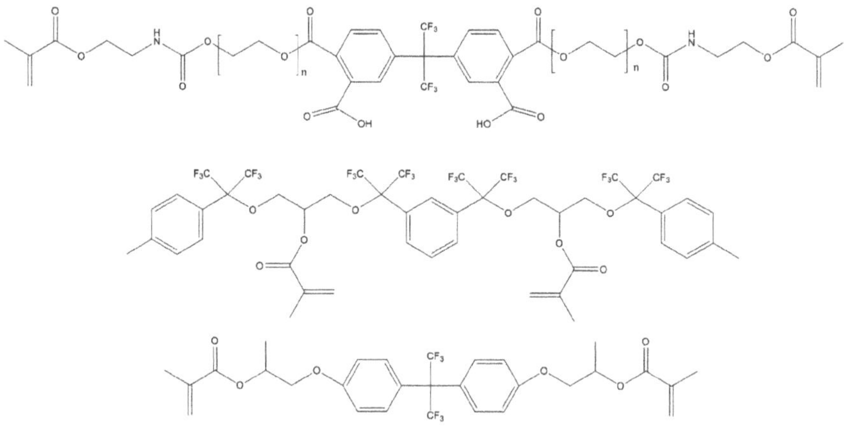

Figure 11. Molecular structure of a few examples of fluorinated monomers proposed for dental applications. Adapted from Refs. [100, 101, 105]

Other examples of increased hydrophobicity include the monomers shown in Figure 11. Those specific examples were designed to reduce stress, respectively, via ring-opening polymerization (silorane, A) and polymerization-induced phase-separation (dimer-acid derivatives, B), as already mentioned. The hydrophobicity of commercial materials containing those monomers has been tested in terms of water sorption and solubility.[42,108,109] Siloranes have demonstrated significantly lower water sorption/solubility values compared to conventional methacrylate controls.[42,108,109] Dimer-acid derivative-containing materials presented water sorption/solubility values comparable with the methacrylate controls.[42] Clinical studies, however, have failed to demonstrate the potential to extend the lifetime of restorations constructed with these materials compared to conventional methacrylates.[49,50]

8. Water- and Enzyme-Stable Monomers

For fluorinated monomers, the rationale for use is to inhibit material interaction with the aqueous environment while still relying on ester-containing methacrylate monomers. Other approaches have focused on replacing methacrylates with other polymerizable functionalities to avoid the presence of the hydrolysable ester bond. One noteworthy example, with commercial application in adhesive systems so far, is the methacrylamide chemistry.[110] Methacrylamides have the general chemical structure shown in Figure 12. In general, they also polymerize via a chain-growth radical mechanism, with reactivity varying according to the substitutions in R1 and R2. In general, acrylamides are more reactive than methacrylamides, and secondary acryl/methacryl-amides are more reactive than tertiary counterparts.[111,112] The latter has been reported to require the use of chain-transfer agents to allow for ambient temperature polymerization via radical-assisted mechanisms.[113] These monomers are attractive for use in dentistry because they have been shown to have enhanced stability in aqueous environments and, for select examples, enhanced stability when subjected to enzymatic challenges.[114] For those reasons, the use of methacrylamides has been proposed for dental composites.[115] One study has demonstrated that composite formulated with a multifunctional methacrylamide presented mechanical properties comparable to the methacrylate counterpart, while presenting much greater stability after storage in aqueous ethanol solutions containing 20 wt.% phosphoric acid at 37°C for 4 months.[116] Under those harsher conditions, the carbamate present in the methacrylamide has shown, as expected,

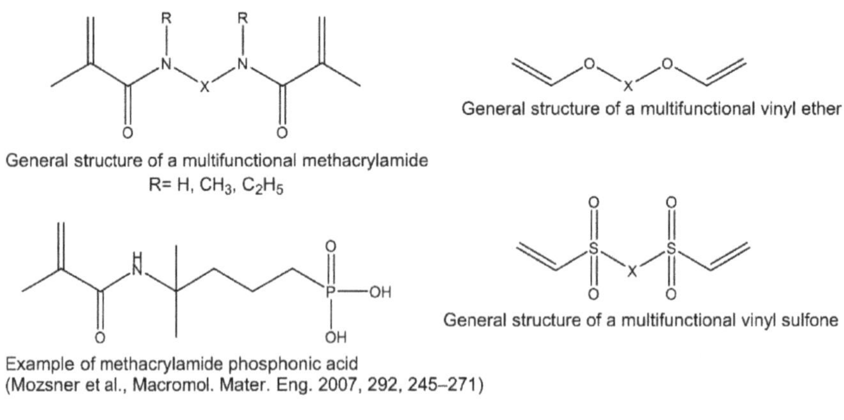

Figure 12. Molecular structure of ester-free monomers.

to be much better able to resist degradation than the methacrylate. In addition, methacrylamide phosphonic acids (Figure 12) have been proposed for dental adhesives. While the phosphonic acid moiety keeps the molecule hydrophilic and imparts self-etching character, the polymerization via the methacrylamide or acrylamide moieties makes the resulting network less prone to degradation.[117] At least one commercial example exists (AdheSE, Ivoclar-Vivadent) that contains methacrylamides in the composition.

Other ester-free monomers include vinyl ethers and vinyl sulfones, whose general chemical structure is shown in Figure 12. Vinyl ethers have demonstrated resistance to hydrolysis in aqueous environments and to degradation by cholinesterase.[118] However, they usually require super-ambient temperatures or cationic initiation mechanisms to homopolymerize to any appreciable extents,[118,119] which can be difficult to impossible to achieve in the oral environment. Viable co-polymerization pairs at room temperature include methacrylates,[120,121] though that option re-incorporates ester bonds into the network, or thiol-ene co-polymerizations,[122] with the disadvantage of low Tgs,[123] or homopolymerization via RAFT initiation mechanisms.[124] Vinyl sulfones have recently been proposed for use as restorative dental materials, mainly because of their expected hydrolytic stability, in turn conveyed by the absence of ester functionalities.[125] Vinyl sulfones were shown to have much greater reactivity toward thiol monomers compared to acrylates due to the greater electron deficiency of the former,[126] and also to form networks presenting much higher glass transition temperature compared to classic thiol-ene networks.[127–128] The good mechanical properties, namely toughness and fracture toughness, have been attributed to strong intermolecular interactions of dipole nature.[125] All of those features make these networks very attractive for use as dental materials. Initiator systems based on photo-base generators allow for the temporal control of polymerization reactions.[129] Combined, these two technologies might make the translation of thiol-vinyl sulfone materials to clinical use more of a reality.

Recently, azide-alkyne networks have been proposed as biomaterials.[130,131] The copper-catalyzed azide-alkyne reaction has first been

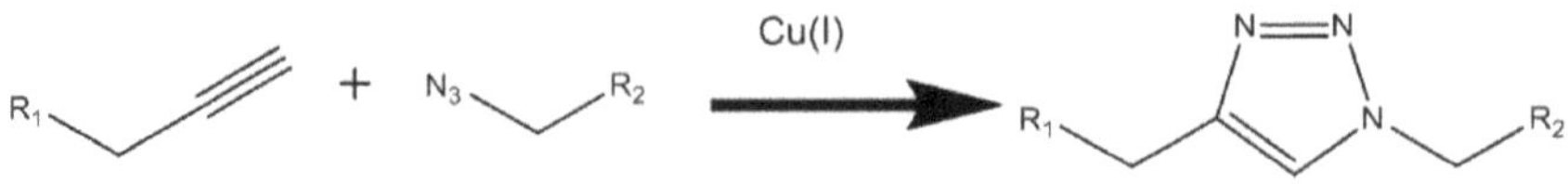

Figure 13. General reaction scheme for alkyne-azides, catalyzed by copper I. Copper I is reduced copper II either by reaction with sodium ascorbate or in the presence of a photoinitiator. Adapted from Refs. [133, 135]

described by Sharpless and collaborators,[132,133] and progresses according to the schematic shown in Figure 13.

These materials have been suggested for potential use in dental composite formulations because they are ester-free, not prone to hydrolysis or enzymatic degradation, and can be photoactivated on demand to produce glassy materials at room temperature.[134] The photochemical reduction of the copper catalyst was a milestone responsible for allowing spatial–temporal control of the polymerization reactions.[135] So far, these materials have shown significant polymerization stress reduction in relation to methacrylate networks, with only modest decrease in flexural strength and modulus.[134] As far as resistance to degradation, at least for use as fluorescent nanospheres for live cell imaging, these materials present good stability in solution.[136] Potential pitfalls include toxicity concerns with the use of the copper catalyst, as well as a blue tint as a result of incomplete copper reduction.

9. Antimicrobial Monomers

The interaction between restorative materials and the oral biofilm has been investigated in great detail. As already mentioned, the action of salivary and dentinal enzymes can lead to degradation of methacrylate monomers and the formation of products such as methacrylic acid and BisHPP. These products may have stimulating or inhibitory effects on caries-forming bacteria, especially at low pH.[137,138] Upregulation of virulence genes in *S. mutans* as a result of exposure to such products also has been shown.[137] Enzymes and acidic hydrolysis originating from the biofilm, however, have also been suggested to accelerate the degradation of dental materials.[6,22] Acquired pellicle formation on the surface of dental materials occurs virtually instantaneously, and mature biofilm can be observed roughly on the same time-scale as in pristine enamel.[16] The presence of the biofilm can potentially accelerate not only the degradation of the composite restoration but also of the bonded interface,[21] and the presence of cariogenic bacteria on stress-induced marginal gaps *in vitro* has also been demonstrated.[18] Even though clinical studies have failed to demonstrate a definitive correlation between stress-induced marginal gaps and secondary decay, the fact that bacteria can penetrate those spaces is definitely a matter of concern. With that in mind, materials based on antimicrobial and antifouling monomers have been developed.[139,140] The largest body of literature for antibacterial monomers for dental applications is on the group of quaternary ammonium methacrylates, or QAMs.[141–151] Examples of QAM monomers proposed for use in dental composites are shown in Figure 14. The quaternization of the tertiary amine moiety renders the molecule positively charged, which promotes interaction with the bacterial cell wall.[152] Several iterations of these monomers have been synthesized, and the charge density and size of the side chain have been correlated with the efficiency of such monomers/polymers to disrupt the integrity of the bacterial wall.[146,151,153] At least for the materials reported so far, however, the action mechanism seems to be contact kill, which means the bactericidal effect is not marked in the bulk of the biofilm layer, unless unreacted monomers or degradation by-products leach into the biofilm.[146] In this case two concerns arise: the sustainability

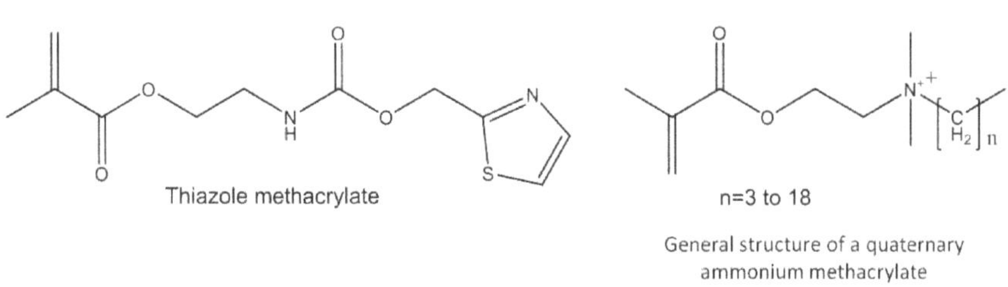

Figure 14. Molecular structure of examples of antibacterial monomers proposed for use in dental materials. Adapted from Refs. [146, 157]

of the bactericidal effect and toxicity to pulpal or epithelial cells. For those reasons, the combination of QAMs with protein-repellent monomers, which would avoid the formation of the acquired pellicle on the surface of the restoration, thus rendering the material antifouling and potentiating the action of QAMs.[154] QAMs have also been included in self-healing material formulations, loaded into vesicles containing healing liquid, which are activated upon crack propagation through a composite material.[155] Potential problems that may arise with this method, however, include decreased mechanical properties with the inclusion of vesicles and incomplete reaction of the healing liquid, posing cytotoxicity concerns.[155] Overall, the use of quaternary ammonium methacrylates in commercial materials is still limited to one product, and long-term clinical studies with this material are still scarce.[156]

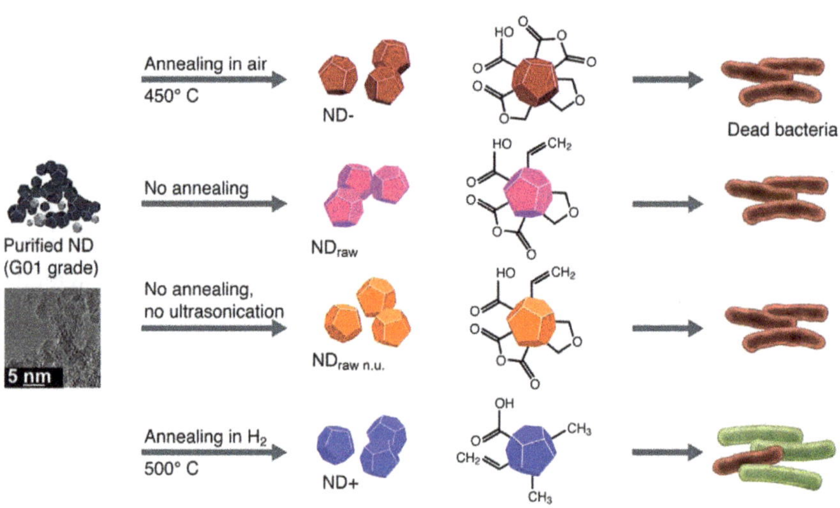

Figure 15. Illustration of nanodiamond powder and the influence of annealing conditions on the bactericidal effect of said particles. Negatively charged ND and NDraw/NDraw n.u were shown to exhibit strong antibacterial properties under aqueous conditions, while NDp caused bacterial death only at high ND concentrations. NDpure, independent of their charge, did not show any bactericidal effects. Adapted from Ref. [159]

More recently, non-quaternary ammonium alternatives have been proposed, such as the use of thiazoles.[157] At least in one study, this system has shown the advantages of increased conversion and decreased water sorption and solubility in relation to un-modified methacrylate, without prejudice to mechanical properties.[157] Biofilm and cytotoxicity studies for thiazole-based dental materials are not available to date.

Finally, the use of oxidized nanodiamond particles has been proposed as an antibacterial alternative in dental materials.[158,159] Surface properties seem to play a key role on the efficacy of the antibacterial effect of these particles, with partially oxidized particles rendering the most potent results against gram positive and gram negative bacteria.[159] Mechanical properties of composites containing these nanoparticles were shown to increase with the concentration of nanodiamonds up to 20 wt.%, concentration at which a two-fold increase in fracture toughness is observed.[158,160] The use of nanodiamonds is yet to be investigated for use in dentistry.

10. Final Considerations

In spite of the effervescent research on alternative chemistries for restorative dental materials, most monomers and organic matrices in commercial products are still based on methacrylates. As previously mentioned, they polymerize under mild conditions to relatively high degrees of conversion and produce glassy materials, with a reasonable lifetime. Compared to amalgams and other metal-based restorations, nevertheless, esthetic composite restorations still fall short. New and improved materials are necessary to avoid costly re-treatments and to preserve natural tooth structure. The future seems to lie with materials that interact well with the environment surrounding them, which means that, besides presenting low polymerization stress and good mechanical properties and chemical stability, the search is for a composition that will simultaneously be able to resist biofilm formation, be antibacterial, and be bioactive, both in terms of mineralization and in terms of epithelial cell attachment (in the case of class II and V restorations, for example). This is an extremely tall order, but progress is underway.

References

1. Pallesen, U.; van Dijken, J. W. V.; Halken, J.; Hallonsten, A. L.; Höigaard, R. *Clin. Oral Invest.* **2014**, *18* (3), 819–827.
2. Feng, L.; Suh, B. I.; Shortall, A. C. *Dent. Mater.* **2010**, *26* (8), 719–729.
3. Fronza, B. M.; Rueggeberg, F. A.; Braga, R. R.; Mogilevych, B.; Soares, L. E. S.; Martin, A. A.; Ambrosano, G.; Giannini, M. *Dent. Mater.* **2015**, *31* (12), 1542–1551.
4. Ferracane, J. L.; Hilton, T. J. *Dent. Mater.* **2016**, *32* (1), 1–10.
5. Nishiyama, N.; Tay, F. R.; Fujita, K.; Pashley, D. H.; Ikemura, K.; Hiraishi, N.; King, N. M. *J. Dent. Res.* **2006**, *85* (5), 422–426.
6. Salz, U.; Zimmermann, J.; Zeuner, F.; Moszner, N. *J. Adh. Dentist.* **2005**, *7* (2), 107–116.
7. Minguez, N.; Ellacuria, J.; Soler, J. I.; Triana, R.; Ibaseta, G. *J. Hist. Dent.* **2003**, *51* (3), 103–105.
8. Eriksen, H. M. *J. Oral Rehabil.* **1974**, *1* (4), 317–321.
9. Leinfelder, K. F.; Sluder, T. B.; Sockwell, C. L.; Strickland, W. D.; Wall, J. T. *J. Prosth. Dentist.* **1975**, *33* (4), 407–416.
10. Smales, R. J. *Aus. Dent. J.* **1975**, *20* (4), 228–234.
11. Mitchem, J. C.; Gronas, D. G. *J. Am. Dent. Assoc.* **1985**, *111* (6), 961–964.
12. Van Dijken, J. W. V. *Acta Odontol. Scand.* **1986**, *44* (6), 357–367.
13. Pfeifer, C. S.; Shelton, Z. R.; Braga, R. R.; Windmoller, D.; MacHado, J. C.; Stansbury, J. W. *Eur. Poly. J.* **2011**, *47* (2), 162–170.
14. Anseth, K. S.; Goodner, M. D.; Reil, M. A.; Kannurpatti, A. R.; Newman, S. M.; Bowman, C. N. *J. Dent. Res.* **1996**, *75* (8), 1607–1612.
15. Cenci, M. S.; Pereira-Cenci, T.; Cury, J. A.; Ten Cate, J. M. *Caries Res.* **2009**, *43* (2), 97–102.
16. Kuper, N. K.; Van De Sande, F. H.; Opdam, N. J. M.; Bronkhorst, E. M.; De Soet, J. J.; Cenci, M. S.; Huysmans, M. C. D. J. N. M. *J. Dent. Res.* **2015**, *94* (1), 62–68.

17. Zhou, Y.; Shimada, Y.; Matin, K.; Sadr, A.; Sumi, Y.; Tagami, J. *Dent. Mater.* **2016**, *32* (9), 1177–1188.
18. Khvostenko, D.; Salehi, S.; Naleway, S. E.; Hilton, T. J.; Ferracane, J. L.; Mitchell, J. C.; Kruzic, J. J. *Dent. Mater.* **2015**, *31* (6), 702–710.
19. Burke, F. J. T.; Crisp, R. J.; James, A.; MacKenzie, L.; Pal, A.; Sands, P.; Thompson, O.; Palin, W. M. *Dent. Mater.* **2011**, *27* (7), 622–630.
20. Rho, Y. J.; Namgung, C.; Jin, B. H.; Lim, B. S.; Cho, B. H. *Operative Dent.* **2013**, *38* (6), 572–582.
21. Bourbia, M.; Ma, D.; Cvitkovitch, D. G.; Santerre, J. P.; Finer, Y. *J. Dent. Res.* **2013**, *92* (11), 989–994.
22. Finer, Y.; Jaffer, F.; Santerre, J. P. *Biomaterials* **2004**, *25* (10), 1787–1793.
23. Finer, Y.; Santerre, J. P. *J. Biomed. Mater. Res. A* **2004**, *69* (2), 233–246.
24. Finer, Y.; Santerre, J. P. *J. Dent. Res.* **2004**, *83* (1), 22–26.
25. Park, J. G.; Ye, Q.; Topp, E. M.; Lee, C. H.; Kostoryz, E. L.; Misra, A.; Spencer, P. *J. Biomed. Mater. Res. B* **2009**, *91* (1), 61–70.
26. Shokati, B.; Tam, L. E.; Santerre, J. P.; Finer, Y. *J. Biomed. Mater. Res. B* **2010**, *94* (1), 230–237.
27. Chen, S.; Öhman, C.; Jefferies, S. R.; Gray, H.; Xia, W.; Engqvist, H. *J. Mech. Behav. Biomed. Mater.* **2016**, *61*, 283–289.
28. Mutluay, M. M.; Zhang, K.; Ryou, H.; Yahyazadehfar, M.; Majd, H.; Xu, H. H. K.; Arola, D. *J. Mech. Behav. Biomed. Mater.* **2013**, *18*, 219–231.
29. Vidhawan, S. A.; Yap, A. U.; Ornaghi, B. P.; Banas, A.; Banas, K.; Neo, J. C.; Pfeifer, C. S.; Rosa, V. *Dent. Mater.* **2015**, *31* (9), 1068–1074.
30. Kostoryz, E. L.; Dharmala, K.; Ye, Q.; Wang, Y.; Huber, J.; Park, J. G.; Snider, G.; Katz, J. L.; Spencer, P. *J. Biomed. Mater. Res. B* **2009**, *88* (2), 394–401.
31. Tay, F. R.; Pashley, D. H. *Am. J. Dent.* **2003**, *16* (1), 6–12.
32. Stansbury, J. W.; Dickens, S. H. *Dent. Mater.* **2001**, *17* (1), 71–79.
33. Rueggeberg, F. A.; Craig, R. G. *J. Dent. Res.* **1988**, *67* (6), 932–937.
34. Odian, G. *Principles of Polymerization*. 4th edn. (Hoboken: Wiley Interscience, **2004**).

35. Lu, H.; Stansbury, J. W.; Bowman, C. N. *Probing the Fundamental Relationship between Polymerization Shrinkage Stress and Degree of Conversion* (Transactions — 7th World Biomaterials Congress, **2004**), p. 956.
36. Lu, H.; Stansbury, J. W.; Dickens, S. H.; Eichmiller, F. C.; Bowman, C. N. *J. Mater. Sci.: Mater. Med.* **2004**, *15* (10), 1097–1103.
37. Cunha, L. G.; Alonso, R. C. B.; Pfeifer, C. S. C.; Correr-Sobrinho, L.; Ferracane, J. L.; Sinhoreti, M. A. C. *J. Dentist.* **2007**, *35* (4), 318–324.
38. Pfeifer, C. S. C.; Braga, R. R.; Ferracane, J. L. *Operative Dent.* **2006**, *31* (5), 610–615.
39. Lovell, L. G.; Lu, H.; Elliott, J. E.; Stansbury, J. W.; Bowman, C. N. *Dent. Mater.* **2001**, *17* (6), 504–511.
40. Patel, M. P.; Braden, M.; Davy, K. W. M. *Biomaterials* **1987**, *8* (1), 53–56.
41. Boaro, L. C. C.; Gonalves, F.; Guimarães, T. C.; Ferracane, J. L.; Versluis, A.; Braga, R. R. *Dent. Mater.* **2010**, *26* (12), 1144–1150.
42. Boaro, L. C.; Gonçalves, F.; Guimarães, T. C.; Ferracane, J. L.; Pfeifer, C. S.; Braga, R. R. *Dent. Mater.* **2013**, *29* (4), 398–404.
43. Yoo, S. H.; Kim, C. K. *Macromol. Res.* **2010**, *18* (10), 1013–1020.
44. Stansbury, J. W. *J. Dent. Res.* **1992**, *71* (7), 1408–1412.
45. Stansbury, J. W. *J. Dent. Res.* **1990**, *69* (3), 844–848.
46. Miller, M. D.; Holder, A. J.; Chappelow, C. C.; David Eick, J. *THEOCHEM* **2005**, *756* (1–3), 185–194.
47. Kanazawa, A.; Kanaoka, S.; Aoshima, S. *Macromolecules* **2014**, *47* (19), 6635–6644.
48. Baracco, B.; Perdigão, J.; Cabrera, E.; Ceballos, L. *Operative Dent.* **2013**, *38* (6), 591–600.
49. Schmidt, M.; Dige, I.; Kirkevang, L. L.; Vaeth, M.; Hørsted-Bindslev, P. *Clin. Oral Invest.* **2015**, *19* (2), 245–251.
50. Yaman, B. C.; Doğruer, I.; Gümüştaş, B.; Efes, B. G. *Clin. Oral Invest.* **2014**, *18* (4), 1071–1079.
51. Hoyle, C. E.; Bowman, C. N. *Angew. Chem. Int. Ed.* **2010**, *49* (9), 1540–1573.
52. Cramer, N. B.; Bowman, C. N. *J. Poly. Sci. A Poly. Chem.* **2001**, *39* (19), 3311–3319.

53. Cramer, N. B.; Couch, C. L.; Schreck, K. M.; Carioscia, J. A.; Boulden, J. E.; Stansbury, J. W.; Bowman, C. N. *Dent. Mater.* **2010**, *26* (1), 21–28.
54. Senyurt, A. F.; Wei, H.; Hoyle, C. E.; Piland, S. G.; Gould, T. E. *Macromolecules* **2007**, *40* (14), 4901–4909.
55. O'Brien, A. K.; Cramer, N. B.; Bowman, C. N. *J. Poly. Sci. A Poly. Chem.* **2006**, *44* (6), 2007–2014.
56. Lu, H.; Carioscia, J. A.; Stansbury, J. W.; Bowman, C. N. *Dent. Mater.* **2005**, *21* (12), 1129–1136.
57. Li, Q.; Zhou, H.; Hoyle, C. E. *Polymer* **2009**, *50* (10), 2237–2245.
58. Boulden, J. E.; Cramer, N. B.; Bowman, C. N. *Thiol-ene-methacrylate Systems as Dental Restorative Materials* (American Chemical Society: Polymer Preprints, Division of Polymer Chemistry, **2008**), pp. 1157–1158.
59. Wei, H.; Senyurt, A. F.; Jönsson, S.; Hoyle, C. E. *J. Poly. Sci. A Poly. Chem.* **2007**, *45* (5), 822–829.
60. Reddy, S. K.; Cramer, N. B.; Bowman, C. N. *Macromolecules* **2006**, *39* (10), 3673–3680.
61. Reddy, S. K.; Cramer, N. B.; Bowman, C. N. *Macromolecules* **2006**, *39* (10), 3681–3687.
62. Lecamp, L.; Houllier, F.; Youssef, B.; Bunel, C. *Polymer* **2001**, *42* (7), 2727–2736.
63. Cramer, N. B.; Couch, C. L.; Schreck, K. M.; Boulden, J. E.; Wydra, R.; Stansbury, J. W.; Bowman, C. N. *Dent. Mater.* **2010**, *26* (8), 799–806.
64. Lee, T. Y.; Smith, Z.; Reddy, S. K.; Cramer, N. B.; Bowman, C. N. *Macromolecules* **2007**, *40* (5), 1466–1472.
65. Pfeifer, C. S.; Wilson, N. D.; Shelton, Z. R.; Stansbury, J. W. *Polymer* **2011**, *52* (15), 3295–3303.
66. Berchtold, K. A.; Hacioglu, B.; Lovell, L.; Nie, J.; Bowman, C. N. *Macromolecules* **2001**, *34* (15), 5103–5111.
67. Berchtold, K. A.; Lovell, L. G.; Nie, J.; Hacioglu, B.; Bowman, C. N. *Polymer* **2001**, *42* (11), 4925–4929.
68. Khire, V. S.; Kloxin, A. M.; Couch, C. L.; Anseth, K. S.; Bowman, C. N. *J. Poly. Sci. A Poly. Chem.* **2008**, *46* (20), 6896–6906.

69. Khire, V. S.; Lee, T. Y.; Bowman, C. N. *Macromolecules* **2007**, *40* (16), 5669–5677.
70. Khire, V. S.; Lee, T. Y.; Bowman, C. N. *Macromolecules* **2008**, *41* (20), 7440–7447.
71. Senyurt, A. F.; Hoyle, C. E.; Wei, H.; Piland, S. G.; Gould, T. E. *Macromolecules* **2007**, *40* (9), 3174–3182.
72. Carioscia, J. A.; Schneidewind, L.; O'Brien, C.; Ely, R.; Feeser, C.; Cramer, N.; Bowman, C. N. *J. Poly. Sci. A Poly. Chem.* **2007**, *45* (23), 5686–5696.
73. Podgórski, M.; Becka, E.; Claudino, M.; Flores, A.; Shah, P. K.; Stansbury, J. W.; Bowman, C. N. *Dent. Mater.* **2015**, *31* (11), 1255–1262.
74. Podgórski, M.; Becka, E.; Claudino, M.; Flores, A.; Shah, P. K.; Stansbury, J. W.; Bowman, C. N. *Dent. Mater.* **2015**, *31* (11), 1263–1270.
75. Cook, W. D.; Brockhurst, P. *J. Dent. Res.* **1980**, *59* (5), 795–799.
76. Chiou, B. S.; Khan, S. A. *Macromolecules* **1996**, *30* (23), 7322–7328.
77. Macosko, C. W. *Rehology: Principles, Measurements and Applications* (Hoboken: John Wiley & Sons, **1994**).
78. Standish, P. M.; Cook, W. D. *Aus. Dent. J.* **1983**, *28* (2), 82–86.
79. Dean, K.; Cook, W. D.; Rey, L.; Galy, J.; Sautereau, H. *Macromolecules* **2001**, *34* (19), 6623–6630.
80. Kloxin, C. J.; Scott, T. F.; Adzima, B. J.; Bowman, C. N. *Macromolecules* **2010**, *43* (6), 2643–2653.
81. Kloxin, C. J.; Bowman, C. N. *Chem. Soc. Rev.* **2013**, *42* (17), 7161–7173.
82. Park, H. Y.; Kloxin, C. J.; Scott, T. F.; Bowman, C. N. *Dent. Mater.* **2010**, *26* (10), 1010–1016.
83. Park, H. Y.; Kloxin, C. J.; Abuelyaman, A. S.; Oxman, J. D.; Bowman, C. N. *Dent Mater.* **2012**, *28* (11), 1113–1119.
84. Lu, H.; Jin, X.; Klee, J. E.; Koltisko, B. Dental composite compositions for reduced stress shrinkage. Google Patents, **2015**.
85. Freilich, M. A.; Goldberg, A. J.; Gilpatrick, R. O.; Simonsen, R. J. *Dent. Mater.* **1992**, *8* (4), 224–228.
86. Nita, L. E.; Chiriac, A. P.; Diaconu, A.; Tudorachi, N.; Mititelu-Tartau, L. *Int. J. Pharm.* **2016**, *515* (1–2), 165–175.

87. Pellizzoni, E.; Tommasini, M.; Marangon, E.; Rizzolio, F.; Saito, G.; Benedetti, F.; Toffoli, G.; Resmini, M.; Berti, F. *Biosens. Bioelectron.* **2016**, *86*, 913–919.
88. Cruz, A.; García-Uriostegui, L.; Ortega, A.; Isoshima, T.; Burillo, G., *Carbohydr. Poly.* **2017**, *155*, 303–312.
89. Morães, R. R.; Garcia, J. W.; Wilson, N. D.; Lewis, S. H.; Barros, M. D.; Yang, B.; Pfeifer, C. S.; Stansbury, J. W. *J. Dent. Res.* **2012**, *91* (2), 179–184.
90. Moraes, R. R.; Garcia, J. W.; Barros, M. D.; Lewis, S. H.; Pfeifer, C. S.; Liu, J.; Stansbury, J. W. *Dent.l Mater.* **2011**, *27* (6), 509–519.
91. Liu, J.; Howard, G. D.; Lewis, S. H.; Barros, M. D.; Stansbury, J. W. *Eur. Poly. J.* **2012**, *48* (11), 1819–1828.
92. Dailing, E. A.; Nair, D. P.; Setterberg, W. K.; Kyburz, K. A.; Yang, C.; D'Ovidio, T.; Anseth, K. S.; Stansbury, J. W. *Polym. Chem.* **2016**, *7* (4), 816–825.
93. Bacchi, A.; Pfeifer, C. S. *Dent. Mater.* **2016**, *32* (8), 978–986.
94. Bacchi, A.; Nelson, M.; Pfeifer, C. S., *Dent. Mater.* **2016**, *32* (2), 233–239.
95. Bacchi, A.; Consani, R. L.; Martim, G. C.; Pfeifer, C. S. *Dent. Mater.* **2015**, *31* (5), 565–574.
96. Bacchi, A.; Dobson, A.; Ferracane, J. L.; Consani, R.; Pfeifer, C. S. *J. Dent. Res.* **2014**, *93* (12), 1320–1325.
97. Shin, J.; Matsushima, H.; Comer, C. M.; Bowman, C. N.; Hoyle, C. E. *Chem. Mater.* **2010**, *22* (8), 2616–2625.
98. Li, H.; Yu, B.; Matsushima, H.; Hoyle, C. E.; Lowe, A. B. *Macromolecules* **2009**, *42* (17), 6537–6542.
99. Li, Q.; Zhou, H.; Wicks, D. A.; Hoyle, C. E.; Magers, D. H.; McAlexander, H. R. *Macromolecules* **2009**, *42* (6), 1824–1833.
100. Stansbury, J. W.; Antonucci, J. M. *Dent. Mater.* **1999**, *15* (3), 166–173.
101. Prakki, A.; Pereira, P. N. R.; Kalachandra, S. *Dent. Mater.* **2009**, *25* (1), 26–32.
102. Prakki, A.; Tallury, P.; Mondelli, R. F. L.; Kalachandra, S. *Dent. Mater.* **2007**, *23* (10), 1199–1204.
103. Yin, M.; Guo, S.; Liu, F.; He, J. *J. Mech. Behav. Biomed. Mater.* **2015**, *51*, 337–344.
104. Kurata, S.; Yamazaki, N. *Dent. Mater. J.* **2011**, *30* (1), 103–108.

105. Buruiana, T.; Melinte, V.; Aldea, H.; Pelin, I. M.; Buruiana, E. C. *Mater. Sci. Eng. C* **2016**, *62*, 96–104.
106. Kadoma, Y. *Dent. Mater. J.* **2010**, *29* (5), 602–608.
107. Kadoma, Y.; Tamaki, Y. *Dent. Mater. J.* **2009**, *28* (5), 642–648.
108. Giannini, M.; Di Francescantonio, M.; Pacheco, R. R.; Boaro, L. C.; Braga, R. R. *Operative Dent.* **2014**, *39* (3), 264–272.
109. Wei, Y. J.; Silikas, N.; Zhang, Z. T.; Watts, D. C. *Dent. Mater.* **2011**, *27* (2), 197–205.
110. Moszner, N. *New Monomers for Dental Application* (Macromolecular Symposia, **2004**), pp. 63–75.
111. Pan, H.; Yang, J.; Kopečková, P.; Kopeček, J. I. *Biomacromolecules* **2010**, *12* (1), 247–252.
112. Xu, X.; Wang, R.; Ling, L.; Burgess, J. O. *J. Poly. Sci. A Poly. Chem.* **2007**, *45* (1), 99–110.
113. Dobson, A. H., V.; Mbyia, W.; Ferracane, J. L.; Pfeifer, C. S. *J. Dent. Res.* **2016**, *95* (B), #0178.
114. Moszner, N.; Zeuner, F.; Rheinberger, V. *Macromol. Symposia* **2001**, *175*, 133–139.
115. Moszner, N.; Fischer, U. K.; Angermann, J. *Macromol. Mater. Eng.* **2016**, *301* (6), 750–759.
116. Moszner, N.; Zeuner, F.; Angermann, J.; Fischer, U. K.; Rheinberger, V., *Macromol. Mater. Eng.* **2003**, *288* (8), 621–628.
117. Moszner, N.; Salz, U. *Macromol. Mater. Eng.* **2007**, *292* (3), 245–271.
118. Gonzalez-Bonet, A.; Kaufman, G.; Yang, Y.; Wong, C.; Jackson, A.; Huyang, G.; Bowen, R.; Sun, J. *Biomacromolecules* **2015**, *16* (10), 3381–3388.
119. Vitale, A.; Cominotti, M.; Ameduri, B.; Bongiovanni, R. *Eur. Poly. J.* **2016**, *82*, 122–131.
120. Patil, Y.; Ameduri, B. *Prog. Polym. Sci.* **2013**, *38* (5), 703–739.
121. Tran, B.; Oladeji, I. O.; Zou, J.; Chai, G.; Zhai, L. *Solid State Ion.* **2013**, *232*, 37–43.
122. Uchiyama, M.; Satoh, K.; Kamigaito, M. *Macromolecules* **2015**, *48* (16), 5533–5542.
123. Hao, Y.; Shih, H.; Muñoz, Z.; Kemp, A.; Lin, C. C. *Acta Biomater.* **2014**, *10* (1), 104–114.

124. Sugihara, S.; Kawamoto, Y.; Maeda, Y. *Macromolecules* **2016**, *49* (5), 1563–1574.
125. Xi, W.; Wang, C.; Kloxin, C. J.; Bowman, C. N. *ACS Macro Letters* **2012**, *1* (7), 811–814.
126. Chatani, S.; Sheridan, R. J.; Podgórski, M.; Nair, D. P.; Bowman, C. N. *Chem. Mater.* **2013**, *25* (19), 3897–3901.
127. Podgórski, M.; Chatani, S.; Bowman, C. N. *Macromol. Rapid Commun.* **2014**, *35* (17), 1497–1502.
128. Podgórski, M.; Wang, C.; Yuan, Y.; Konetski, D.; Smalyukh, I.; Bowman, C. N. *Chem. Mater.* **2016**, *28* (14), 5102–5109.
129. Xi, W.; Peng, H.; Aguirre-Soto, A.; Kloxin, C. J.; Stansbury, J. W.; Bowman, C. N. *Macromolecules* **2014**, *47* (18), 6159–6165.
130. Nimmo, C. M.; Shoichet, M. S. *Bioconjugate Chem.* **2011**, *22* (11), 2199–2209.
131. Hardy, M. D.; Konetski, D.; Bowman, C. N.; Devaraj, N. K. *Org. Biomol. Chem.* **2016**, *14* (24), 5555–5558.
132. Rostovtsev, V. V.; Green, L. G.; Fokin, V. V.; Sharpless, K. B. *Angew. Chem. Int. Ed.* **2002**, *41* (14), 2596–2599.
133. Sharpless, K. B. *Angew. Chem. Int. Ed. n* **2002**, *41* (12), 2024–2032.
134. Song, H. B.; Sowan, N. *Dent. Mater.* **2016**, *32* (11), 1332–1342.
135. Adzima, B. J.; Tao, Y.; Kloxin, C. J.; DeForest, C. A.; Anseth, K. S.; Bowman, C. N. *Nat. Chem.* **2011**, *3* (3), 256–259.
136. Pu, K. Y.; Li, K.; Shi, J.; Liu, B., *Chem. Mater.* **2009**, *21* (16), 3816–3822.
137. Khalichi, P.; Singh, J.; Cvitkovitch, D. G.; Santerre, J. P. *Biomaterials* **2009**, *30* (4), 452–459.
138. Singh, J.; Khalichi, P.; Cvitkovitch, D. G.; Santerre, J. P. *J. Biomed. Mater. Res. A* **2009**, *88* (2), 551–560.
139. Lewis, J. S.; Gittard, S. D.; Narayan, R. J.; Berry, C. J.; Brigmon, R. L.; Ramamurti, R.; Singh, R. N. *ASME* **2010**, *132* (3), 0309191–0309197.
140. Watanabe, T.; Tateishi, T.; Sakai, T.; Toyama, K.; Hayakawa, Y.; Ono, T. *Kobunshi Ronbunshu* **2013**, *70* (4), 166–174.
141. Cheng, L.; Zhang, K.; Weir, M. D.; Melo, M. A. S.; Zhou, X.; Xu, H. H. K. *Nanomedicine* **2015**, *10* (4), 627–641.
142. Ge, Y.; Wang, S.; Zhou, X.; Wang, H.; Xu, H. H. K.; Cheng, L. *Materials* **2015**, *8* (6), 3532–3549.

143. Gong, T.; Adzima, B. J.; Baker, N. H.; Bowman, C. N. *Advanced Mater.* **2013**, *25* (14), 2024–2028.
144. Hoshika, T.; Nishitani, Y.; Yoshiyama, M.; Key, W. O.; Brantley, W.; Agee, K. A.; Breschi, L.; Cadenaro, M.; Tay, F. R.; Rueggeberg, F. *et al. Dent. Mater.* **2014**, *30* (11), 1213–1223.
145. Hoshika, T.; Nishitani, Y.; Yoshiyama, M.; Key, W. O.; Brantley, W.; Agee, K. A.; Breschi, L.; Cadenaro, M.; Tay, F. R.; Rueggeberg, F.; Pashley, D. H. *Dent. Mater.* **2014**, *30* (11), 1213–1223.
146. Li, F.; Weir, M. D.; Xu, H. H. K. *J. Dent. Res.* **2013**, *92* (10), 932–938.
147. Liu, N.; Li, F.; Chen, Y. J.; Zhang, L.; Lu, S.; Kang, J. J.; Chen, J. H. *J. Dentist.* **2013**, *41* (11), 1101–1108.
148. Tezvergil-Mutluay, A.; Agee, K. A.; Mazzoni, A.; Carvalho, R. M.; Carrilho, M.; Tersariol, I. L.; Nascimento, F. D.; Imazato, S.; Tjäderhane, L.; Breschi, L.; Tay, F. R.; Pashley, D. H. *Dent. Mater.* **2015**, *31* (2), e25–e32.
149. Tezvergil-Mutluay, A.; Agee, K. A.; Uchiyama, T.; Imazato, S.; Mutluay, M. M.; Cadenaro, M.; Breschi, L.; Nishitani, Y.; Tay, F. R.; Pashley, D. H. *J. Dent. Res.* **2011**, *90* (4), 535–540.
150. Zhang, K.; Cheng, L.; Weir, M. D.; Bai, Y. X.; Xu, H. H. K. *Int. J. Oral Sci.* **2016**, *8*, 45–53.
151. Zhou, H.; Li, F.; Weir, M. D.; Xu, H. H. K. *J. Dentist.* **2013**, *41* (11), 1122–1131.
152. He, J.; Söderling, E.; Lassila, L. V. J.; Vallittu, P. K. *Dent. Mater.* **2015**, *31* (5), 575–582.
153. Li, F.; Weir, M. D.; Chen, J.; Xu, H. H. K. *Dent. Mater.* **2014**, *30* (4), 433–441.
154. Zhang, N.; Ma, J.; Melo, M. A. S.; Weir, M. D.; Bai, Y.; Xu, H. H. K. *J. Dentist.* **2015**, *43* (2), 225–234.
155. Wu, J.; Weir, M. D.; Zhang, Q.; Zhou, C.; Melo, M. A. S.; Xu, H. H. K. *Dent. Mater.* **2016**, *32* (2), 294–304.
156. Pupo, Y. M.; Farago, P. V.; Nadal, J. M.; Simão, L. C.; Esmerino, L. A.; Gomes, O. M. M.; Gomes, J. C. *Int. J. Mol. Sci.* **2014**, *15* (5), 8998–9015.
157. Luo, W.; Huang, Q.; Liu, F.; Lin, Z.; He, J. *J. Mech. Behav. Biomed. Mater.* **2015**, *49*, 61–68.

158. Haleem, Y. A.; Liu, D.; Chen, W.; Wang, C.; Hong, C.; He, Z.; Liu, J.; Song, P.; Yu, S.; Song, L. *Compos. B Eng.* **2015**, *78*, 480–487.
159. Wehling, J.; Dringen, R.; Zare, R. N.; Maas, M.; Rezwan, K. *ACS Nano* **2014**, *8* (6), 6475–6483.
160. Haleem, Y.; Song, P.; Liu, D.; Wang, C.; Gan, W.; Saleem, M.; Song, L. *Mater.* **2016**, *9* (7), 507.

Chapter 12

Development of Polymerization Contraction Stresses in Resin-Based Composites

Roberto Ruggiero Braga*, Marcela Charantola Rodrigues, and Yvette Alania

Department of Biomaterials and Oral Biology, School of Dentistry, University of São Paulo, Av. Prof. Lineu Prestes, 2227 — São Paulo, Brazil

**rrbraga@usp.br*

Photoactivated dimethacrylate-based composites have become the material of choice for direct tooth restorations due to their aesthetics, virtually unlimited working time, cure on command, and adhesiveness to tooth structure, which requires minimal cavity preparation. During polymerization, the transition from a viscous paste to a glassy polymer is accompanied by substantial shrinkage. As volumetric change is restrained by the composite adhesion to the walls of the cavity preparation and cannot be compensated by plastic deformation due to the material's increasing stiffness, stresses build up at the tooth–restoration interface. Furthermore, being a localized state and not a material-intrinsic property, stress magnitude depends on how compliant the bonding substrate is to shrinkage forces. Polymerization stress can potentially be related to several clinically undesirable outcomes, such as post-operative sensitivity, development of white lines around the restoration margins, tooth cracking, and, ultimately, new caries lesions. Several strategies were proposed to reduce polymerization stress magnitude, with limited success. They include the development of "low-shrinkage" composites, light-curing protocols with modulated irradiance, low modulus liners, incremental placement techniques, and composite pre-heating.

1. Introduction

Resin-based composites have become the material of choice for direct restorations, both in anterior and posterior teeth. Besides being aesthetically appealing, it presents the advantage of "cure on command". Moreover, despite the lack of sound scientific evidence on health-related issues caused by dental amalgams, resin composites have virtually replaced them in posterior restorations. However, the use of resin composites is not without its limitations. Its placement technique is more time consuming and technique sensitive, and longitudinal clinical studies report higher annual failure rates compared to amalgam.[1] One of the main causes of composite restoration failure is the recurrence of caries lesions at the tooth–restoration interface.[2] Though caries development has multiple causes, there is some scientific evidence linking this occurrence to the presence of gaps at the tooth–restoration interface.[3] Interfacial debonding may occur due to deficiency in the adhesive system application, degradation of the adhesive layer, or as a consequence of polymerization stress development.

During polymerization, stresses arise as a result of composite shrinkage and elastic modulus development.[4] Though its occurrence has been reported by Bowen, the inventor of dimethacrylate-based composites, in 1967,[5] it was not until the late 1980s with the studies by Feilzer *et al.* that this topic gained wider attention.[6] To date, there is no definite evidence linking polymerization stress with the clinical performance of resin composite restorations. However, the abundance of laboratory studies relating polymerization stress with failure of the bonded interface makes it almost impossible to deny its importance in this process.[7] In this chapter, the factors involved in polymerization stress development are described, as well as the testing methods and the approaches proposed to reduce stress magnitude.

2. Experimental Methods for Polymerization Stress Determination

Stress is a vectorial entity, and therefore cannot be directly measured. Stresses are calculated, for example, using recorded force values, as well as the geometry and dimensions of the specimen. Specimen boundary conditions are also important, as they affect its behavior during the test. Polymerization stress can be assessed by different methods, the most ubiquitous being those using load cells mounted on rigid frames to record the axial shrinkage force. Other mechanical tests use more complex mathematical solutions to calculate stress from variables affected by composite shrinkage forces, such as the ring-slitting method and the crack analysis method. Finite element analysis (FEA) and photoelasticity are useful tools to observe stress distribution within the composite and support experimental findings. Other methods, such as the use of strain gauges to determine cuspal deflection caused by shrinkage forces, are used as an indirect assessment of polymerization stress magnitude. Obviously, every method has advantages and limitations. Unfortunately, due to the lack of standardization, the comparison of data from different studies must be conducted very judiciously.

2.1. *Mechanical Tests*

2.1.1. *Systems Using Rigid Frames for Axial Force Detection*

Load cells connected to rigid frames can be used to record the axial force generated by composite shrinkage. In the basic setup, the composite is applied between two rods, one of them connected to the load cell of a universal testing machine or custom-built rigid framework. When the composite shrinks, it pulls both rods toward each other and the load cell records the force development over time.

A feedback loop is normally used to monitor the approximation of the rods and command the crosshead to re-establish the initial distance between the rods. Force values are divided by the cross-sectional area of the specimen to obtain the nominal (average) shrinkage stress. With photoactivated composites, specimen thickness is usually lower than 1 mm to ensure a homogeneous curing. The choice of rod material has a definite effect on stress magnitude. Stiffer rods (e.g. steel or glass) reduce the compliance of the testing system, resulting in higher stress values. On the other hand, with less stiff substrates, such as acrylic, the recorded values are lower because a fraction of the shrinkage force causes elongation of the rod and, consequently, is not detected by the load cell.[8] When testing a series of materials, their relative rankings may change according to the compliance of the testing system,[9] meaning that one must be aware of its influence on composite behavior.

2.1.2. *Systems Based on Cantilever Deflection*

Testing methods using single cantilever devices rely on its length, elastic modulus, and deflection to calculate shrinkage stress.[10] Alternatively, a cantilever load cell can be used to record the force directly.[11] In both cases, a disc-shaped specimen is made by inserting the composite between two opposing rods close to the free extremity of the beam. The compliance of the system can be modulated by changing the cantilever beam length (i.e. the shorter the beam, the lower is the compliance).

2.1.3. *Crack Analysis*

In this method, Vickers indentations are made on soda-lime glass discs (approximately 1 mm in thickness) with a central perforation, at a predefined distance from the hole margin. The corner cracks developed from the indentation are measured under a light microscope and the perforation is filled with the tested composite. After polymerization, the corner cracks are remeasured and stress at the glass substrate around the indentation is calculated based on crack growth and glass fracture toughness.[12] Stress at various distances from the glass/composite interface can be calculated by changing the indentation site.[13]

2.1.4. *Ring Slitting Method*

Different from the previous methods, where it is possible to monitor stress development, the ring slitting method is used to determine residual stresses in the composite. Composite rings (internal diameter: 15 mm, external diameter: 18 mm, thickness: 1 mm) are made using a metallic mold. After curing, two reference marks 3 mm apart are made in the specimen. Digital images of the ring are obtained before and after sectioning between the reference marks with a rotating diamond blade. The residual stress in the composite ring is calculated based on the change in distance between the marks, ring dimensions, and composite elastic modulus. The elapsed time between curing and sectioning is critical because of post-cure polymerization. Likewise, the interval between sectioning and imaging also affects the stress values obtained due to stress relaxation.[14]

2.2. *Methods used for Assessing Stress Distribution*

2.2.1. *Photoelasticity*

Mechanical testing provides an average stress value for the entire specimen. However, polymerization stresses are not uniformly distributed along the composite/substrate interface or within the bulk of the material, and knowing how stresses are distributed in a composite-filled cavity is important to understand some of the failure mechanisms found with adhesive restorations. Photoelastic analysis uses a transparent resin material that when stressed shows what is called "interference fringes" under polarized light.[15] A higher number of fringes at a particular site indicates the photoelastic resin is under higher stress. Stress levels can also be quantified if the photoelastic resin's stress optical coefficient is previously determined. The photoelastic resin can be used as the substrate where a box or cylindrical cavity is prepared and filled with composite. Therefore, what is actually being measured is the stress at the bonding substrate resulting from composite polymerization.[16]

2.2.2. *Finite Element Analysis*

The FEA uses computer-generated models to evaluate polymerization stress magnitude and distribution. A mesh is applied to the model (using, for example, tetrahedral elements) and the magnitude of the stress vector on each node is calculated. Results are expressed based upon "failure criteria". For brittle materials, such as resin composites and the tooth structure, the maximum principal stress criteria (i.e. maximum tensile stress) is more appropriate.[9] Another frequently found failure criteria is Von Mises. However, it seems less appropriate for the problem in question, since it is based on the distortion energy theory, more suitable for ductile materials. The accuracy of the method is highly dependent on the parameters used in modeling, such as elastic modulus and Poisson's coefficient (both of the composite and the substrate), composite shrinkage, and boundary conditions. Usually, simplified representations such as two-dimensional axisymmetric models are preferred to reduce computational costs.[8] Ideally, FEA results should be validated by data obtained experimentally. In fact, the association of both methods allows for a much more consistent interpretation of the results of either test alone.[17]

2.3. *Influence of Test Parameters on Stress Results*

The previous section represents an overview of the most frequently used testing methods according to the literature. Due to the lack of a standardized method, stress values from different studies are not comparable. In fact, even among seemingly similar methods direct comparisons may be problematic due to variations in the compliance of the testing system. Compliance is the reciprocal of stiffness (unit: mm/N). As a general rule, testing systems with high compliance result in low recorded forces because part of the force generated by composite shrinkage causes elongation of the system components and, consequently, is not detected by the load cell.[8] There has been some debate on which compliance level provides the most clinically meaningful results. While low-compliance systems represent the most critical situation in terms of stress generation — in other words, the composite "full stress-generating potential" — the biological substrates on which composites are applied (enamel, dentin, cement) are relatively compliant. Therefore, in theory, data gathered from high-compliance systems would be more representative. In any scenario, the elements of the testing system with a direct effect on compliance and, consequently, on stress magnitude must be taken into consideration when comparing data from different studies. They are described in the following sections.

2.3.1. *Specimen Dimensions*

Testing methods based on load cells mounted on stiff frames use disc-shaped specimens, with the diameter following the perimeter of the rods used as bonding substrate (usually between 3 mm and 5 mm). Specimen height is around 1 mm, which is important to ensure a homogeneous curing of the composite in cases where the rod material is transparent (glass or acrylic) and photoactivation is accomplished with the tip of the curing unit at the opposite end of one of the rods. When metal rods are used as substrate, keeping the thickness low is less of an issue, as photoactivation must be conducted with the light tip perpendicularly to the long axis of the specimen. In case of self-cure composites, specimen height is limited by the possibility of shaping the cylinder between the rods without slumping.

Specimen radius and height define its level of confinement, usually expressed as the ratio between both dimensions (see C-factor, below). In low compliance systems, there is a direct relationship between radius-to-height and nominal stress.[18] On the other hand, in high compliance systems, stress is directly related to the specimen's volume.[19]

2.3.2. *Bonding Substrate*

The bonding substrate for the composite is the most influential variable defining polymerization stress magnitude. The first reports of mechanical tests for stress determination used steel rods.[6] However, bonding composite to metal relies solely on the irregularities created on the metal surface by sandblasting. As a consequence, debonding is a likely event under relatively high shrinkage forces, and if it happens, the specimen is lost. Glass can be sandblasted and coated with a silane primer to improve the bond strength to composite. An additional advantage of using glass rods is the possibility of light curing through one of the rods, which allows for a more homogeneous curing compared to positioning the light guide perpendicularly to the specimen long axis.[20] However, debonding or even glass fracture may occur under high shrinkage forces. The use of acrylic (polymethyl methacrylate, PMMA) rods increases the compliance of the testing system considerably. That, along with a strong bonding to the composite and the possibility of light curing through the rod, makes this substrate the most convenient of the three.[21] Depending on the properties of the composites tested, their relative rankings may differ according to the bonding substrate (i.e. compliance level) of the testing system.[22]

2.3.3. *Feedback Loop*

The longitudinal compliance of a testing system can also be modulated by the use of a transducer to monitor the relative distance between both upper and lower rods. When the transducer registers an approximation between its fixation points caused by shrinkage forces, the software controlling the testing machine can command the actuator to return the transducer reading to zero (with a resolution as low as 0.1 μm). This continuous elongation of the specimen restricts the compliance of the testing system to the elongation taking place between the transducer fixation points. Therefore, the use of a transducer significantly lowers the system's compliance.

2.4. *Relationship Between Polymerization Stress Tests and In Vitro Tests for Assessing Quality of the Bonded Interface*

Significant correlations were observed between polymerization stress values obtained in low compliance testing systems and *in vitro* microleakage, suggesting that higher interfacial stresses were responsible for the debonding of the interface.[23,24] However, when a series of commercial composites were tested for polymerization stress in both low and high compliance systems and the results were compared with bond strength to dentin, microleakage, and marginal gaps, stronger correlations were observed with data obtained in the high compliance system. Also, no relationship was observed between stress determined in the low compliance system and bond strength to dentin.[25] Therefore, the use of high compliance testing systems for polymerization stress determination seems to be more representative of the possible effects on the quality of tooth–composite interfaces.

3. Polymerization Stress Determinants Related to Composite Formulation

Resin composites are composed of an organic matrix, constituted by the combination of different monomers, and an inorganic fraction, usually constituted by silanated glass fillers. Also, photoinitiators such as camphorquinone and a tertiary amine are also present. Its polymerization reaction can be described as having two different phases: the pre-gel phase, when the material still presents a low elastic limit, allowing for plastic deformation of the growing polymer chains under relatively low stress values,[26] and the post-gel phase, when the establishment of a polymer network impedes the mobility of free radicals and other reactive species. In the post-gel phase, the reaction rate decreases and the material develops a glassy character.[27]

Polymerization reaction of resin-based composites occurs by chain growth, where monomers are successively added to the reactive site (free radical polymerization). During the reaction, the addition of monomers to the growing chain results in a volumetric shrinkage. The fraction of shrinkage occurring prior to gelification (pre-gel or non-rigid shrinkage) does not have any clinical consequences.[28] The post-gel shrinkage, on the other hand, is clinically relevant, as at this stage the material cannot compensate the reduction in shrinkage by viscous flow, and stress starts to build.[29,30]

At this point, it is important to point out that polymerization stress development is not determined only by volumetric shrinkage. Composite elastic modulus is also an important determinant of stress magnitude. Is possible to state that, as a rule of thumb, the higher the composite shrinkage and the elastic modulus, the higher its polymerization stress will be. However, these two characteristics are not necessarily related in a direct manner. For example, if two composites with different filler fractions are compared, the material with higher filler content will present lower shrinkage and higher modulus than the other. Moreover, as will be discussed in this chapter, there are several other modulating factors in polymerization stress development. These factors can be intrinsic (i.e. related to composite formulation) or extrinsic (related to the substrate on which the composite is applied). Among the intrinsic factors, those related to the organic and inorganic components of the material will be discussed in the following sections.

3.1. *Polymerization Shrinkage*

Polymerization shrinkage is a time-dependent phenomenon that takes place throughout the entire polymerization reaction.[31] During the pre-gel phase, the stress generated due to shrinkage is relieved by plastic deformation. At the onset of gelation (gel point), there is a sudden increase in viscosity and the polymer transitions from a liquid to a gel. The polymer network is established, and polymer cross-linking density keeps increasing concomitantly to the increase in stiffness. During this phase, the material already presents some stiffness and is not capable of plastic deformation. Therefore, the shrinkage that takes place during this phase is responsible for the development of polymerization stress.[29,32]

Post-gel shrinkage represents a percentage varying between 17% and 32% of the total shrinkage, indicating that for the most part volumetric shrinkage occurs during the pre-gel phase. Moreover, when different materials are compared for pre-gel shrinkage (using the strain gauge method) and total shrinkage (using a mercury dilatometer), no linear correlation between both variables are observed, meaning that the characteristics of polymer network formation vary as a function of material composition and reaction kinetics. The strong correlation observed between polymerization stress and post-gel shrinkage and the lack of correlation between stress and total shrinkage confirm that volumetric shrinkage occurring prior to vitrification has very little effect on polymerization stress development.[33]

Composite shrinkage is determined by its inorganic fraction and the composition of its organic matrix. Commercially available materials present filler fractions between 46% and 74% by volume.[34] Barium, strontium, zirconia, and silica glasses are the inorganic fillers most often found in commercial composites, and are added to the material with the purpose of reducing shrinkage, improving mechanical properties, and to make them radiopaque.[35]

In general, polymerization shrinkage of commercial composites vary between 1% and 4%,[34] and the volumetric filler fraction is inversely related to the magnitude of shrinkage.[36] That occurs because the increase in filler fraction reduces the concentration of carbon double bond per unit volume in the material.[37] However, incorporating high percentages of particles with the purpose of reducing the volume of organic matrix does not seem an effective approach to reduce post-gel shrinkage and polymerization stress,[33] since the increase in inorganic content, besides promoting an increase in elastic modulus, also reduces monomer mobility during polymerization.[38]

Organic matrix formulation also influences the polymerization shrinkage of resin-based composites. Dental composites usually present in their formulation the monomers BisGMA (bisfenol-A glycidyl methacrylate or 2,2-bis[4-(2-hydroxy-3-methylacryloxypropoxy)-phenyl]propane) and TEGDMA (triethylene glycol dimethacrylate or 2-methyl-2-propenoic acid). Other monomers, such as BisEMA (ethoxylated bisphenol-A dimethacrylate) and UDMA (urethane dimethacrylate) can also be found in several commercial composite formulations. These monomers are combined in different ways and proportions with the objective of optimizing mechanical properties and reducing composite shrinkage, warranting a high degree of conversion and suitable handling characteristics for the material.

BisGMA is a high molecular weight and high viscosity monomer (512 g/mol). Its viscosity is due to the presence of two hydroxyl groups that favor the establishment of intermolecular hydrogen bonds. It also presents two aromatic rings that reduce molecular rotation. Such characteristics preclude Bis-GMA as a homopolymer to reach high degrees of conversion. TEGDMA (286 g/mol) is a highly flexible molecule due to the presence of ether groups which, associated with its low molecular weight and absence of intermolecular interactions, allows for a high degree of conversion. However, these characteristics are associated with a high volumetric shrinkage of polymers containing high amounts of this monomer,[27,39] which also increases polymerization stress development.[8] For example, in unfilled resins, a 20 wt.% increase in TEGDMA concentration doubled polymerization stress values.[40]

TEGDMA can be partially or totally replaced by BisEMA or UDMA to reduce shrinkage.[41] However, the lower viscosity of TEGDMA is responsible for a higher degree of conversion of BisGMA/TEGDMA copolymers, in comparison to BisGMA/BisEMA.[36]

3.2. *Elastic Modulus*

Elastic modulus shows a direct relationship with the inorganic content of resin composites. This property is defined by the stiffness of the particles and the way these particles interact among themselves within the material.[42] In experimental materials with similar organic contents, the elastic modulus increased by approximately four times between 25 wt.% and 60 wt.% of fillers.[36]

The composition of the organic phase may also influence the elastic modulus of resin composites. High BisGMA concentrations reduce polymer stiffness by lowering its degree of conversion and cross-linking density. On the other hand, its rigid molecular structure and the establishment of intermolecular hydrogen bonds contribute to the stiffness of the formed polymer.[39,43,44] Low-viscosity monomers are usually employed to reduce the material's viscosity and increase the molecular mobility of the organic matrix, therefore increasing its degree of conversion.[45]

The elastic modulus has an important role in the development of composite polymerization stress.[31,33,36,38] According to Hooke's law, stress is determined by the stiffness of the material when subjected to a given strain. Therefore, assuming the resin composite as a perfectly elastic material, the higher its elastic modulus and polymerization shrinkage, the higher the contraction stress will be. In fact, during polymerization the composite changes from a viscous paste to a viscoelastic (albeit predominantly elastic) material, and therefore stress cannot be calculated simply as the product of both variables.

However, the relationship between elastic modulus and stress development can differ depending on the testing system used.[22,36] An inverse relationship between elastic modulus and polymerization stress was observed when high-compliance testing systems were used; however, a direct relationship between both variables is found in low compliance systems, for example, using glass or metal as bonding substrates.[8,22]

3.3. *Degree of Conversion*

Degree of conversion is defined as the percentage of carbon double bonds present in the uncured material that were consumed in the polymerization reaction. Therefore, it indicates the quality of the formed polymer. A high degree of conversion is necessary to optimize mechanical properties and reduce degradation of resin-based composites.[46] However, the relationship between degree of conversion and mechanical properties is not linear and above a certain threshold increases in conversion are not followed by improvements in mechanical behavior.[47]

In the polymerization of linear dimethacrylate monomers, the establishment of a covalent single bond between the carbon atom with an unpaired electron (i.e. the free radical) and a monomer with a carbon double bond results in a reduction in the distance between them. For this reason, degree of conversion is linearly related to volumetric shrinkage.[48] Degree of conversion is directly related to the viscosity of the initial monomer mixture. This is explained by the fact that conversion stops when the glass transition temperature (Tg) of the forming polymer reaches the temperature of the reaction. The Tg of the initial monomer mixture is related with their viscosity in a way that less viscous mixtures have low glass-transition temperature.[49] High filler contents may reduce degree of conversion, probably due to an increase in light attenuation and a reduction in monomer mobility.[37]

Though a linear, direct relationship between degree of conversion and total volumetric shrinkage exists, the same is not true for the relationship between polymerization stress and shrinkage. As previously mentioned, not all shrinkage causes stress. Moreover, stress is also determined by the development of elastic properties by the polymer, restricting stress relief by viscous flow. Therefore, initially, stress levels do not raise considerably with conversion, until approximately a degree of conversion of approximately 40% is reached. Beyond that conversion level, polymerization stress increases dramatically with small increments in conversion.[30]

3.4. *Polymerization Kinetics*

The free-radical polymerization of dimethacrylate composites is diffusion-controlled, meaning its progress (in terms of reaction rate and ultimate conversion) is defined by the mobility of the reacting species in the developing network. Initially, propagation and termination are chemically controlled, meaning that the availability of monomers and free radicals make both events equally likely to occur. At this stage, polymerization proceeds at relatively low rates. As the reaction continues, the viscosity of the reaction medium increases and propagation becomes more prevalent, which leads to a sudden increase in reaction rate (known as "auto-acceleration", or "gel effect"). Further increases in viscosity hinders the mobility of the reactive species and reduces the availability of monomers close to the reactive end of the free radical, causing the reaction to proceed at progressively lowers rates (auto-deceleration) until the material reaches vitrification.[27] The occurrence of gelation is very important in terms of stress development because it is after the so-called "gel point" (i.e. the degree of conversion corresponding to the onset of auto-acceleration) that stresses start to build up.

Reaction rate does not seem to have a strong influence on polymerization stress development. Significant reductions in stress of photoactivated composites were observed only in cases where reaction rate was reduced below a certain threshold value.[30] Clinically, it is unlikely that reaction rate of light-cured materials can be reduced to the appropriate values without compromising the degree of conversion. On the other hand, the lower reaction rate displayed by self-cured composites seem to favor lower polymerization stress values.[50]

4. Local Factors Associated to Stress Development

As mentioned before, stress is not a basic material property, but a local physical state.[51] Therefore, its magnitude and distribution are not defined only by the composite intrinsic characteristics (e.g. volumetric shrinkage, elastic modulus, and reaction rate). The geometry and dimensions of the tooth cavity, as well as the stiffness (or its reciprocal, compliance) of the bonding substrate are extremely influential. In fact, depending on the local conditions, composite properties may have opposite effects on stress development, as explained in the following sections.

4.1. *Composite Confinement and Volume*

One of the first variables identified as having a definite influence on stress magnitude was the confinement conditions imposed on the composite during polymerization. If a mass of composite had total freedom to shrink, no stress would be generated. However, polymerization always take place with the composite bonded to a substrate, for example, the tooth cavity walls. It has been demonstrated that in a typical load cell testing setup, polymerization stress is directly related to the composite bonded-to-unbonded surface ratio, termed "cavity configuration factor" or C-factor.[6,18] This relationship was confirmed by microleakage[23,24] and bond strength studies.[52] Due to its simplicity, the C-factor was rapidly assimilated by researchers and clinicians. For example, restorations with a high C-factor were "doomed to failure" due to the high interfacial stresses. The reduction of C-factor was the justification for inserting the composite into the cavity in small increments.[53] However, this idea was challenged by *in vitro* investigations showing that interfacial integrity was associated with cavity volume, and not its C-factor.[54,55] Moreover, the efficacy of the incremental placement technique was shown to increase final tooth deflection.[56] In fact, a 12-year longitudinal study did not find a particularly high annual failure rate for class I restorations with high C-factor.[57] This contradiction was explained by the fact that the effect of composite volume and C-factor on stress development depends upon the compliance of the surrounding structures. The relationship between nominal stress and C-factor was observed in low compliance testing systems, using either steel (elastic modulus: 207 GPa) or glass (elastic modulus: 64 GPa) as bonding substrate. However, when PMMA (elastic modulus: 3 GPa) rods were used instead of glass, the increase in compliance resulted in a linear direct relationship between the normalized nominal stress (i.e. nominal stress divided by the system's longitudinal compliance) and specimen volume. Interestingly, by varying specimen height and diameter it was possible to compare conditions with similar volumes and different C-factors. In such cases, experimental groups corresponding to higher confinement displayed higher stress values.[19]

4.2. *Substrate Compliance*

The compliance of the structures surrounding the composite, either represented by the bonding substrate in the testing system or the cavity preparation in a tooth, is determined by the elastic modulus of the substrate and amount of deformation presented by the structure when subjected to shrinkage forces (cuspal deflection, for example). The influence of compliance on polymerization stress development cannot be underestimated. In fact, it is the reason why results from different studies can lead to quite divergent conclusions. FEA revealed that depending on the level of compliance, stress may be directly related to composite shrinkage or its elastic modulus. For example, if a group of composites with different filler concentrations (and, therefore, opposite characteristics in terms of shrinkage and modulus) are tested in a low compliance scenario, those with the highest elastic modulus, but not necessarily the highest shrinkage will develop the highest stress. On the other hand, if the same group of materials is tested in a high compliance system, the highest stress levels will be displayed by the composites also with the highest shrinkage, but with the lowest elastic modulus. This happens because even though only the shrinkage forces manifesting in the longitudinal direction are actually recorded by the load cell, radial stresses also build up at the composite/rod interface. If the composite has a high elastic modulus, the ratio between the elastic modulus of the rod and the composite ($E_{rod}/E_{composites}$) diminishes, and radial shrinkage stress causes bending of the rod interface away from the composite center, counteracting the axial shrinkage forces and reducing the load cell reading. With less stiff composites, this phenomenon does not occur and, consequently, load cell reading is not reduced.[9] It is important to point out that if variations in shrinkage and modulus occur *in tandem* (for example, if one composite is tested at different conversion levels), stress will be directly related to both shrinkage and modulus, regardless of the testing system compliance. In testing systems using rigid frames and a feedback loop (see Section 2.3.3), longitudinal compliance due to rod elongation is directly related to the rod initial length (i.e. from the bonding surface to the point where the transducer sensor is attached) and inversely related to the rod's cross-sectional area and elastic modulus.[18] Radial (transversal) compliance cannot be analytically calculated. However, rod deformation due to radial forces can be estimated by FEA.

In vitro studies revealed that the amount of remaining tooth structure affects residual stress distribution in restored teeth. In small cavities, due to the larger volume of tooth structure, the compliance is reduced and higher stresses are developed at the tooth/restoration interface. Conversely, in large cavities, the relatively thin cavity walls yield to the shrinkage forces and, as a consequence, higher stresses are predicted in the tooth structure.[51]

5. Strategies for Minimizing Polymerization Stress Development

Over the last decades, several attempts were made to reduce the stress developed in composite restorations. Variations in the restorative technique, as well as the development of low-shrinkage composites have been proposed to reduce the magnitude and effects of contraction stress. These methods include the use of low-modulus intermediate layers, light irradiation protocols, and incremental layering technique. The development of new low-shrinkage materials through modifications of current formulations or by the introduction of new filler technologies and monomer chemistries have also been the subject of several studies.

5.1. *Low-Modulus Liners*

The application of an intermediate low-modulus liner between the tooth structure and the resin composite is the basis for the technique known as the "elastic wall concept".[58,59] Theoretically, a low modulus liner could contribute to reduce the shrinkage stress generated by the subsequent layer of high-modulus material by increasing the compliance of the bonding substrate where the restorative composite will be applied. The shrinkage force generated by the restorative composite would cause the elongation of the low-modulus liner and, consequently, reduce the stress developed at the bonded interface.[60]

Flowable composites are one example of intermediate material used in this technique. These low-viscosity resin-based restorative materials differ from conventional resin composites in their lower filler load and/or higher content of low viscosity monomers. They were developed to simplify the placement procedure and improve the adaptation to the cavity. Their low elastic modulus (granted by the relatively low filler content) would make them suitable to be applied as an intermediate "stress relieving" layer.[61] However, the results in the literature are contradictory. While there are reports stating the use of flowable as a liner improves marginal seal,[62] other studies reported no improvement in marginal integrity.[63–66]

Undoubtedly, there is a wide spectrum of products with a broad range of physical characteristics.[66,67] Besides, despite having a lower elastic modulus than non-flowable (high viscosity) composites, it may not be low enough to counteract the effects of their high volumetric shrinkage. Actually, flowable composites presented higher polymerization shrinkage[68] when compared with non-flowable composites, and both type of materials presented similar contraction stress values.[21,67,69] Furthermore, significant stress relief was only observed when an unfilled resin was used as intermediate layer.[69,70]

The thickness of the liner is also an important parameter, with thicker layers providing a higher stress reduction.[61] Reductions in contraction stress between 24% and 37% have been verified for composites tested in a low-compliance rigid frame system with multiple adhesive layers (up to 276 μm) in comparison with the stress registered when only one layer of unfilled resin was applied (maximum thickness: 68 μm). These results were also confirmed by the reduced microleakage along the tooth/restoration interface when adhesive thickness was increased.[71] A disadvantage of this technique is that an adhesive layer too thick usually shows an increased porosity,[72] it is more susceptible to wear and hydrolytic degradation, and if the adhesive is radiolucent, a thick layer can provide a false diagnosis on future examinations.[71]

The use of glass ionomer or resin-modified glass ionomer as an intermediate layer, called "sandwich technique", was proposed with the intention of achieving a better dentinal surface sealing.[73] The use of resin-modified glass-ionomer cements underneath the composite was shown to improve marginal adaptation when compared to composite-only restoration, built either by layering or by bulk insertion.[74] Also, cuspal deflection due to composite shrinkage was significantly reduced when glass ionomer was used as liner (approximately 1 mm of thickness).[75] This can be attributed to the glass ionomer's slow curing rate, which allows for stress relaxation when subjected to shrinkage forces from the subsequent composite layer.[76] Indeed, stress reduction ranging from 18% to 50% was verified when a 0.15–0.30 mm layer of glass ionomer was applied to the bonding substrate in a low-compliance testing system.[70]

5.2. *"Soft-start" Photoactivation*

Alternative curing routines were developed with the intent of reducing composite curing rate at early stages of photoactivation, increasing its flow capacity before gelation and, consequently, reducing the shrinkage forces exerted by the hardening material on the bonded interface.[77] Low curing rates are attained either by using low irradiances (i.e. light power per unit area, mW/cm^2) during the first few seconds of photoactivation or by applying an initially low energy dose to the composite (i.e. irradiance over a period of time, mJ/cm^2) using a short pulse, followed by an interval "in the dark". By doing so, less free radicals are generated and the reaction proceeds at lower rates, allowing more time for the curing composite to flow (i.e. undergo plastic deformation) under shrinkage forces and postponing stress build-up before the gel point conversion is reached. The recommended energy dose is delivered by complementing the irradiation using a high irradiance for the necessary time period. In order to be effective, soft-start curing protocols should be able to reduce contraction stress without compromising the degree of conversion or mechanical properties.[32,78,79]

There are different soft-start curing protocols described in the literature. The "ramped" protocol consists of initial light exposure with reduced irradiance for a certain period of time, gradually increasing to a maximum irradiance value.[80] "Step-curing" uses an initially low irradiance for a few seconds, immediately increasing to the maximum irradiance,[81] and the "pulse-delay" curing protocol consists of initial light exposure at very low irradiance, a subsequent delay (of seconds or even minutes) without irradiance followed by a second exposure at full irradiance.[60] When a two-step curing routine is adopted, three aspects should be observed: the initial light intensity, the exposure duration of the initial low-intensity irradiation, and the time interval between the two irradiations.[32] Previous studies agree that an initial pulse with exposures up to 1 J/cm^2 and less than 100 mW/cm^2 for a period no longer than 7 s seems to be the most efficient curing setting for reducing shrinkage stress.[82] However, the benefit of using lower initial light intensity to relieve the shrinkage stress prior to the vitrification stage has a limited action,[40,83,84] and yet the irradiance of the initial pulse remains a controversial matter among authors.[82]

Photopolymerization protocols often show a variable effect on polymerization stress, because it is dependent on material composition and the energy densities applied to the samples.[85,86] Those observations may lead to the misinterpretation of positive results in investigations on polymerization stress.[21] Indeed, the literature is inconsistent regarding the reduction of shrinkage stress when different soft-start curing methods are used. Some results have shown that the exponential ramp polymerization model reduced the maximum shrinkage stress (up to 20%) when compared to stepped and continuous curing model.[21,80] Reductions in shrinkage stress between 19% and 33% were observed using pulse-delay (up to 5 min delay) when compared to continuous light-curing methods.[77] Nonetheless, some clinical and *in vitro* studies refer to a lack of benefit from soft-start methods regarding polymerization shrinkage, evaluated through marginal seal and the modified Ryge/USPHS criteria.[87–89] Notwithstanding, it seems consensual among researchers that longer delay periods between pulses would increase possibility for chain relaxation. Indeed, dark periods ranging from 1 to 5 min have demonstrated significant reductions in shrinkage stress.[77,82,83] Those findings reveal that longer delay times are needed in order to achieve a reasonable amount of shrinkage stress, which is unrealistic in the clinical practice.[83]

A major concern when using soft-start irradiation protocols is related to a possible reduction in degree of conversion. Also, there is evidence showing that the pulse-delay protocol resulted in lower polymer cross-linking density compared to the continuous, high irradiance curing method.[90] Low degrees of conversion are associated with poor mechanical properties and higher degradation. Therefore, is very important to deliver the recommended energy dose to the composite, regardless of the curing protocol.[91,92] In fact, one must not assume that a preset energy application sequence for photopolymerization is optimal for all composites, since chemical composition varies and may strongly influence degree of conversion and shrinkage stress values.[21,80,83,85] Polymerization kinetics is also material dependent. Finally, it must be considered that the viscous flow of the material during an extended pre-vitrification stage may have minimal consequences because most shrinkage stress is developed during and after the vitrification stage.[83] Therefore, opportunities for polymer relaxation would be restricted during a very short period during light activation.[21]

5.3. *Incremental Technique*

Composite incremental layering was first suggested by Lutz.[53] The rationale is to direct the polymerization vectors favorably to reduce the risk of interfacial debonding[93] and decrease the C-factor, allowing a larger surface for the composite of flow and partially dissipate the shrinkage stress.[59] Incremental techniques may vary according to layer orientation, i.e. the horizontal, oblique, facio-lingual, U-oriented, or the cusp-oriented layering technique.[93] Among those, oblique increments were shown to improve the marginal integrity because the occlusal-most layer would never be tied simultaneously to both facial and lingual enamel margins. The use of an incremental technique resulted in significantly less microleakage than the use of a bulk technique,[94] and cuspal deflection.[95]

As usual, literature on this topic is controversial, as other studies did not find any difference between filling techniques.[96,97] Moreover, through FEA it has been reported that incremental composite restoration actually results in higher polymerization shrinkage stresses than bulk fillings, contrary to the widely accepted evidence. The criticism is based on the finding that the contraction of each individual layer would cause the deformation of the cavity and the displacement of the cusps, decreasing the cavity volume, which result in a higher stress state.[56,98] Cavity depth is a possible reason why incongruent results are reported. As the depth of the cavity increases, bulk insertion may prevent the resin composite from been appropriately cured at the bottom surface as the irradiance decreases. This gradient in conversion may favor some stress relief.[99]

5.4. *Composite Pre-Heating*

Composite pre-heating was introduced as an alternative to lower its viscosity and, consequently, improve adaptation to cavity walls.[100] An additional benefit is that the higher temperatures allow for increased mobility of the reactive species with consequent increase of degree of conversion[27,101–104] and hardness of the resin composite.[105] This is explained by the fact that the increased molecular vibration forces the monomers further apart, allowing them to slide by each other more readily[106] leading to the delay of auto-deceleration and postponing vitrification, allowing the reaction to continue for longer times.[27,100] Indeed, if preheated, it is possible to reduce the energy dose without compromising the degree of conversion.[102,103,107] However, increased polymerization rate also associated with curing at high temperatures may lead to an increased polymerization stress, unless the low viscosity (induced by preheating the composite) permits chain relaxation and, therefore, lower shrinkage stress.[103]

Although some studies have not demonstrated relevant benefits, since no significant reduction on shrinkage stress nor reduced microleakage was observed when compared with non-heated resin composite,[100,108,109] another study reported a significant relaxation percentage and a 55% reduction on final stress when composite is heated up to 40°C or 60°C.[103] A commercially available heating device has shown limited efficacy in terms of stress reduction, explained by the fact that the temperature of the pre-heated composite drops rapidly once it is removed from the heating device.[103,110] Another important factor to consider is the composite heat that will be transferred to the dentin–pulp complex and its consequence on pulpal response. Literature shows a 15% risk of induced necrosis when the intra-pulpal temperature is increased by 5.5°C and a 60% chance when there is an increase of 11°C.[111] Preheating the composite as well as the heat generated by the curing light may increase heat buildup, which was shown to reach 8°C at the pulpal floor.[112]

5.5. *Low Shrinkage Composites*

Over the years, several modifications in resin composites formulations have been proposed in order to reduce polymerization shrinkage. Marketed as "low shrinkage" materials, most of them are dimethacrylate-based with modifications in the filler phase. Changes in the photoinitiator systems and polymerization inhibitors have also been reported.[113] Manufacturers and researchers are continuously investigating new alternative monomers with reduced shrinkage.

5.5.1 *Low-Modulus Fillers*

The use of silica particles without any surface treatment (non-bonded) or functionalized with non-functional silane was proposed aiming to minimize the interaction between the filler surface and the forming polymer, therefore providing sites for stress relief. Stress reductions between 30% and 50% were obtained compared to a composite with silane-treated microfillers. Unfortunately, the handling characteristics were negatively affected by increasing its viscosity.[20]

The addition of high-density polyethylene (HDPE) spheres in composites was another approach attempting to reduce contraction stress with minimal effect on mechanical properties. The incorporation of porosity or microvoids between the spheres and the polymer matrix is expected to produce areas for stress relief.[114] A 23–29% stress reduction was achieved by adding 20% of HDPE spheres on both hybrid and nanofilled composites. The less-rigid nature of the spheres helped reduce the contraction stress but negatively affected the mechanical properties. Fracture toughness, flexural strength, and flexural modulus were reduced with the incorporation of HDPE spheres, limiting the efficacy of this approach.[115]

High molecular weight polymeric nanoparticles, or nanogels, were tested as additives to reduce the reactive group concentration and, therefore, the polymerization shrinkage. When a high nanogel content is incorporated on a resin matrix, viscosity changes dramatically.[116]. Polymeric fibers produced by electrospinning processes represent another way to add pre-polymer particles into resin composites.[117]

5.5.2 *Commercial Low-Shrinkage Composites*

A new monomer system, named silorane, was made commercially available in the last decade. Silorane is a cationic ring-opening monomer synthesized from the combination of a hydrophobic siloxane backbone and an oxirane ring. It is characterized by its biocompatibility, hydrophobicity, insensitivity to oxygen, high reactivity, and low shrinkage. Silorane pre-gel time is 7.6 s, which is significantly higher when compared with dimethacrylate-based composites.[118] Its volumetric shrinkage stress was reported as being as low as 1.34%, and significant stress reductions (from 82% to 95%) were observed when compared with other low-shrinkage commercial products.[94,119,120] Part of its low shrinkage can be attributed to its low degree of conversion, which is expected because of the tetrafunctionality of the silorane molecules.[19]

Other attempts to reduce shrinkage include modifications in a urethane-based methacrylate resin that led to a reduction of 60–70% in shrinkage stress, explained by a reduction in polymerization rate. In this material, shrinkage stress was reduced by plastic flow occurring during the pre-gelation phase.[121] Also, the use of a high molecular weight (MW = 895) reactive oligomer (DX-511, DuPont) with a stiff structural core and flexible arms,[122] a high molecular weight monomer was derived from dimer acid methacrylates (dimer dicarbamate dimethacrylate — DADMA) with high reactivity with BisEMA and UDMA.[123] A highly filled, BisGMA-based composite containing 74 vol% of glass fillers was also developed, However, its contraction stress was not significantly reduced due to the high elastic modulus granted by the filler fraction.[34] Overall, these new formulations exhibited polymerization shrinkage similar to those of traditional composites,[34] except by the silorane-based material which showed half of the total shrinkage developed by a nanohybrid composite.[34] However, a severe reduction (75%) in elastic modulus was seen for the silorane composite after 4-month storage in ethanol.[34]

Recently, materials with improved photoinitiator dynamics, controlled polymerization contraction stress, and increased translucency were developed for insertion in bulk. In fact, the use of bulk-fill materials on extensive cavities has demonstrated lower cuspal deflection and contraction stress.[121,124] However, other studies found that bulk-fill composites presented a much higher shrinkage when compared with conventional resin composites.[125–127]

5.5.3 *Experimental Composite Materials*

Much interest has been focused on the development of low-shrinkage materials, either by introducing new filler technologies or changing monomer chemistry. Several alternatives to conventional dimethacrylate monomers have been proposed. The first approach was the use of spiro orthocarbonates (SOCs), an ester of orthocarboxylic acid, characterized by the presence of bicyclic compounds in a ring opening polymerization. In such monomers, for every van der Waals bond converted to a covalent bond, at least two rings are opened during polymerization, inducing a local volumetric expansion in order to compensate for volumetric shrinkage.[128] Initially, reductions in polymerization shrinkage (38% reduction with copolymer containing 33 wt.% SOCs) were minimal, probably due to insufficient ring opening rate.[41] However, when SOCs were mixed with epoxy resin, a considerably higher reduction in polymerization shrinkage was obtained.[129] Nonetheless, several drawbacks were observed: the polymerization reaction did not occur with visible light, SOCs-containing composites exhibited poor mechanical strength, and volumetric expansion was insufficient to counteract for the polymerization shrinkage.[130]

Developmental silicon-containing tetraoxaspiroundecane monomer (TOSU) belongs to the spiroorthocarbonates-type monomers reported to undergo polymerization with expansion in volume due to double ring opening. A 10% mol addition of TOSU monomer to a silorane gives a dramatic reduction in polymerization stress with only a modest reduction in physical properties. It had 90% less shrinkage stress than silorane.[119] Experimental monomer FIT-852 is a nonlinear difunctional methacrylate with molecular weight of 1200. Based on a modification of UDMA and very similar to the DuPont monomer structure, this FIT-852 monomer is expected to achieve higher conversion, lower shrinkage values, and also improve the toxicity observed with Bis-GMA. Despite its lower shrinkage, its mechanical performance still needs to be improved.[131]

The thiol-ene photopolymerization has also gained much attention as a different approach to formulate novel materials. Due to the step growth evolution of the network, the thiol and ene monomers are quickly consumed, while low molecular weight species participate in early stages of polymerization. Thus, this mechanism causes a delay on gel point conversion lowering induced shrinkage and shrinkage stress.[132]

Despite continuous improvements on techniques and development of new materials, no method has been shown to be totally effective in abating the effects of polymerization shrinkage.[95] Although little or no clinical evidence sustains the hypothesis that composite materials with greater polymerization shrinkage have poorer clinical performance, laboratory data from several studies support this belief; however, effectiveness must come from clinical outcomes,[78] and such data rarely come to light. In the meantime, as a better understanding emerges regarding the complex process of network formation and the relationships between materials and its properties, further advances are certain to follow.[113] Surely, it is likely that new materials with proved low polymerization shrinkage will dominate the market before a complete understanding of this clinically important phenomenon is achieved.[78]

6. Composite Water Sorption as a Means for Polymerization Stress Reduction

Water uptake by dimethacrylate-based composites is considered a clinical problem because it is associated with chemical degradation, loss in mechanical properties, staining, and hydrolysis of the tooth/restoration interface.[133] Notwithstanding, hygroscopic expansion of resin composites may reverse tooth deformation caused by polymerization shrinkage stress, as verified after immersion periods varying from 4 weeks to 6 months.[134–136] Such a finding seems contradictory based on the fact that polymerization shrinkage is not completely offset by hygroscopic expansion.[137] However, only the post-gel shrinkage is responsible for stress development, and therefore it is this fraction of the total shrinkage that must be compensated.[134] This reduction in cuspal deflection overtime cannot be ascribed to composite stress relaxation by viscoelastic deformation because no reduction in tooth deformation was recorded when the restored teeth were kept in silicone oil instead of water.[138] The relaxation of residual stresses by water uptake was also verified using the ring-slitting method. The calculated residual stress in composite rings kept in water for seven days was approximately 30% lower compared to those kept dry.[139] It is important to remember that water uptake cannot avoid clinical problems usually related to polymerization stress development such as post-operative sensitivity, enamel cracking, and interfacial debonding but, still, it seems to compensate for the residual stresses responsible for cuspal deflection.

References

1. Rasines Alcaraz, M. G.; Veitz-Keenan, A.; Sahrmann, P.; Schmidlin, P. R.; Davis, D.; Iheozor-Ejiofor, Z. *Cochrane Database Syst. Rev.* **2014**, *3*, CD005620.
2. Brunthaler, A.; Konig, F.; Lucas, T.; Sperr, W.; Schedle, A. *Clin. Oral Investig.* **2003**, *7* (2), 63–70.
3. Nedeljkovic, I.; Teughels, W.; De Munck, J.; Van Meerbeek, B.; Van Landuyt, K. L. *Dent. Mater.* **2015**, *31* (11), e247–e77.
4. Ferracane, J. L. *Oper. Dent.* **2008**, *33*(3), 247–257.
5. Bowen, R. L. *J. Am. Dent. Assoc.* **1967**, *74* (3), 439–445.
6. Feilzer, A. J.; De Gee, A. J.; Davidson, C. L. *J. Dent. Res.* **1987**, *66* (11), 1636–1639.
7. Ferracane, J. L.; Hilton, T. J. *Dent. Mater.* **2016**, *32* (1), 1–10.
8. Goncalves, F.; Pfeifer, C. S.; Meira, J. B.; Ballester, R. Y.; Lima, R. G.; Braga, R. R. *Dent. Mater.* **2008**, *24* (5), 645–652.
9. Meira, J. B.; Braga, R. R.; Ballester, R. Y.; Tanaka, C. B.; Versluis, A. *J. Dent. Res.* **2011**, *90* (3), 365–370.
10. Chiang, M. Y.; Giuseppetti, A. A.; Qian, J.; Dunkers, J. P.; Antonucci, J. M.; Schumacher, G. E.; Gibson, S. L. *Dent. Mater.* **2011**, *27* (9), 899–905.
11. Watts, D. C.; Marouf, A. S.; Al-Hindi, A. M. *Dent. Mater.* **2003**, *19* (1), 1–11.
12. Yamamoto, T.; Ferracane, J. L.; Sakaguchi, R. L.; Swain, M. V. *Dent. Mater.* **2009**, *25* (4), 543–550.
13. Yamamoto, T.; Nishide, A.; Swain, M. V.; Ferracane, J. L.; Sakaguchi, R. L.; Momoi, Y. *Acta Biomater.* **2011**, *7* (1), 417–423.
14. Park, J. W.; Ferracane, J. L. *Dent. Mater.* **2005**, *21* (9), 882–889.
15. Kinomoto, Y.; Torii, M. *J. Dentist.* **1998**, *26* (2), 165–171.

16. Kinomoto, Y.; Torii, M.; Takeshige, F.; Ebisu, S. *J. Dentist.* **1999**, *27*(5), 383–389.
17. Braga, R. R.; Koplin, C.; Yamamoto, T.; Tyler, K.; Ferracane, J. L.; Swain, M. V. *Dent. Mater.* **2013**, *29*(10), 1026–1033.
18. Witzel, M. F.; Ballester, R. Y.; Meira, J. B.; Lima, R. G.; Braga, R. R. *Dent. Mater.* **2007**, *23*(2), 204–210.
19. Boaro, L. C.; Meira, J. B.; Ballester, R. Y.; Braga, R. R. *Dent. Mater.* **2013**, *29*(10), 1034–1039.
20. Condon, J. R.; Ferracane, J. L. *Dent. Mater.* **1998**, *14*(4), 256–260.
21. Charton, C.; Colon, P.; Pla, F. *Dent. Mater.* **2007**, *23*(8), 911–920.
22. Boaro, L. C.; Goncalves, F.; Braga, R. R. *Acta Biomater.* **2010**, *6*(2), 547–551.
23. Ferracane, J. L.; Mitchem, J. C. *Am. J. Dent.* **2003**, *16*(4), 239–243.
24. Calheiros, F. C.; Sadek, F. T.; Braga, R. R.; Cardoso, P. E. *J. Dentist.* **2004**, *32*(5), 407–412.
25. Boaro, L. C.; Froes-Salgado, N. R.; Gajewski, V. E.; Bicalho, A. A.; Valdivia, A. D.; Soares, C. J.; Miranda Junior, W. G.; Braga, R. R. *Dent. Mater.* **2014**, *30*(9), 984–992.
26. Feilzer, A. J.; de Gee, A. J.; Davidson, C. L., *J. Dent. Res.* **1990**, *69*(1), 36–39.
27. Lovell, L. G.; Newman, S. M.; Bowman, C. N., *J. Dent. Res.* **1999**, *78*(8), 1469–1476.
28. Bowen, R. L., *J. Am. Dent. Assoc.* **1963**, *66*, 57–64.
29. Davidson, C. L.; Feilzer, A. J., *J. Dentist.* **1997**, *25*(6), 435–440.
30. Braga, R. R.; Ferracane, J. L., *J. Dent. Res.* **2002**, *81*(2), 114–118.
31. Watts, D. C.; Cash, A. J. *Dent. Mater.* **1991**, *7*(4), 281–287.
32. Braga, R. R.; Ferracane, J. L. *Crit. Rev. Oral Biol. Med.* **2004**, *15*(3), 176–184.
33. Boaro, L. C.; Goncalves, F.; Guimaraes, T. C.; Ferracane, J. L.; Versluis, A.; Braga, R. R. *Dent. Mater.* **2010**, *26*(12), 1144–1150.
34. Boaro, L. C.; Goncalves, F.; Guimaraes, T. C.; Ferracane, J. L.; Pfeifer, C. S.; Braga, R. R. *Dent. Mater.* **2013**, *29*(4), 398–404.
35. Tarumi, H. T. M.; Tsuchitani, Y. *Dent. Mater. J.* **1995**, *14*(1), 8.
36. Goncalves, F.; Kawano, Y.; Braga, R. R. *Dent. Mater.* **2010**, *26*(7), 704–709.

37. Goncalves, F.; Azevedo, C. L.; Ferracane, J. L.; Braga, R. R. *Dent. Mater.* **2011**, *27* (6), 520–526.
38. Helvatjoglu-Antoniades, M.; Papadogiannis, Y.; Lakes, R. S.; Dionysopoulos, P.; Papadogiannis, D. *Dent. Mater.* **2006**, *22* (5), 450–459.
39. Floyd, C. J.; Dickens, S. H. *Dent. Mater.* **2006**, *22* (12), 1143–1149.
40. Charton, C.; Falk, V.; Marchal, P.; Pla, F.; Colon, P. *Dent. Mater.* **2007**, *23* (11), 1447–1159.
41. Peutzfeldt, A. *Eur. J. Oral Sci.* **1997**, *105* (2), 97–116.
42. Braga, R. R.; Yamamoto, T.; Tyler, K.; Boaro, L. C.; Ferracane, J. L.; Swain, M. V. *Dent. Mater.* **2012**, *28* (6), 632–641.
43. Goncalves, F.; Pfeifer, C. S.; Ferracane, J. L.; Braga, R. R. *J. Dent. Res.* **2008**, *87* (4), 367–371.
44. Goncalves, F.; Pfeifer, C. C.; Stansbury, J. W.; Newman, S. M.; Braga, R. R. *Dent. Mater.* **2010**, *26* (7), 697–703.
45. Dickens, S. H.; Flaim, G. M.; Takagi, S. *Dent. Mater.* **2003**, *19* (6), 558–566.
46. Ferracane, J. L.; Greener, E. H. *J. Biomed. Mater. Res.* **1986**, *20* (1), 121–131.
47. Calheiros, F. C.; Daronch, M.; Rueggeberg, F. A.; Braga, R. R. *J. Biomed. Mater. Res.* **2008**, *84* (2), 503–509.
48. Braga, R. R.; Ballester, R. Y.; Ferracane, J. L. *Dent. Mater.* **2005**, *21* (10), 962–970.
49. Stansbury, J. W.; Dickens, S. H. *Dent. Mater.* **2001**, *17* (1), 71–79.
50. Braga, R. R.; Ferracane, J. L.; Condon, J. R. *J. Dentist.* **2002**, *30* (7–8), 333–340.
51. Versluis, A.; Tantbirojn, D.; Pintado, M. R.; DeLong, R.; Douglas, W. H. *Dent. Mater.* **2004**, *20* (6), 554–564.
52. Yoshikawa, T.; Burrow, M. F.; Tagami, J. *J. Adh. Dentist.* **2001**, *3* (2), 177–183.
53. Lutz, E.; Krejci, I.; Oldenburg, T. R. *Quintessence Int.* **1986**, *17* (12), 777–184.
54. Costa Pfeifer, C. S.; Braga, R. R.; Cardoso, P. E. *J. Am. Dent. Assoc.* **2006**, *137* (2), 197–202.
55. Braga, R. R.; Boaro, L. C.; Kuroe, T.; Azevedo, C. L.; Singer, J. M. *Dent. Mater.* **2006**, *22* (9), 818–823.

56. Bicalho, A. A.; Pereira, R. D.; Zanatta, R. F.; Franco, S. D.; Tantbirojn, D.; Versluis, A.; Soares, C. J. *Oper. Dent.* **2014**, *39* (2), E71–E82.
57. van Dijken, J. W. *J. Dentist.* **2010**, *38* (6), 469–474.
58. Van Meerbeek, B.; Willems, G.; Celis, J. P.; Roos, J. R.; Braem, M.; Lambrechts, P.; Vanherle, G. *J. Dent. Res.* **1993**, *72* (10), 1434–1442.
59. Armstrong, S. R.; Keller, J. C.; Boyer, D. B. *Dent. Mater.* **2001**, *17* (3), 268–276.
60. Mantri, S. P.; Mantri, S. S. *J. Esthet. Restor. Dentist.* **2013**, *25* (5), 305–313.
61. Alster, D.; Feilzer, A. J.; de Gee, A. J.; Davidson, C. L. *Dent. Mater.* **1997**, *13* (3), 146–150.
62. Peutzfeldt, A.; Asmussen, E., *Oper. Dent.* **2002**, *27* (6), 569–575.
63. Jain, P.; Belcher, M. *Am. J. Dent.* **2000**, *13* (5), 235–238.
64. Ernst, C. P.; Canbek, K.; Aksogan, K.; Willershausen, B. *Clin. Oral Investig.* **2003**, *7* (3), 129–134.
65. Lindberg, A.; van Dijken, J. W.; Horstedt, P. *Clin. Oral Investig.* **2005**, *9* (2), 77–83.
66. Bayne, S. C.; Thompson, J. Y.; Swift, E. J., Jr.; Stamatiades, P.; Wilkerson, M. *J. Am. Dent. Assoc.* **1998**, *129* (5), 567–577.
67. Cadenaro, M.; Marchesi, G.; Antoniolli, F.; Davidson, C.; De Stefano Dorigo, E.; Breschi, L. *Dent. Mater.* **2009**, *25* (5), 649–654.
68. Labella, R.; Lambrechts, P.; Van Meerbeek, B.; Vanherle, G. *Dent. Mater.* **1999**, *15* (2), 128–137.
69. Braga, R. R.; Hilton, T. J.; Ferracane, J. L. *J. Am. Dent. Assoc.* **2003**, *134* (6), 721–728.
70. Kemp-Scholte, C. M.; Davidson, C. L. *J. Dent. Res.* **1990**, *69* (6), 1240–1243.
71. Choi, K. K.; Condon, J. R.; Ferracane, J. L. *J. Dent. Res.* **2000**, *79* (3), 812–817.
72. Alster, D.; Feilzer, A. J.; De Gee, A. J.; Davidson, C. L. *J. Dent. Res.* **1995**, *74* (11), 1745–1748.
73. McLean, J. W.; Powis, D. R.; Prosser, H. J.; Wilson, A. D. *British Dent. J.* **1985**, *158* (11), 410–414.
74. Kemp-Scholte, C. M.; Davidson, C. L. *J. Prosthetic Dentist.* **1990**, *64* (6), 658–664.

75. Alomari, Q. D.; Reinhardt, J. W.; Boyer, D. B. *Oper. Dent.* **2001**, *26* (4), 406–411.
76. Dauvillier, B. S.; Feilzer, A. J.; De Gee, A. J.; Davidson, C. L. *J. Dent. Res.* **2000**, *79* (3), 818–823.
77. Lim, B. S.; Ferracane, J. L.; Sakaguchi, R. L.; Condon, J. R. *Dent. Mater.* **2002**, *18* (6), 436–444.
78. Ferracane, J. L. *Dent. Mater.* **2005**, *21* (1), 36–42.
79. Silikas, N.; Eliades, G.; Watts, D. C. *Dent. Mater.* **2000**, *16* (4), 292–296.
80. Bouschlicher, M. R.; Rueggeberg, F. A. *J. Esthet. Dentist.* **2000**, *12* (6), 328–339.
81. Bouschlicher, M. R.; Rueggeberg, F. A.; Boyer, D. B. *J. Esthet. Dentist.* **2000**, *12* (1), 23–32.
82. Pfeifer, C. S.; Braga, R. R.; Ferracane, J. L. *Oper. Dent.* **2006**, *31* (5), 610–615.
83. Lu, H.; Stansbury, J. W.; Bowman, C. N. *Dent. Mater.* **2004**, *20* (10), 979–986.
84. Chan, D. C.; Browning, W. D.; Frazier, K. B.; Brackett, M. G. *Oper. Dent.* **2008**, *33* (3), 265–271.
85. Ernst, C. P.; Kurschner, R.; Rippin, G.; Willershausen, B. *Am. J. Dent.* **2000**, *13* (2), 69–72.
86. Witzel, M. F.; Calheiros, F. C.; Goncalves, F.; Kawano, Y.; Braga, R. R. *J. Dentist.* **2005**, *33* (9), 773–779.
87. Aguiar, F. H.; Ajudarte, K. F.; Lovadino, J. R. *Oper. Dent.* **2002**, *27* (6), 557–562.
88. Brackett, W. W.; Covey, D. A.; St Germain, H. A., Jr. *Oper. Dent.* **2002**, *27* (3), 218–222.
89. Hofmann, N.; Siebrecht, C.; Hugo, B.; Klaiber, B. *Oper. Dent.* **2003**, *28* (2), 160–167.
90. Asmussen, E.; Peutzfeldt, A. *Acta Odontol. Scand.* **2002**, *60* (3), 146–150.
91. Sakaguchi, R. L.; Berge, H. X. *J. Dentist.* **1998**, *26* (8), 695–700.
92. Goncalves, F.; Calheiros, F. C.; Witzel, M. F.; Kawano, Y.; Braga, R. R. *J. Biomed. Mater. Res.* **2007**, *82* (1), 89–92.
93. Deliperi, S.; Bardwell, D. N., *J. Am. Dent. Assoc.* **2002**, *133* (10), 1387–1398.

94. Yamazaki, P. C.; Bedran-Russo, A. K.; Pereira, P. N.; Wsift, E. J., Jr., *Oper. Dent.* **2006**, *31* (6), 670–676.
95. Park, J.; Chang, J.; Ferracane, J.; Lee, I. B., *Dent. Mater.* **2008**, *24* (11), 1501–1505.
96. Tjan, A. H.; Bergh, B. H.; Lidner, C. *J. Prosth. Dentist.* **1992**, *67* (1), 62–66.
97. Wilson, J. *Oper. Dent.* **1993**, *18* (4), 155–159.
98. Versluis, A.; Douglas, W. H.; Cross, M.; Sakaguchi, R. L. *J. Dent. Res.* **1996**, *75* (3), 871–878.
99. Losche, G. M. *J. Adh. Dentist.* **1999**, *1* (1), 31–39.
100. Lohbauer, U.; Zinelis, S.; Rahiotis, C.; Petschelt, A.; Eliades, G. *Dent. Mater.* **2009**, *25* (4), 514–519.
101. Bagis, Y. H.; Rueggeberg, F. A. *Dent. Mater.* **1997**, *13* (4), 228–232.
102. Daronch, M.; Rueggeberg, F. A.; De Goes, M. F. *J. Dent. Res.* **2005**, *84* (7), 663–667.
103. Calheiros, F. C.; Daronch, M.; Rueggeberg, F. A.; Braga, R. R. *Dent. Mater.* **2014**, *30* (6), 613–618.
104. Daronch, M.; Rueggeberg, F. A.; De Goes, M. F.; Giudici, R. *J. Dent. Res.* **2006**, *85* (1), 38–43.
105. Lucey, S.; Lynch, C. D.; Ray, N. J.; Burke, F. M.; Hannigan, A. *J. Oral Rehabil.* **2010**, *37* (4), 278–282.
106. Blalock, J. S.; Holmes, R. G.; Rueggeberg, F. A. *J. Prosthet. Dentist.* **2006**, *96* (6), 424–432.
107. Froes-Salgado, N. R.; Silva, L. M.; Kawano, Y.; Francci, C.; Reis, A.; Loguercio, A. D. *Dent. Mater.* **2010**, *26* (9), 908–914.
108. Tantbirojn, D.; Chongvisal, S.; Augustson, D. G.; Versluis, A. *Quintessence Int.* **2011**, *42* (3), e51–e9.
109. Karaarslan, E. S.; Usumez, A.; Ozturk, B.; Cebe, M. A. *European J. Dentist.* **2012**, *6* (1), 87–94.
110. Rueggeberg, F. A.; Daronch, M.; Browning, W. D.; MF, D. E. G. *J. Esthet. Restor. Dentist.* **2010**, *22*(5), 314–322.
111. Zach, L.; Cohen, G. *Oral Surg. Oral Med. Oral Path.* **1965**, *19*, 515–530.
112. Daronch, M.; Rueggeberg, F. A.; Hall, G.; De Goes, M. F. *Dent. Mater.* **2007**, *23* (10), 1283–1288.
113. Stansbury, J. W. *Dent. Mater.* **2012**, *28* (1), 13–22.

114. Alster, D.; Feilzer, A. J.; De Gee, A. J.; Mol, A.; Davidson, C. L. *J. Dent. Res.* **1992**, *71* (9), 1619–1622.
115. Ferracane, J. L.; Ferracane, L. L.; Braga, R. R. *J. Biomed. Mater. Res.* **2003**, *66* (1), 318–323.
116. Moraes, R. R.; Garcia, J. W.; Barros, M. D.; Lewis, S. H.; Pfeifer, C. S.; Liu, J.; Stansbury, J. W. *Dent. Mater.* **2011**, *27* (6), 509–519.
117. Tian, M.; Gao, Y.; Liu, Y.; Liao, Y.; Hedin, N. E.; Fong, H. *Dent. Mater.* **2008**, *24* (2), 235–243.
118. Ilie, N.; Jelen, E.; Clementino-Luedemann, T.; Hickel, R. *Dent. Mater. J* **2007**, *26* (2), 149–155.
119. Eick, J. D.; Kotha, S. P.; Chappelow, C. C.; Kilway, K. V.; Giese, G. J.; Glaros, A. G.; Pinzino, C. S. *Dent. Mater.* **2007**, *23* (8), 1011–1017.
120. Papadogiannis, D.; Kakaboura, A.; Palaghias, G.; Eliades, G. *Dent. Mater.* **2009**, *25* (12), 1509–1516.
121. Ilie, N.; Hickel, R. *Dent. Mater.* **2011**, *27* (4), 348–355.
122. Sideridou, I. D.; Vouvoudi, E. C.; Keridou, I. V. *Dent. Mater.* **2015**, *31* (9), e179–e189.
123. Bracho-Troconis, C.; Trujillo-Lemon, M.; Boulden, J.; Wong, N.; Wall, K.; Esquibel, K. *Compendium Contin. Edu. Dentist.* **2010**, *31* (Special Issue 2), 5–9.
124. Moorthy, A.; Hogg, C. H.; Dowling, A. H.; Grufferty, B. F.; Benetti, A. R.; Fleming, G. J. *J. Dentist.* **2012**, *40* (6), 500–505.
125. El-Damanhoury, H.; Platt, J. *Oper. Dent.* **2014**, *39* (4), 374–382.
126. Benetti, A. R.; Havndrup-Pedersen, C.; Honore, D.; Pedersen, M. K.; Pallesen, U. *Oper. Dent.* **2015**, *40* (2), 190–200.
127. Zorzin, J.; Maier, E.; Harre, S.; Fey, T.; Belli, R.; Lohbauer, U.; Petschelt, A.; Taschner, M. *Dent. Mater.* **2015**, *31* (3), 293–301.
128. Bailey, W. J. *J. Macromol. Sci. Chem. A* **1975**, *9*, 16.
129. Eick, J. D.; Byerley, T. J.; Chappell, R. P.; Chen, G. R.; Bowles, C. Q.; Chappelow, C. C. *Dent. Mater.* **1993**, *9* (2), 123–127.
130. Stansbury, J. W. *J. Dent. Res.* **1992**, *71* (7), 1408–1412.
131. Manojlovic, D.; Dramicanin, M. D.; Milosevic, M.; Zekovic, I.; Cvijovic-Alagic, I.; Mitrovic, N.; Miletic, V. *Mater. Sci. Eng. C* **2016**, *58*, 487–494.
132. Podgorski, M.; Becka, E.; Claudino, M.; Flores, A.; Shah, P. K.; Stansbury, J. W.; Bowman, C. N. *Dent. Mater.* **2015**, *31* (11), 1255–1262.

133. Santerre, J. P.; Shajii, L.; Leung, B. W. *Crit. Rev. Oral Biol. Med.* **2001**, *12* (2), 136–151.
134. Suiter, E. A.; Watson, L. E.; Tantbirojn, D.; Lou, J. S.; Versluis, A. *J. Dent. Res.* **2016**, *95* (5), 543–549.
135. Versluis, A.; Tantbirojn, D.; Lee, M. S.; Tu, L. S.; DeLong, R. *Dent. Mater.* **2011**, *27* (2), 126–133.
136. Segura, A.; Donly, K. J. *J. Oral Rehabil.* **1993**, *20* (5), 495–499.
137. Ruttermann, S.; Kruger, S.; Raab, W. H.; Janda, R. *J. Dentist.* **2007**, *35* (10), 806–813.
138. Meriwether, L. A.; Blen, B. J.; Benson, J. H.; Hatch, R. H.; Tantbirojn, D.; Versluis, A. *Dent. Mater.* **2013**, *29* (5), 573–579.
139. Park, J. W.; Ferracane, J. L. *J. Dent. Res.* **2014**, *93* (2), 195–200.

Chapter 13

Flexible Impression Materials

Charlene S. Solomon

Department Restorative Dentistry, University of Manitoba, 780 Bannatyne Avenue, Winnipeg, MB, R3E 0W2, Canada

charlene.solomon@umanitoba.ca

Flexible dental impression materials form an integral part of daily clinical practice. It allows for the making of accurate impressions or a negative replica of the mouth and oral structures. These flexible impression materials are mostly selected based on their physicochemical properties and applications. A thorough knowledge of impression material classifications and their respective properties allows for an educated and evidenced-based decision for impression materials selection. The various classes of flexible impression materials commercially available allow for a wide range of clinical practice applications from routine diagnostic impressions to precision impression for intricate fixed restorative procedures. Although the desirable physicochemical properties of flexible impression materials are well researched and documented, impression materials continue to evolve to meet the demands of improved and advanced dental and clinical practice technologies. Newer contemporary hybrid impression materials emerged in the early 2000s combining the best properties of an economical alginate impression material with the accuracy of an elastomeric impression material. This chapter focuses on the history and development of the different flexible impression materials, elaborating on specific physicochemical properties for each class of flexible impression material.

1. Introduction

Flexible impression material forms a foundational and integral component of everyday clinical dental practice. Dental practitioners use flexible impression materials to make accurate impressions of the oral tissues to make a gypsum stone model, which serves as a positive replica of the oral structures. The gypsum stone models can be easily and conveniently manipulated on a bench top to evaluate, modify, and be used to fabricate an indirect oral prosthesis. Indirect prostheses can be fixed, meaning crowns or bridges that are permanently fixated to the natural teeth or implants or it can be removable referring to complete or partial dentures, mouth guards, bruxism splints, and orthodontic appliances.

Impression materials have evolved over time as the esthetic and implant realm of dentistry saw new technologies and techniques emerge for the fabrication of intricate and often complex indirect prostheses. More specifically, dental impressions evolved from labor-intensive, technique-sensitive procedures to simplified-impression techniques with user-friendly and accurate impression materials. Clinical practice demands impression materials with high accuracy, dimensional stability, and hydrophilicity. In addition, the clinical practice setting benefits from materials that can be manipulated and handled with efficiency. This relates to the dispensing technique, patient acceptance, and ease of cleanup of the materials.

Research on flexible impression materials has focused mainly on *in vitro* material properties testing as a function of its clinical requirements.[1–4] This chapter provides a broad overview of flexible impression materials, its classification, history, and its physical properties as it relates to impression making in clinical dental practice.

1.1. *History*

The history and development of flexible dental impressions started in the 20th century, known as the era of innovations and technology.

This era in the dental realm started with the introduction of the porcelain jacket crown by Charles Land in 1903, and the introduction of the lost wax technique by William Taggart in 1907. This was the start of fabrication of direct and indirect fixed restorations. The historical development of impression materials was founded in the development of impression materials for mostly complete dentures.[5]

The first successful flexible impression materials introduced to dentistry were the aqueous reversible agar hydrocolloids in the 1930s. The agar material sets in a flexible gel form and allowed for accurate recording of undercuts. The agar hydrocolloids were an improvement to the waxes, plaster, and compound materials that were available at the time.[6–8] Sears introduced agar hydrocolloids into fixed prosthodontics in 1937,[9,10] and it became the standard of excellence for impression making. The agar material was the same material that bacteriologists used in their petri dishes.[6] The making of an agar hydrocolloid impression requires equipment such as a conditioning unit[9] to convert the agar gel form to a liquid state and special water cooling impression trays.[6] Its clinical application was initially limited to removable partial dentures until Sears introduced a different technique whereby reversible hydrocolloids can be used for inlays, crown, and bridges.[7]

A second aqueous, but irreversible alginate hydrocolloid flexible impression material was introduced during World War II, at a time when agar hydrocolloids were scarce. This was due to the fact that most of the processing of the algae used for the manufacturing of agar-agar at the time was done in Japan.[5–7] The processing of a native brown algae yielded a new flexible aqueous impression material with an alginate base. The introduction of alginate impression materials became a desirable and convenient alternative impression material. In contrast to agar hydrocolloids, the making of an alginate impression requires no special equipment or special impressions trays, and it involves a simple mixing of powder and liquid components. Its physical properties allowed a controlled setting process with the material exhibiting toughness and resiliency.[7]

The first non-aqueous flexible material introduced was the polysulfides in 1953.[11] It provided greater strength and stability than the hydrocolloids and was popular in its application for completed denture impressions. The 1960s saw the introduction of two more non-aqueous impression materials in fixed prosthodontics, namely the condensation silicones and polyethers. These non-aqueous materials had a rubber-like consistency, were user-friendly, and easier to manipulate and clean up than the polysulfides. The polyethers provided a significant improvement in dimensional stability and accuracy by means of its improved mechanical properties. The significance of this material is that it maintained its high accuracy and competitiveness with other elastomers well into the 21st century with improvement in delivery mechanisms. The condensation silicones were less stable than polyethers as it polymerized by means of a condensation reaction, forming a by-product affecting the accuracy of the final set material (see Table 1).

The next significant development in the history of flexible impression materials was the development of addition type silicones (vinyl-polysiloxanes or VPS) as part of the Apollo space program[7] in the 1970s. The VPS impression materials became the impression material of choice for fabrication of high-precision prosthesis such as crowns and bridges. It has superior dimensional stability compared to its predecessors, but comparative to polyethers.

The 21st century saw the introduction of flexible hybrid impression materials, specifically alginate–silicone and VPS–polyether combinations. These hybrid materials provide unique impression properties that combine the benefits of a low-cost impression material with the high-dimensional accuracy of another.

Currently, the alginate hydrocolloids, addition-type silicone, and polyethers are the most common flexible materials used for advanced restorative procedures in clinical dental practice.

Table 1. History timeline for flexible dental impression materials

1937	Reversible hydrocolloids, agar
1943	Irreversible hydrocolloids, alginates
1953	Polysulfides
1960s	Condensation Silicone
1965	Polyether
1970	Addition Silicone
2000s	Hybrid Impression materials

2. Classification

Flexible dental impression materials can be classified according to its chemistry, mechanical properties, viscosity, or applications. Dentists learn and identify dental materials mainly by their chemical composition. Different chemistries bring about a specific set of characteristics that may be suitable for a specific dental application. Figure 1 categorizes flexible materials by chemistry, broadly classified into aqueous and non-aqueous impression materials including the newer hybrid impression material varieties.

The aqueous impression materials are natural polymers and consist of two main groups, the reversible and irreversible hydrocolloids. The non-aqueous impression materials are synthetic polymers and also referred to as elastomers. The term elastomer refers to a polymer that has viscoelastic properties. Both aqueous and non-aqueous impression materials groups are elastic and flexible, but only the synthetic polymers are referred to as elastomers.

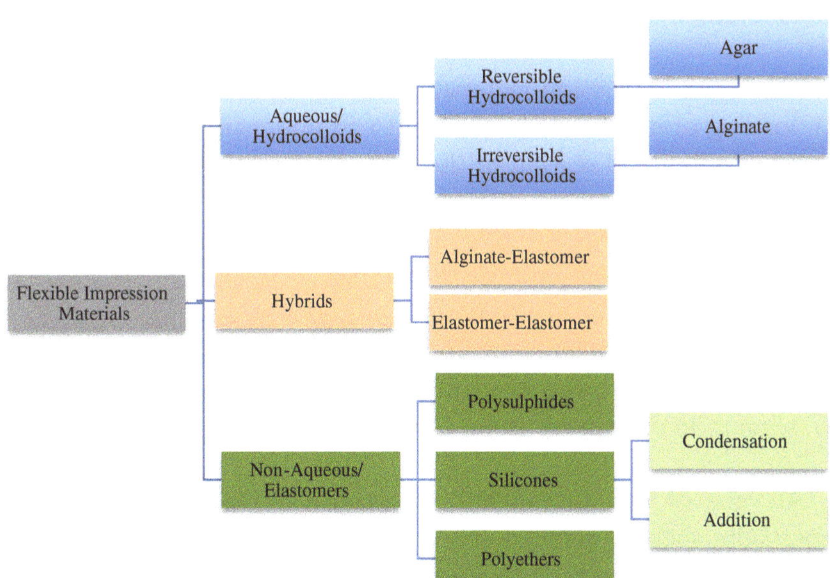

Figure 1. Classification of flexible impression materials

Hybrid impression materials are grouped into two main chemistries. One hybrid group consists of an alginate–elastomer combination, and a second hybrid group consists of exclusively elastomer combinations.

3. Flexible Impression Material Properties

The most important characteristics for flexible impression materials are its accuracy and elasticity. The accurate recording of the contours of teeth and supporting structures demands a material that flows into cervices and over contours, capturing intricate tooth preparation details and sets without distortion. Similarly, the material should flow and engage to the full depth of tooth and soft tissues undercuts and withdraw from those undercuts without distortion or tearing. It should also be capable of being disinfected without affecting its set properties and must maintain its dimensional accuracy.

A thorough knowledge and understanding of impression material properties at every stage of the clinical and laboratory processes is key for an accurate final outcome of the clinical procedure. The life of a flexible dental impression involves the following sequenced clinical and laboratory steps:

(1) mixing of impression material,
(2) loading of impression material into an impression tray,
(3) positioning and seating of the loaded impression tray inside the mouth,
(4) setting of the impression material,
(5) removal of the set impression material,
(6) disinfection,
(7) transportation to a dental laboratory,
(8) pouring of a gypsum stone into dental impression,
(9) separation of gypsum stone cast from dental impression.

At each of the aforementioned stages in the life of a dental impression, specific material characteristics and qualities are desired to achieve an overarching goal of making an exceptionally accurate final prosthesis on the final gypsum stone model. Table 2 summarizes

Table 2. Desirable impression material properties at impression making

Stages of impression making	Desired material properties
Mixing	Ease of manipulation
Loading of impression tray	Biocompatibility Suitable viscosity Flow & Flexibility
Intraoral positioning and seating of the loaded impression tray	Flow and flexibility Hydrophilicity/Wettability Accuracy Biocompatible
Setting	Accuracy Dimensional stability
Removal of the set material	Elastic recovery Flexibility Tear strength Dimensional stability
Disinfection	Biocompatibility Dimensional stability
Transportation/Delayed pouring	Dimensional stability
Pouring of a stone model	Wettability Accuracy Biocompatibility Dimensional stability
Removal of set stone model	Elastic recovery Flexibility Tear strength Dimensional stability

the desired properties of the impression material at every stage in the clinical and laboratory processes.

3.1. *Ease of Manipulation*

The ease by which flexible impression materials can be handled and manipulated plays a crucial role in the everyday dynamics of a busy dental office. Manufacturers continue to improve formulations and dispensing methods for maximum efficiency at the chairside.

Irreversible hydrocolloids are powder and liquid systems that are mainly hand mixed, but semi-automatic mixing techniques are available to enhance mixing and provide a smoother material consistency. These powder formulations may be color-coded; the material changes color during mixing to indicate timing of tray loading and prevents the overspatulation of material.

Most elastomeric impression materials are dispensed with automated systems and mixing tips for efficiency and void-free mixes.[12] Its benefits include reduced contamination, and it eliminates voids,[12–14] and produces less wastage[15] as is often seen with spatulation methods. The auto-mixing allow ease of dispensing by injecting material directly around critical tooth preparations and into the custom tray. Auto-mixing saves time by eliminating the need for cleaning of mixing bowls and spatulas. Auto-mixing is the preferred mixing technique for dentists, dental students, and dental assistants[16] allowing an improved workability compared to hand mixing.

3.2. *Accuracy*

Accuracy of dental impressions is measured in two ways. First, it has to meet a specific standard as determined by the American Dental Association (ADA) and the International Standards Organization (ISO). The ADA specification #19 for elastomeric materials states that this materials should be able to record fine details of up to 25 μm.[17] The International Standards Organization (ISO) for dental elastomeric materials classifies a Type III impression material as one that can produce a line of 0.020 mm in width.[18]

Second, accuracy is measured as a function of dimensional stability by measuring tooth-to-tooth dimensions within the same arch and in the cross-arch.[17] This is a function of how accurate the material can produce a copy of the oral structures. The majority of impression materials today provide excellent accuracy when used correctly.

3.2.1. *Elastic Recovery*

Dental impressions are typically subjected to compressive and tensile forces upon seating and removal of the impression. This is inevitable as impression material often engages into soft or hard tissue undercuts. The maximum tensile strain tend to be greater than the maximum compressive force.[19] The ISO 4823 standard for elastomeric material specifies elastic recovery from a 30% compressive strain, although the validity of using compressive strain rather than tensile strain has been questioned.[19] This is termed as elastic recovery, and no impression material has absolute 100% elastic recovery.[17]

3.2.2. *Dimensional Stability*

The ability of a dental impression to be accurate and maintain its form and dimension over a period of time is critical to provide an accurate and predictable final impression. Dental practitioners who discerningly embrace contemporary dental manufacturing technology and materials may need to courier their dental impressions to out of province or out of state locations to access specific technologies. Courier services could involve more than a 24 h delay in pouring of the impression. This clinical reality demands an impression material with high dimensional stability.

Dimensional change can be affected by: (1) polymerization shrinkage, (2) loss of a condensation reaction by-product such as water or alcohol, (3) thermal contraction from oral temperature to room temperature, (4) absorption of water or disinfectant over time, (5) incomplete recovery of deformation.[20] Vinyl polysiloxane impression material possesses ideal dimensional stability as it forms no by-product upon setting, and pouring of impressions can be delayed for hours, days, and even weeks after making the final impression.[17]

3.3. *Flow Properties/Rheological Properties*

The ability of an impression material to flow is referred to as its rheological properties. Flow properties allow impression materials to move into microspaces in the oral cavity and record minute details such as grooves, tooth–gingiva interfaces, and beveled tooth margins. A low viscosity impression material flows readily to accurately capture intricate details. A medium body or heavy viscosity impression materials flows less, but accurately captures macrostructures such as tooth contour and arch form. When used in combination, the medium or heavy viscosity materials provide the overall support for the impression, while the light body records finer details.

3.4. *Flexibility*

Flexibility refers to the stiffness or rigidity of a material. Ideal flexibility allows the dental impression material to be easily removed from undercuts in the mouth without any discomfort. It should also have sufficient rigidity to withstand any tearing or distortion. At the same time, it should support the ease of removal of the gypsum stone cast when separated from the impression.

3.5. *Wettability/Hydrophilicity*

The mouth is a moist environment, and the properties of wettability and hydrophilicity are important for accurate impressions. Hydrophilicity is the affinity for water, and the wettability of an impression material is the ability to flow and adhere onto solid surfaces. Wettability allows for ease of flow and an intimate contact between tooth structures and the impression material.[21] At the same time, also allow ease of wettability by water-containing gypsum material when pouring a stone cast. Inadequate wetting of an impression is characterized by the incorporation of voids and bubbles in stone casts.[22,23] Voids are typically seen on critical areas of stone cast such as preparation margins and grooves.

Wettability of an impression material is a function of the contact angle formed between the surface of the wetted solid and tangential to the curved drop at the point of contact. A small angle (less than 90°C) indicates good wettability[22] and large angles indicate a poor affinity[24] or low wettability.

3.6. *Biocompatibility*

Biocompatibility refers to a material's ability to maintain accuracy and dimensional stability when coming into contact with other materials. This would include operator gloves, disinfection products, gypsum stone, and clinical medicaments.

3.7. *Tear Strength*

For dental impression making, the material that engages in interdental and subgingival areas are often thin and of a low viscosity variety. This makes it particularly prone to tearing upon removal. The amount of force needed to tear a specific material divided by the thickness of the material is termed tear strength.[20]

4. Aqueous Hydrocolloid Impression Materials

The two main groups of aqueous materials are the reversible agar hydrocolloids and the irreversible alginate hydrocolloids. The reversible agar impression material has largely been replaced with irreversible alginate materials today, but is included here for completeness.

4.1. *Agar/Reversible Hydrocolloids*

When Sears introduced reversible hydrocolloids in 1937,[9,10] it soon became the standard of care for impressions for indirect restorations.[6] At that time, it was regarded as the best impression material for detailed and precision impressions. Its applications were for full arch or quadrant impressions without deep undercuts.[25]

4.1.1. *Composition*

Agar hydrocolloids are complex polysaccharides that are extracted from seaweed. The agar hydrocolloid materials exist in two forms; a gel and a sol form. The sol form comprises a random arrangement of polysaccharide chains, and the gel form represents organized and aligned polysaccharide chains. Agar impression materials are supplied in tubes in a gel form, which is viscous and flexible. The sol state is fluid with a low viscosity. Its main ingredients are agar as a gelling agent, borax to improve strength, potassium sulfate for dental stone compatibility, and alkylbenzoates as preservatives.[25] The water content is as high as 80%, and the agar content on average may be 15%.[6]

4.1.2. *Manipulation and Properties*

Heat applied to agar hydrocolloid converts its gel form to a sol state with a consistency suitable for dental impressions. Cooling of the sol state reverts the material back to a viscous gel state. Special temperature-controlled water baths are needed for the liquefaction of the gel state, and special water-cooling impression trays are needed to solidify the sol agar intraorally. The water baths have three sections that accommodate three different temperatures for liquefaction, storage, and tempering of the agar. The water cooling metal stock trays consist of narrow-diameter metal tubing attached to the outside of the tray, which in turn can be attached to a water supply inlet. The gel is converted to a liquid state by boiling it at 100°C for about 10 min. The agar is then placed in the storage unit of the water bath at 65–68°C for a ready-to-use consistency. At impression making, the material is tempered at 46°C for two minutes and loaded into the impression cooling trays. The flow of cold water (18–21°C) around the periphery of the tray cools the material and supports the conversion from sol to gel state. Bear in mind that this water-cooling effect takes place while the impression tray is seated intraorally, making this a more complex impression technique.

Agar hydrocolloid impressions exhibit a high degree of accuracy and detail, producing a high quality and precise indirect dental casting. This can be attributed to its fluid sol state and true hydrophilic property,[17] allowing it to flow better and record fine details more accurately.

Agar impressions should be poured immediately to avoid the loss of water during storage (syneresis) or absorption of water (imbibition). The minimum storage time for agar impressions is 1 h in 100%

relative humidity. It has poor mechanical properties and low tear resistance. It is an inexpensive material with no unpleasant taste or odor. The main drawbacks of agar impression materials are that they need specialized equipment, are dimensionally unstable, and the dental impression can only be used for single casts.[25] In addition, the water cooling trays are fairly bulky to place due to the additional metal water channels attached.

4.2. *Alginate/Irreversible Hydrocolloids*

Alginate hydrocolloids are the workhorse impression material for routine diagnostic impressions in most dental practices. It is generally well tolerated by patients and economical.[26] It is mostly supplied as a powdered alginate material mixed with water to produce a creamy consistency for dental impressions. It is supplied in a two-paste system too,[26] also known as modified alginates.[20] Based on its composition, the consistency, setting time, color, and taste may vary between manufacturers. It is available in both regular and fast setting times.

4.2.1. *Composition*

Alginates are extracted from seaweed and supplied in a powder form. The alginate powder is the sodium or potassium salt of alginic acid that is easily soluble in water. It has calcium sulfate as a reacting agent and sodium phosphate as a retarder. The bulk of the powder contains inorganic fillers (zinc, talc, diatomaceous earth), which determines the flow properties and strength of the set alginate. The diatomaceous earth contains silica particles that can become airborne during fluffing of the powder, risking inhalation of fine silica particles.[20] A dustless alginate is available with additional glycol components that make the alginate powder denser and less able to become airborne.

The final alginate impressions consist of approximately 80% of water, which makes it susceptible to distortion if water is lost (by syneresis) or water is absorbed (by imbibition).[27] The time delay between making the impression and pouring a gypsum cast and the manner of storage is critical to avoid these two phenomena of syneresis or imbibition from occurring.

4.2.2. *Manipulation and Properties*

The alginate powder tends to settle with storage and may affect the final water:powder ratios at the time of mixing. It is recommended that stored alginate powder be shaken or fluffed before mixing to aerate and allow for an even distribution of its constituents. Special powder scoops and water measuring cups are used to ensure accurate powder:water ratios. Mixing of the powder and water is done at room temperature, with the wet alginate mixture being pressed against the side of a rubber mixing bowl to eliminate any air entrapment during mixing. Automated rotating mixing bowls can provide an automated mixing technique producing less air bubbles in the set material.[28] Automated mixing techniques also produce a more homogenous mix with a reduced working time.[28] Slower or faster setting times can also be manipulated by using either cooler or warmer water, respectively.[29]

Alginate impression material demonstrate maximum accuracy when it has a cross-sectional thickness of 4–6 mm.[17] The use of appropriate sized stock trays allows for this bulk of thickness for alginate impression material. A perforated impression tray further secures the impression material to avoid separation of the set material from the tray during impression removal. Alginate tray adhesive is recommended for non-perforated trays.[20]

Setting of alginate impression material occurs within two minutes, and upon removal, the saliva is rinsed off under running water and then disinfected by means of a spray technique. Traditionally, these impressions are to be poured immediately or within 30 min of making the impression. The extended-time alginates were shown to exhibit dimensional stability for up to 100 h.[27]

The dimensional stability of alginate impression materials is a key function of its chemical composition. Aqueous impression materials contain 80% water and are particularly sensitive to distortion by either evaporation of its water content (syneresis) or the absorption of water (imbibition). Therefore, the general recommendation is that alginate impression material be poured immediately to avoid the phenomena of syneresis or imbibition to occur. There is no clear evidence on the dimensional stability of alginate impression materials as a function of the pouring time[30] and storage time for that matter. However, casts produced from alginate impressions stored in 100% relative humidity at different storage times for up to 5 days showed no difference in surface detail production and dimensional accuracy.[31]

4.3. *Hybrids/Alginate Alternatives*

Alginate impression material has been modified by the incorporation of silicone polymers[32] to function as alginate alternatives (AA) with comparable function and applications of alginates, but with improved stability and ease of mixing and dispensing of silicones. These materials have been referred to as alginate alternatives, alginate substitutes, or a hybrid impression material.

There appear to be conflicting terminologies based on properties of the AA, with some describing it as a superior alginate alternative and others describing it as a low-cost VPS alternative. Although described as an AA, it is classified as a Type II addition silicone.[34] It is available in one viscosity only, a medium-body addition-type polyvinyl siloxane-based material.[35]

Its cost is considerably more than that of conventional alginates[35] and less than that of vinyl polysiloxanes. A probable explanation for its lower cost is explained by the omission of palladium in the chemical formula.[33] Palladium is an expensive component in conventional vinyl polysiloxanes impression materials that acts as a scavenger for excess hydrogen gas during the setting process.

4.3.1. *Composition*

The term hybrid denotes the combination of alginate and silicone elastomers, providing the ease and economics of alginates but with the quality and stability of an elastomer. Due to the presence of vinyl polysiloxane in alginate alternatives, the testing of the physical properties of AA is measured and assessed in accordance with American National Standards Institute and American Dental Association (ANSI/ADA) No. 19 for elastomeric impression materials.[33] It has shown to reproduce detail (25 μm line) as required by specification No.19 for elastomeric materials, but demonstrating deformation properties of alginates.[36] Although referred to as an alginate alternative, its properties are closely aligned to that of elastomeric materials.

4.3.2. *Manipulation and Properties*

Alginate alternatives are dispensed with auto-mixing technologies that provide a predictable and even consistency with a precise setting time. The additional features of ease of impression making with reduced mixing times, reduced intraoral setting times, and less cleaning-up time compared to traditional alginates are added benefits.

In vitro investigation on the physical properties of AA shows superior performance as regards detail reproduction, gypsum compatibility, and linear dimensional change.[33,34] The improved rheological properties of this material allow it to better capture surface detail when compared to conventional alginates.[34] This property is suggested to be a function of the flow properties of the VPS constituent.[33]

The earlier reports on the first alginate alternatives available showed a material with improved tear and compressive strength but with no improvement in dimensional stability.[37] Subsequent tear strength testing showed AA to reproduce thin intrasulcular and interproximal areas, suggesting higher tear strengths than traditional alginates.[33]

Impressions made with AA exhibit excellent dimensional stability with a 4 h delayed pour when compared to conventional alginate impression material.[35] Some manufactures suggest pouring can be delayed for up to 14 days without loss of accuracy (Alginot by Kerr). The stability of AA impressions not only allows for a delayed pour of the impression but also allows for the making of multiple, accurate diagnostic casts from one impression.[20] The recommendation is that AA be poured 60 min after mixing as the material shows more outgassing with cast porosity when poured immediately.[33]

4.3.3. *Clinical Applications*

Alginate alternative impression material has similar but more widespread clinical applications to the traditional alginate materials. This is mainly due to its properties of increased accuracy and prolonged dimensional stability. It is often marketed as a stable and reliable preliminary impression material for improved productivity. Other applications include opposing dentition models for full arch crown-and-bridge cases, case study models, orthodontic models, retainers and splints, sports guards, and whitening trays. In particular, its function as an accurate template for crown-and-bridge provisional crowns are highlighted.[38]

Due to its stiffness, it may not be suitable for making impression in areas of severe soft tissue undercuts, such as maxillofacial impressions or for teeth that show signs of mobility.

5. Non-Aqueous Elastomeric Impression Materials

Where the aqueous hydrocolloid groups of flexible impression materials are natural polymers, the non-aqueous elastomers are synthetic polymers. Both are elastic and flexible, though the non-aqueous groups are referred to as elastomeric impression materials or elastomers. The elastomers are rubber-like impression materials produced by cross-linked polymers of silicone and oxygen and addition of long chains. This gives it a unique chemistry with superior properties to the aqueous impression materials. It is supplied as two components, a base and catalyst system, that are mixed for impression taking. They are formulated in various consistencies and setting times giving them a wide range of clinical applications. The elastomers attempt to address two main shortcomings associated with hydrocolloid impression materials, namely poor tear resistance and poor dimensional stability. In addition to being easily handled, mostly odorless, and tasteless, elastomers gained quick acceptance within the dental community and became the gold standard for precision impressions.

Chemically, there are three main groups of polymer-based elastomeric impression materials namely (1) Polysulfides (PS), (2) Silicones/ Vinylpolysiloxanes (VPS), both condensation and addition type, and (3) Polyethers (PE). Elastomeric hybrid impression materials are available too, namely vinylpolyether silicone (VPES).

5.1. *Polysulfides*

Polysulfide impression material was the first elastomeric impression material to be introduced in the 1950s and was also referred to as mercaptan or thymol.

5.1.1. *Composition*

The base of this two-paste system contains a polysulfide polymer that contains a multifunctional mercaptan (–SH) polymer, a suitable filler to provide strength, a plasticizer to provide appropriate viscosity, and a small quantity of sulfur (0.5%) to accelerate the reaction. The catalyst paste contains an inert oil to form the paste, sulfur as a catalyst, and lead dioxide that allows for cross-linking and polymerization reaction.[20]

5.1.2. *Manipulation and Properties*

Its clinical advantages include long working time, accuracy, high tear strength, economical, less hydrophobicity, and a longer shelf life. It records details of 25 μm and less, meeting the standard of accuracy as set by the American Dental Association. Polysulfide impression materials have the highest resistance to tearing; however, it is more susceptible to permanent distortion.[20] It exhibits significant radiopacity due to its lead dioxide content.[18,39] This also makes polysulfide one of the most radiopaque impression materials in the market. The radiopacity may be beneficial for the radiographic identification of accidentally swallowed or aspirated impression material.

Polysulfide impression material is a reasonably accurate impression material that provides excellent detail when used with a customized impression tray. However, it needs to be poured within 24 h as there is a significant potential for shrinkage and distortion. Multiple pours are not recommended. A significant drawback is its unpleasant odor due to the lead dioxide content. The base and catalyst pastes are hand mixed, and so it is often described as being messy. It tends to stain clothes due to the presence of the lead dioxide.

5.2. *Silicones*

Silicones are the vinyl polysiloxanes (VPS) of the elastomeric impression materials group. Silicones are generally hydrophobic by nature, and its chemical structure exhibits hydrophobic aliphatic hydrocarbon groups surrounding the siloxane bonds. The addition of surfactants to the elastomeric impression materials changed it from a hydrophobic to a hydrophilic material.[23,40] There are two main types of silicone materials; a condensation-type silicone referred to as C-silicones and an addition-type silicone also referred to as A-silicones.

5.2.1. *Condensation-Type Silicones*

The most important difference between condensation and addition silicones is their dimensional stability. Condensation silicones exhibit dimensional changes after setting due to the formation of by-products. Although not meeting the standard for accurate impression making, C-silicones nonetheless are widely used in other clinical and laboratory procedures.

5.2.1.1. Composition

The formation of condensation silicones (C-silicones) occurs through cross-linking between terminal groups of silicone polymers and an alkyl silicate to form a three-dimensional network.[20] The polymerization process of C-silicones produces ethyl alcohol as a by-product of the condensation setting reaction. The evaporation of the ethyl alcohol is responsible for most of the contraction that occurs during the setting reaction.

5.2.1.2. Manipulation and properties

Condensation silicones are available in a base and catalyst system, which involves a viscous base and a catalyst paste. Accurate dispensing of the base and catalyst components together with vigorous hand mixing by means of folding in of the two components and finger molding produces a smooth rubberlike consistency. Upon setting polymerization, there is some contraction that occurs as a result of the formation of by-products. This make the C-silicones less accurate than its A-silicone counterpart. In addition, C-silicones are hydrophobic in nature, making it less wettable and not advocated for precision impressions in a moist oral environment. Its clinical applications include duplication procedures, the making of customized matrices to make provisional restorations, and its use in a variety of dental laboratory procedures.

5.2.2. *Addition-Type Silicones*

Addition or A-silicones are the most common elastomeric impression material used for precision impressions in dental practice. Its superior properties of accuracy and dimensional stability have significantly increased its use and demand, with it now constituting a significant component of the dental impression material market. Addition silicones are also termed as polyvinyl siloxanes (PVS) or vinyl polysiloxanes (VPS).

5.2.2.1. Composition

Addition silicones (A-silicones) set by means of an addition reaction with no by-product formation. The base paste contains a polymethylhydrosiloxane and a divinylpolysiloxane. The catalyst paste contains divinylpolysiloxane and a platinum salt. The addition reaction occurs between a siloxane with a terminal hydrogen and a siloxane with a terminal vinyl group, forming a cross-linked silicone rubber. Therefore, based on its chemical composition, the commonly used alternative term polyvinylsiloxanes (or VPS) is incorrect.[29]

Hydrogen gas forms during the addition reaction, but does not affects its dimensional stability.[20] This hydrogen gas can produce minute voids in the gypsum model, especially if the impression is poured immediately. Manufacturers add a noble metal such as palladium that acts as a scavenger for the hydrogen gas. A delayed pour of 30 min will allow sufficient time for the hydrogen gas to escape and reduce the risks of potential voids in the gypsum model.

Silicones generally are hydrophobic in nature. To improve its clinical performance, manufactures add a non-ionic surfactant to provide hydrophilic-like properties to the A-silicones. This allows improved wettability of the impression material.

5.2.2.2. Manipulation and properties

The A-silicones are considered to be the most accurate impression material, and apart from the putty viscosity, all other A-silicone viscosities can reproduce fine detail of 0.020 mm in width.[18] The addition silicone impression material is a more dimensional stable material when compared to polysulfide, condensation silicones, and polyether.

Addition silicones are manufactured and available in four different consistencies namely:

(1) Low viscosity
(2) Medium viscosity
(3) High viscosity
(4) Very high viscosity/Putty

The viscosity of an impression material increases with the proportion of filler content,[18,41] meaning low viscosity silicone materials will have a higher flow property.[41] Less filler content and higher flow records fine detail more accurately, but has greater polymerization shrinkage.[17] Higher viscosity impression materials are therefore used in combination with low-viscosity varieties to provide the best outcome for the final impressions. The higher viscosity material is injected into an impression tray and forms the bulk of the impression and provides support for low viscosity material. The low viscosity and higher flow impression material is injected around the intricate tooth preparations and forms the wash that records fine detail. The impression tray with higher viscosity material is then seated intraorally over the preparations covered with low viscosity material and is allowed to set. The high viscosity impression material also pushes the lower viscosity material into the sulcular area and due to its higher filler content, has less polymerization shrinkage.[17] A combination of medium and low viscosity impression material is more accurate than a putty and low viscosity combination.[18]

Silicones are available in regular and fast setting times. Fast set materials have less retarder and results in a shorter setting time.[41] Silicone materials are mainly hydrophobic in nature. However, their wettability has been improved by the incorporation of a non-ionic surfactant.[17,29]

Like any other dental impression material, VPS undergoes small amounts of contraction upon setting due to polymerization shrinkage. This occurs as the impression cools from mouth to room temperature.[29] An appropriate VPS-matched adhesive painted on the custom tray will support impression material shrinkage toward the tray[17] and potentially reduce the polymerization shrinkage. A-silicone impression materials typically undergo a 0.15–0.2% polymerization shrinkage[42] that is compensated by an equal compensatory setting expansion of the high-strength gypsum material used for the stone model.

Addition silicones exhibit similar radiopaque characteristics to polysulfides. The radiopacity of a material can be expressed as a function of the radiopacity of a certain thickness of aluminum. It is estimated that a minimum radiographic value equal to 1.5 mm thickness of aluminum is needed for a material to be detected radiographically.[39] Addition silicone exhibit falls within this category. Used in combination with selected radiographic stents, it can assist with implant treatment planning.

Of all the elastomeric impression materials, vinyl polysiloxanes exhibit the most elastic recovery, with the possibility of distortion being almost non-existent.[20]

Sulfur-containing clinical latex gloves can inhibit the setting of A-silicones, and so alternative glove varieties are recommended for use during A-silicone usage.

5.3. *Polyethers*

Polyether impression material is another popular elastomeric impression material for precision impressions. It terms of accuracy and dimensional stability, it is often compared to VPS in many research papers. Polyethers and A-silicones are the only two elastomeric impression materials recommended for implant impressions.[43]

Polyether impression material is a single consistency impressioning system. It is available as a two-paste base and catalyst system that can be hand mixed or it can be delivered by means of a cartridge system or automixing devices for consistent results.

5.3.1. *Composition*

The baste paste contains liquid polyether and fillers with inert oils. The activator paste contains a sulfonate ester in hydrocarbons.

5.3.2. *Manipulation and Properties*

Polyether has been developed and evolved over the years with improved flow properties, wettability, better taste, and improved elasticity.[44] Unlike VPS impression materials, polyethers are truly hydrophilic[17] and allow for void-free impressions in moist conditions. Its hydrophilicity is due to the presence of functional groups such as carbonyl and ether groups that enable the water molecule to interact through hydrogen bonding.[21]

Although a single-consistency impression material, it has excellent flow properties allowing for the capture of fine detail for precision impressions. It is also known for its low tear strength and rigidity.

The rigidity of PE is twice that of VPS, and greater force is needed to remove the PE impression from the mouth.[44] It has a snap-set behavior, meaning the material sets quickly as soon as the working time has passed. Removal may be especially difficult in dentate patients with larger interdental embrasures or undercuts around pontics. It is beneficial to rather block out any potential undercuts with soft dental wax to facilitate ease of removal of the impression. Its high rigidity is a common cause for gypsum stone fractures when the impression and stone cast is separated.[17] In contrast, handling properties of PE demonstrates superior accuracy and predictable in implant impressions.

Drawbacks with polyethers are its poor taste, relatively low tear strength, and rigidity upon removal. Unlike VPS materials, polyether should be poured within an hour[17] or at least 25 h. The recommendation is that polyether be stored in a dry and cool environment (relative humidity below 50%) and not be left in disinfectant solution for extended periods of time.[20] This will reduce the risk of potential water absorption and leaching of its water-soluble plasticizer.

5.4. *Hybrid Vinylpolyether Silicones*

Vinylpolyether silicone (VPES) is a hybrid impression material introduced in 2008 with the intent to combine the best properties of polyether and polyvinylsiloxane impression materials. Another term used for this hybrid combination is vinylsiloxanether.[45]

5.4.1. *Composition*

The exact formulations of this impression material is proprietary, but it is suggested to consist of 5–20% of PE content.[46] As both component materials are elastomers, this hybrid material allows for a chemical bond between VPES and VPS.[45]

5.4.2. *Manipulation and Properties*

This hybrid impression material were introduced to exhibit the high tear strength and dimensional stability of VPS and the intrinsic hydrophilic nature and improved flow of polyether.[19] The end result is a predictable impression with high accuracy and dimensional stability and improved wettability. It is available in multiple viscosities and different setting times for different clinical applications.

Current evidence-based information on the properties of this material is not readily available. One study compared the dimensional stability of a conventional heavy-body VPS to that of the hybrid VPES material.[46] VPES were found to function within the limits of ADA Specification No.19 for VPS materials, and showed stability after disinfection and a 2-week storage time. The VPES demonstrated less dimensional change after 2 weeks, and this finding is thought to be a function of its rigidity. The casts produced from monophasic VPES impressions after a 2-week storage period showed excellent and comparable dimensional stability to monophasic VPS and PE.[47]

This material shows promise as it combines the best properties of VPS and PE impression materials. It is suggested to be a good alternative to PE for implant impressions[45] based on its accuracy and rigidity. Of note is that the PVES material was reported to have a better taste rating than PE.[45]

6. Disinfection Procedures

Disinfection of impression materials forms a critical component in the clinical and laboratory use of flexible impression materials. Disinfection of impression material received a more urgent focus more so in the late 20th century with the outbreak of AIDS[48] and the realities of cross-contamination. Contaminated dental impressions can produce contaminated casts by means of cross-infections.[49,50] Disinfection of dental impressions therefore prevents cross-contamination between the dental clinic and laboratory, and between dental professionals and any staff who may be handling or transporting the impression. It is the responsibility of the dental healthcare provider to disinfect impressions prior to sending it to the laboratory.

The disinfection process typically involves an immersion in a chemical disinfectant solution for a specific period of time. Some impression materials are sensitive to immersion, and a spray technique for disinfection is then recommended. Spraying is not as effective as immersion as complete contact of the disinfectant on all the impression surfaces is not always possible. In addition, spray disinfection can create aerosols and increase the risk of staff exposure.[51] An immersion technique is therefore the preferred choice of disinfection. Disinfection of a dental impression most appropriately starts with rinsing under running water to remove all saliva and possible blood contaminants. This initial rinse removes a significant amount of the microorganisms.[17] This is followed by exposure to a chemical disinfectant for a known period of time, by means of an immersion or a spray.

Most impression materials can be disinfected with Environmental Protected Agency (EPA)-registered solutions. Table 3 summarizes appropriate chemical solutions and disinfection techniques for flexible impression materials. Glutaraldehyde is the preferred solution for disinfection, but chlorine compounds and iodophors are suitable too.

Alginate impressions harbor three times more microorganisms than silicone impression materials.[52] Suitable disinfectant solutions include glutaraldehyde, chlorine-based, and iodophor solutions. Immersion disinfection of alginates were shown to produce dimensional changes.[53] Others believed that a 10-min imbibition may be beneficial to alginates to counteract the syneresis-associated shrinkage.[48] Contrary to the belief that alginates tend to expand on immersion with water, alginates generally shrink after a short period of expansion.[54] Immersion demonstrates more shrinkage for alginates[54] and potential distortion. The recommended disinfection technique for alginate impression materials are spraying rather than immersion to avoid potential imbibition, the absorption of water.[53] Spray disinfection has no effect on the surface detail and the accuracy of stone models made from alginate impressions.[31,52]

The elastomeric impression materials, particularly vinyl polysiloxanes and polyethers can be immersed in chemical solutions without affecting its surface properties or accuracy.[20] Disinfectant solutions typically do not affect the accuracy or dimensional stability

Table 3. Recommended disinfection protocols

Material	Method	Disinfectant
Agar	Short exposure <10 min	Chlorine compounds or idodophors
Alginates	Spray Immerse with caution	Chlorine compounds or idodophors Gluteraldehyde
Hybrid Alginate-VPS		Gluteraldehyde, idodophors, phenolics
Polysulfide	Immersion	Gluteraldehyde, chlorine compounds, idodophors, phenolics
Condensation VPS	Immersion	Gluteraldehyde, chlorine compounds, idodophors, phenolics
Addition VPS	Immersion	Gluteraldehyde, chlorine compounds, idodophors, phenolics
Polyether	Immerse with caution	Chlorine compounds or idodophors
Hybrid VPES	Immersion	Gluteraldehyde

of impression materials.[55,56] The recommended disinfectants for VPS and PE include sodium hypochlorite, gluteraldehyde-, and alcohol-based solutions. Both sodium hypochlorite and gluteraldehyde disinfectant solutions do not affect the wettability VPS and PE impressions.[57] The new VPES impression material demonstrated stability after immersion in a 2.5% gluteraldehyde solution for 20–30 min.[46,47] Casts produced from VPES show excellent dimensional stability and are comparable to VPS and PE.[47]

Polyether is the one impression material that is susceptible to extended immersion times (>10 min). This is due to its true hydrophilic nature, which causes it to absorb moisture from the environment.[20]

References

1. Nayar, S.; Mahadevan, R. *J. Pharm. Bioallied. Sci.* **2015**, *7* (Suppl 1), S213–S215.
2. Cho, S. H.; Schaefer, O.; Thompson, G. A.; Guentsch, A. *J. Prosthet. Dent.* **2015**, *113* (4), 310–315.
3. Menees, T. S.; Radhakrishnan, R.; Ramp, L. C.; Burgess, J. O.; Lawson, N. C. *J. Prosthet. Dent.* **2015**, *114* (4), 536–542.
4. Nowakowska, D.; Raszewski, Z.; Saczko, J.; Kulbacka, J.; Wieckiewicz, W. *J. Prosthet. Dent.* **2014**, *112* (2), 168–175.
5. Starcke, E. N., Jr. *J. Am. Dent. Assoc.* (*1939*) **1975**, *91* (5), 1037–1041.
6. Reed, H. V. *Quintessence Int.* **1990**, *21* (3), 225–229.
7. Hansson, O.; Eklund, J. *Swed. Dent. J.* **1984**, *8* (2), 81–95.
8. Hamalian, T. A.; Nasr, E.; Chidiac, J. J. *J. Prosthodont.* **2011**, *20* (2), 153–160.
9. Nemetz, H.; Tjan, A. H., *J. Prosthet. Dent.* **1988**, *60* (3), 267–270.
10. Sears, A. W. *Sci. Edu. Bull.* **1970**, *3* (1), 55–62.
11. Schulein, T. M. *J. Hist. Dent.* **2005**, *53* (2), 63–72.
12. Keck, S. C. *J. Prosthet. Dent.* **1985**, *54* (4), 479–483.
13. Soh, G.; Chong, Y. H. *J. Oral Rehabil.* **1991**, *18* (6), 547–553.
14. Chong, Y. H.; Soh, G.; Wickens, J. L. *Int. J. Prosthodont.* **1989**, *2* (4), 323–326.
15. Wilson, N. H.; Cowan, A. J.; Crisp, R. J.; Wilson, M. A. *SADJ* **2001**, *56* (5), 233–236.
16. Nam, J.; Raigrodski, A. J.; Townsend, J.; Lepe, X.; Mancl, L. A. *J. Prosthet. Dent.* **2007**, *97* (1), 12–17.
17. Donovan, T. E.; Chee, W. W. *Dent. Clin. North Am.* **2004**, *48* (2), vi–vii, 445–470.
18. Mandikos, M. N. *Aust. Dent. J.* **1998**, *43* (6), 428–434.
19. Lawson, N. C.; Burgess, J. O.; Litaker, M. S. *J. Prosthet. Dent.* **2008**, *100* (1), 29–33.
20. Anusavice, K. J.; Shen, C.; Rawls, H. R. *Phillips' Science of Dental Materials*, 12th ed. (Amsterdam: Elsevier Health Sciences, **2013**).
21. Rupp, F.; Axmann, D.; Jacobi, A.; Groten, M.; Geis-Gerstorfer, J. *Dent. Mater.* **2005**, *21* (2), 94–102.
22. Pratten, D. H.; Craig, R. G. *J. Prosthet. Dent.* **1989**, *61* (2), 197–202.

23. Cullen, D. R.; Mikesell, J. W.; Sandrik, J. L. *J. Prosthet. Dent.* **1991**, *66* (2), 261–265.
24. Vassilakos, N.; Fernandes, C. P. *J. Dent.* **1993**, *21* (5), 297–301.
25. O'Brien, W. J. *Dental Materials and their Selection*, 4th ed. (Quintessence Publishing Co, Inc., **2008**).
26. Murata, H.; Kawamura, M.; Hamada, T.; Chimori, H.; Nikawa, H. *J. Oral Rehabil.* **2004**, *31* (11), 1115–1122.
27. Walker, M. P.; Burckhard, J.; Mitts, D. A.; Williams, K. B., *Angle Orthod.* **2010**, *80* (6), 1110–1115.
28. Inoue, K.; Song, Y. X.; Kamiunte N. O.; Oku, J.; Terao, T.; FujiI, K., *J. Oral Rehabil.* **2002**, *29* (7), 615–619.
29. Combe, E. C. B., F. J. T; Douglas W. H. *Dental Biomaterials* (Massachusetts: Kluwer Academic Publishers, **1999**), p. 476.
30. Nassar, U.; Aziz, T.; Flores-Mir, C. *J. Prosthet. Dent.* **2011**, *106* (2), 126–133.
31. Guiraldo, R. D.; Borsato, T. T.; Berger, S. B.; Lopes, M. B.; Gonini-Jr, A.; Sinhoreti, M. A. *Braz. Dent. J.* **2012**, *23* (4), 417–421.
32. McCabe, J. F. W. A. W. G. *Applied Dental Materials*, 9th ed. (Hoboken: Wiley-Blackwell, **2008**), p. 312.
33. Baxter, R. T.; Lawson, N. C.; Cakir, D.; Beck, P.; Ramp, L. C.; Burgess, J. O. *Operative Dent.* **2012**, *37* (5), 540–547.
34. Patel, R. D.; Kattadiyil, M. T.; Goodacre, C. J.; Winer, M. S. *J. Prosthet. Dent.* **2010**, *104* (5), 325–332.
35. Nassar, U.; Hussein, B.; Oko, A.; Carey, J. P.; Flores-Mir, C. *J. Canad. Dent. Assoc.* **2012**, *78*, c2.
36. Suchak, A.; Fan, P. L.; Stanford, J. W.; Rhodes, C. *J. Am. Dent. Assoc.* (*1939*) **1984**, *108* (2), 210–211.
37. Eames, W. B.; Litvak, C. S. *J. Prosthet. Dent.* **1984**, *52* (4), 479–484.
38. Shannon, A. AlgiNot: A Stable, Reliable Preliminary Impression Material for Improved Productivity *Inside Dentistry* [Online], 2006. Available at: https://www.dentalaegis.com/id/2006/10/alginot-a-stable-reliable-preliminary-impression-material-for-improved-productivity.
39. Parissis, N.; Iakovidis, D.; Chirakis, S.; Tsirlis, A. *Aust. Dent. J.* **1994**, *39* (3), 184–187.
40. Re, D.; De Angelis, F.; Augusti, G.; Augusti, D.; Caputi, S.; D'Amario, M.; D'Arcangelo, C. *Int. J. Dent.* **2015**, *2015*, 428286.

41. Lawson, N. C.; Cakir, D.; Ramp, L.; Burgess, J. O. *J. Esthet. Restor. Dentist.* **2011**, *23* (3), 171–176.
42. Lampe, I.; Hegedus, C. *Fogorvosi szemle* **2002**, *95* (6), 249–252.
43. Lee, H.; So, J. S.; Hochstedler, J. L.; Ercoli, C. *J. Prosthet. Dent.* **2008**, *100* (4), 285–291.
44. Perakis, N.; Belser, U. C.; Magne, P. *Int. J. Periodont. Restorat. Dent.* **2004**, *24* (2), 109–117.
45. Enkling, N.; Bayer, S.; Jöhren, P.; Mericske-Stern, R. *Clin. Implant Dent. Relat. Res.* **2012**, *14* (1), 144–151.
46. Nassar, U.; Chow, A. K. *J. Prosthodont.* **2015**, *24* (6), 494–498.
47. Nassar, U.; Oko, A.; Adeeb, S.; El-Rich, M.; Flores-Mir, C. *J. Prosthet. Dent.* **2013**, *109* (3), 172–178.
48. Kotsiomiti, E.; Tzialla, A.; Hatjivasiliou, K. *J. Oral Rehabil.* **2008**, *35* (4), 291–299.
49. Connor, C. *Int. J. Prosthodont.* **1991**, *4* (4), 337–344.
50. Owen, C. P.; Goolam, R. *Int. J. Prosthodont.* **1993**, *6* (5), 480–494.
51. Miller, C. H, *Infection Control and Management of Hazardous Material for the Dental Team*, 5th ed. (Amsterdam: Elsevier Mosby: St. Louis, Missouri, **2014**).
52. Demajo, J. K.; Cassar, V.; Farrugia, C.; Millan-Sango, D.; Sammut, C.; Valdramidis, V.; Camilleri, J. *Int. J. Prosthodont.* **2016**, *29* (1), 63–67.
53. Hamedi Rad, F.; Ghaffari, T.; Safavi, S. H. *J. Dent. Res.* **2010**, *4* (4), 130–135.
54. Muzaffar, D.; Braden, M.; Parker, S.; Patel, M. P. *Dent. Mater.* **2012**, *28* (7), 749–755.
55. Kwon, J. S.; Lee, S. B.; Kim, K. M.; Kim, K. N. *Acta Odontol. Scand.* **2014**, *72* (8), 618–622.
56. Shetty, S. R.; Kamat, G.; Shetty, R. *Eur. J. Prosthodont. Restor. Dent.* **2013**, *21* (3), 98–104.
57. Lad, P. P.; Gurjar, M.; Gunda, S.; Gurjar, V.; Rao, N. K. *J. Int. Oral Health: JIOH* **2015**, *7* (6), 80–83.

Chapter 14

Resilient Liners for Removable Prosthesis

Igor J. Pesun

Division of Prosthodontics, Department of Restorative Dentistry, College of Dentistry, University of Manitoba, 780 Bannatyne, Winnipeg, MB, R2E1J6, Canada

Igor.Pesun@umanitoba.ca

Resilient or soft liners for removable prosthesis are used to improve the comfort of the existing denture, treat denture stomatitis, and allow for the functional impressioning of the soft tissues to reline dentures. The resilient denture liners are made up of silicone elastomer materials or plasticized acrylic resin. These materials are modified in such a way to achieve the desired elastic properties and resilience when they are bonded to the removable prosthesis. It is also important that resilient liners have properties that allow for their use in the harsh oral environment. The resilient material needs to have adequate elastic properties and have adequate resilience that can be maintained over time. Patients who have difficulty adapting to their prosthesis due to thin mucosa, sharp bony ridges, persistent sore mouth, or significant oral defect benefit from the use of resilient liners.

1. Introduction

In the United States, one out of every five person in the age group of 18–74 years wears some type of removable prosthetic appliance. The population of the United States has a complete edentulism rate of 10.5%. Current demographics indicate that nearly 61 million people in the United States will wear some sort of removable appliance by the year 2020.[1] The dental profession has advanced in restoring the function and esthetics of the completely edentulous, but 60% of the patients who wear dentures have some problem with them.[2–5] Statistically, there is no difference between males and females when comparing satisfaction of their prosthesis.[2]

The use of resilient denture liners started as early as 1943, but only since the 1960s have resilient liners been effective.[6] Resilient denture liners are often used in the hope of minimizing pressure and reducing trauma to denture-supporting mucosa.[7] These patients have difficulty in adapting to the hard surface of the denture material due to: (1) bony ridges with thin, non-resilient soft tissue coverage, (2) persistent denture-sore mouth, (3) knife-edge ridges resulting from advanced resorption of the residual alveolar ridges, (4) ridges with tissue undercuts where surgical intervention is contraindicated due to medical history, (5) relief for maxillary tori or other heavy bony prominences, and (6) prosthetic restorations for congenital or acquired oral defects.

As such, these materials should exhibit a low level of plastic deformation and elasticity, and their level of rigidity should be such as to enable them to act as and energy-absorbing layer during usage. The ideal resilient liner should have the following properties: (1) ease of processing, (2) cushioning effect upon the mucosa, (3) no adverse effects on the denture base, (4) inhibit mycotic growth, and (5) ridge adaptability. The physical properties should include, (1) permanent resilience, (2) dimensional stability during and after processing, (3) low water sorption and solubility, (4) adequate bond strength to the polymethyl methacrylate, (5) high abrasion resistance, (6) color stability, and (7) no changes over different temperatures.

The processing of resilient denture liners should have the criteria suggested by Lewis and Castleberry.[8]

Certain biological requirements are also desirable: (1) no burning or irritation of the oral tissues, (2) no bad taste or odor, (3) inhibitory action on fungal growth (mycotic), (4) non-toxic, (5) durability in the oral environment, and (6) stability in the oral environment.

Ideal mechanical properties for resilient denture liners includes (1) ease of processing, (2) ease of finishing, (3) ease of polishing, and (4) adhesion to, but without an effect on, denture resin properties.

Clinical properties include (1) no staining or discoloration, (2) adequate thickness of the resilient liner without weakening of the denture base, and (3) ease of finishing and polishing.[6,9–11]

Quality	Desired outcome
Viscosity	The material reproduces the details of the mold, and colorants remain suspended
Bubbles	There are no bubbles in the cured material
Shrinkage	There is no shrinkage, or any shrinkage that occurs is subclinical
Working time	The working time is long enough to carefully fill the mold
Curing temperature	The curing temperature is low enough so that the mold is not damaged
Recovery	The material is easily removed from the mold without damaging either
Trimability	The material is capable of being trimmed

2. Composition of Resilient Denture Liners

The earliest resilient liners were natural rubbers. The first synthetic materials were plasticized polyvinyl chlorides. Currently, there are two types of materials that are used as resilient denture liners; plasticized acrylic resins and silicone elastomers. Plasticized acrylic resin-based materials are higher methacrylate homologs and hydrophilic acrylics that were developed with plasticizers to allow for these materials to be resilient. The plasticizers are found in the liquid and may contain ethyl alcohol, ethyl acetate, and an aromatic plasticizer (e.g. butyl phthalyl butyl glycolate). When the polymethyl methacrylate cures, the plasticizers situate themselves between the polymer chains. They are not chemically attached to the polymer chains but behave like molecular lubricants. The polymer chains do not cross over each other with the plasticizer, they slide over each other more easily. The type and volume of plasticizer incorporated into the material determines the properties of the material. All of these plasticizers can dissolve or evaporate over time. The loss of the various plasticizers in the oral environment results in the material hardening over time. By controlling the chemistry of the resilient liner, the useful life can range from as little as several days or weeks to several years. The biggest clinical advantage of these materials is their excellent adhesion to the polymethyl methacrylate denture bases.

Silicone elastomers are materials available in two forms; a two-component base/catalyst that is a cold cure material or as a one-component heat-cured material. Silicone elastomer materials stay resilient longer than the plasticized acrylic resin materials. The silicone elastomers molecule is very resilient and stable overtime. As silicone elastomers are chemically different from the polymethyl methacrylates, they have poor adhesion. Silicone elastomers require the use of an adhesive bonding agent to prevent delamination of the material over time.

3. Physical Properties

Ideal physical properties are achieved by having a polymer that has an appropriate glass transition temperature (T_g). Temperature plays a significant role in the observed physical properties of a polymer used in the formation of a resilient denture liner. Glass transition temperature is defined as: a range of temperature for each individual polymer where the behavior of the material changes from hard and brittle to soft and flexible. A glass transition temperature needs to be lower than mouth temperature. Mouth temperature is approximately 32°C (range 0–55°C). Acrylic-based polymers have a glass transition temperature that can be modified by the addition of plasticizers to the polymer's molecule.

Dependant on the plasticizers added to the polymer's molecule, the desired properties of resilient are modified to provide higher elasticity during mastication and then behave viscously to accommodate functional and non-functional forces. This resilient material is then able to minimize and relieve pain during function for denture wearers.

An ideal resilient denture liner does not permanently deform and lose resilience over time. If a material does not permanently deform and it returns to its pre-deformation state, it is said to be elastic. Elasticity is an evaluation of a materials' ability to recover and return to its original form after having a strain applied to it. The ability of a material to absorb energy without undergoing permanent deformation is known as resilience.

There are several examples of successful use of mandibular denture-resilient liner materials to reduce the symptoms of discomfort beneath acrylic dentures.[12] Resilient denture liners have the ability to adapt to the patient's ridge, which can only be attained if the material's behavior has a time-dependent component. Unfortunately, a material that returns to its original shape almost instantly after the load has been removed does not comply as well as a more viscous material.[13] This indicates the difficulty in attaining all the requirements of a good resilient liner from one type of material. The ideal characteristics of a resilient liner material are higher elasticity during mastication and then behaving viscously to accommodate functional and non-functional forces to relieve pain, in addition to durability and stability in the oral environment over long periods of time.

Although these prostheses go a long way toward helping these individuals cope with the discomfort of wearing dentures, the prostheses are not perfect. The life expectancy of the liner is 4–6 years, but can be as little as 1 year, although some have shown to be serviceable even after the denture needs to be replaced due to wear on the acrylic teeth.[14–18] Most of the material on the market today are acrylic resin polymers or copolymers of the powder liquid type that when processed have some resiliency to them. These remain soft by the use of ethyl or butyl methacrylate in combination with methyl methacrylate to produce the soft copolymer. Another technique involves the addition of external plasticizers to the monomer. These materials did have the disadvantage of the plasticizer leaching out, especially in the presence of alcohol, thus resulting in hardening of the resilient liner.[9,19]

Silicone elastomers materials are also available for lining denture prosthesis. They have been found to be significantly more stable and are currently the material of choice for a permanent soft lining material. Silicone elastomer resilient denture liners are more elastic than liners made of soft acrylics. Tests on the wear of silicone elastomer-based materials showed that elastic materials, especially heat-cured single-component materials are less likely to deform and lose resilience over time, with no changes over different temperatures, or after prolonged soaking.[20–22] Heat-cured single-component materials have long-lasting serviceability for their physical and mechanical properties. Molloplast-B is a methacryloxy propyl trimethoxy silane heat polymerized silicone elastomers rubber. The curing agent reacts with reactive groups of the polymer, leaving methacrylate groups available to bond with the PMMA denture base material, (e.g. Lucitone199).[23] The chemical properties of heat-cured silicone elastomer rubbers account for compatibility with oral tissues, dimensional stability, resiliency, and compliance. However, there are still problems reported with the clinical use of silicone elastomer rubber resilient liners. For instance, Molloplast-B has shown some loss of compliance with long periods of use in the oral environment.[24]

The resilient liners fail because of the degradation of the material, which leads to both hardening and color changes, sorption of odors, bacterial growth, and breakdown of the bond between the resilient liner and the polymethyl methacrylate.[15,25] Considering the cost involved in replacing these materials and the harm that a degraded material inflicts on the soft tissue, there is a compelling need for improved soft lining material.

Researchers have concentrated on improving the tensile strength; tear strength, percent elongation, and Shore-A hardness of the resilient liners.[6,12,26,27] The process of accelerated aging is used to measure the physical properties and color of soft denture liners. This process exposes the materials to an environment with controlled heat, humidity, and periodic spraying with distilled water. Accelerated aging dramatically affected the physical and mechanical properties of the resilient liners.[21,28] Other environmental factors that can affect the physical properties of soft denture liners include functional wear, time, exposure to adhesives, and cleaning agents. Food stains can also cause significant changes in the color of the elastomers.

4. Viscoelastic Properties and Compliance

Masticatory forces are mainly compressive and delivered cyclically. The force for a mastication cycle is characterized by a rapid closure of the mandible, followed by a deceleration just before tooth contact. In the case of denture wearers, the mastication load is believed to be close to 2.17 N mm^{-2}. These factors are responsible for the shortened life expectancy of the prosthesis. Reproducing all of these factors in a laboratory is very difficult, if not impossible, therefore, full evaluation of the performance of resilient liners requires that it be evaluated *in situ*. One problem with *in situ* evaluation of resilient lined dentures is that there are no standard tests for measuring the physical properties of the resilient liner. The tests for tensile strength, tear strength, and percent elongation require standardized samples that are destroyed during testing. The Shore-A hardness test requires a 6 mm minimum thickness for material. The amount of resilient liner that can be placed within a denture is limited to 2–3 mm; therefore, the Shore-A hardness cannot be used.

The general consensus is that the resilient liner material should undergo minimal changes during use. A balance must exist between the underlying mucosa and the denture-resilient liner. According to previous studies, the resilient liner will not act as a shock absorber based solely on its viscoelastic properties; instead, it functions as a spring in series with the oral mucosa.[29] The resilient liner will absorb the energy applied to the denture only if its elastic modulus is lower than the soft tissue,[23] meaning a softer, more compliant resilient liner would be appropriate for a patient whose ridge is extremely thin and sore. On the other hand, if the case requires improvement of masticatory function, or relief during parafunctional habits, a stiffer resilient liner would be preferable due to its effectiveness in distributing stress more uniformly.[30]

An essential requirement for a soft lining material is its ability to recover elastically following compression during mastication and to retain its elasticity over fairly long periods of time. A good resilient liner material must also be characterized by a relative degree of viscoelasticity. The viscoelastic properties of a material have been effective in determining the serviceability of permanent soft lining materials and their apparent softness when comparing acrylic resins and silicone elastomers materials.[31] An elastic behavior has been attributed to silicone elastomer-based resilient denture liners; whereas acrylic-based liners behave more viscously.[32] Of the physical properties of resilient liner materials investigated, resiliency can best predict the effectiveness of a material. An effective resilient liner material can absorb the impact forces during mastication with minimal deformation and deterioration over time. The definition of resiliency cannot be literally applied to the materials used as resilient denture liners, but only to perfectly elastic materials. A material that is perfectly elastic is not very compliant. Compliance is a measurement of the softness or flexibility of a material. A more general definition of compliance is the strain of an elastic body expressed as a function of the force producing the strain.

Compliance is a physical property which defines a solid material that deforms as easily as it recovers.[23] Resilient materials are used to give dentures a cushioning effect upon the oral mucosa of patients with chronic alveolar ridge and tissue soreness, pathological changes, and bone loss. A viscoelastic material behaves elastically while having a dissipating component of deformation. The efficiency of a resilient liner is dependent on the viscoelastic properties and durability of the material. The silicone elastomers rubbers are the best materials for maintaining their resiliency over time and resisting initial water absorption. Resilient liners are viscoelastic materials and as they age and absorb water they may become more elastic and less viscous, which can lead to failure of strength.[33] This reduction in compliance is inversely related to a material's baseline softness, i.e. the higher the baseline compliance is, the more the reduction in compliance with use.[34] This behavior is more commonly found in acrylic-based resilient liners, and the research is less constant in reference to the silicone elastomers-based resilient liners.

Evaluation of resilient lined denture prostheses *in situ* requires non-destructive tests. If resilient liner materials are to protect the soft mucosal tissues, then the dynamic nature of these tissues must be considered. Force displacement plots for human tissues are generally nonlinear, indicating that these tissues behave like viscoelastic material.[35] The force displacement curves for elastomers are also non-linear.[27] This non-linear relationship implies that the physical properties are time dependent. The viscoelastic nature of these materials occurs under low loads on the order of those experienced during function. The applied stress associated with this load has not been quantified, though an average stress of 1.5 Nmm^{-2} used with the load cell seems close to the stress observed clinically.[36] The maximum stress seen by these materials occurs during eating or parafunctional habits. The magnitude of the stress on the appliance depends on the oral habits of the patient. One method for testing time dependent physical properties of viscoelastic materials is to produce a force displacement curve with a low maximum force. This is a non-destructive test that can be done by applying the force at a specific rate then measuring the displacement of the material with time.[12,22]

Investigators have used direct and non-destructive techniques to determine compliance.[20,27,32,34,36] Many of the methods described apply static loads to the material.[20,34,36] Several studies do accurately reproduce the cyclical force experience during mastication.[27,32] Another common method for measuring softness of resilient liner materials is Shore-A testing. The Shore-A durometer's operating instructions recommend a minimum specimen thickness of 6 mm. Measurements of thinner samples tend to reveal characteristics of the surface beneath the resilient denture liners.[37] This is not clinically applicable because resilient liner material thickness in dentures rarely exceeds 3 mm.

Very few clinical studies have quantified and characterized the viscoelastic properties of resilient liner materials using a dynamic technique. Dynamic mechanical analysis (DMA) measures the shear storage modulus G', the shear loss modulus G'', and the phase angle (ë). G' defines the material's stiffness and is the ratio of the applied stress to strain.[27] Another technique tests materials with a modified Instron 1185 Tensile-testing machine. This machine measures strain semi-continuously during cyclic loading, and a linear voltage displacement transducer (LVDT) obtains displacement.[22] Both of these studies used extensive mathematical calculations to conclude, from the deformation behavior of the tested materials that silicone elastomers resilient denture liners behave nearly elastically, while acrylic resins are more compressible and better in absorbing energy.

The force–displacement curves for silicone elastomers and mucosa are non-linear with time, thus dynamic testing should be used to evaluate the physical properties of these materials.[38] Because of this time-dependent nature and the need for a non-destructive test, a preliminary investigation was done to determine if the force–displacement curves measured by applying a cyclic square wave force to a sample could measure changes in the physical properties of the elastomer. This is the square wave compliance test. Compliance testing with the closed-loop servo hydraulic system dynamically reproduces the stresses a resilient liner experiences *in vivo* during rapidly applied forces due to mastication, swallowing, and speech. The MTS closed-loop servo hydraulic testing system of the MDRCBB (MTS Systems, Eden Prairie, MN) was used for the compliance test.[39] A sample is mounted on the moveable base of the hydraulic actuator, Figure 1. The actuator was moved up until the sample contacted the 5 mm diameter steel ball bearing mounted on the 100 lb. load cell attached to the rigid cross-member of the MTS system. Contact was indicated by an increase in force measured by the load cell. The actuator is run in a load control mode and programmed to apply a compressive force to the test sample following a square wave pattern (force on–force off, etc.). The load cell measures the force transferred through the sample. The displacement is measured using the internal LVDT (Linearly Variable Displacement Transducer) mounted on the servo hydraulic actuator. The force–displacement curve is recorded using a Nicolet 310 Storage Oscilloscope (Nicolet Instrument Corporation, Madison, WI), then saved for future analysis. Force and displacements are given in volts. Preliminary results indicated that for strains below 20% this method could non-destructively measure the stiffness of an elastomer sample.[39]

An important consideration for a proper resilient liner is its thickness. Excessively thick resilient denture liners result in a denture with an increased risk of fracturing, while if the resilient liner is too thin it is ineffective. In a clinical situation, a resilient liner cannot exceed 3.0 mm and it is rarely made to a constant thickness throughout the denture. The thickness of the resilient denture liner should then be kept between 2.5 and 3.5 mm. If it is thinner than this, it will bottom out and result in the denture feeling just as hard on the soft tissue as if there was no soft liner. This thickness restricts the use of the liners to the mandibular dentures as if the maxillary denture was to be 4 mm thick it would impede the patients overall function. As such, most liners are only used to improve the comfort of mandibular dentures.

Resilient liner materials are used to reduce impact forces on denture-bearing mucosa. Studies have found silicone elastomers-base liners behave well during impact absorption and display good serviceability. One of the problems of silicone elastomer resilient liner materials is their apparent hardness upon initial insertion of the lined denture. The instantaneous pressure tissues experience during mastication is better withstood and less damaging when the resilient liner is highly resilient or almost perfectly elastic. A more viscous material may be desirable in response to slowly applied forces like those during parafunctional habits and speech.

Durability of permanent resilient lined dentures is relevant to their clinical success. Longitudinal studies have reported the serviceability of heat-cured single component materials-lined dentures as being as long as 9 years. Heat-cured single component materials, the gold standard of permanent resilient liners has some drawbacks, in particular, ease of processing has been indicated to be low due to its more viscous state before curing. MPDS-SL is a more fluid material, thus making its distribution over the denture base easier and more even. Heat-cured single-component materials like most other resilient liners tend to change in color and display fungal growth after relatively short periods of use.

Data indicated a slight decreased or unchanged compliance value of silicone elastomer-based liner materials, in particular heat-cured single-component materials.[7,12,22] In the cases where no change was observed, the duration of the study was less than 6–12 months and the methods used the Shore-A hardness test.[24]

The increase in compliance of heat-cured single-component materials could be due to the cleaning regimen used by the patients.[40] A parallel study found that patients' dentures cleaned with denture paste tended to have a more positive compliance change, while those cleaned by soak tablets tended to have more negative compliance change.[40]

5. Color

Color stability is a required characteristic of denture soft lining materials, with national and international standards specified by the ADA as Specification No. 12 (American Dental Association 1975). The ADA recommends the use of the CIE Lab color differential system. In this system, all colors are obtained from the blend of three basic colors; red, blue, and green at varying proportions. Patients are more satisfied when their denture resilient liners are indistinguishable from the acrylic base, and the motivation to maintain the dentures is dependent on the ease of cleaning of the materials and the design of the denture. Maintaining color stability of the resilient liner is not often a problem with silicone elastomer-based liners, yet a displeasing liner color may constitute a reason for its replacement.[23] Unlike most other soft lining materials, the silicone elastomers-based liners are not easily discolored, though they can incorporate colorants from ingested foods, drinks, or tobacco products.

Color analysis is normally done using a reflectance spectrophotometer; however, because of the size of most dental prostheses, this technique is not practical. A second method of color analysis was reported by Haug *et al.*[41] The Minolta Chromameter (Minolta

Camera Co. Ltd., Osaka, Japan) was used to measure the color of elastomer samples. It used the CIE Lab tristimulus values: L*, a*, and b*. In the L*a*b* color system L* is the Value of the sample, a* is the red–green axis, and b* is the yellow–blue axis. Color change (ΔE) is calculated with the formula $\Delta E = (\Delta L^{*2} + \Delta a^{*2} + \Delta b^{*2})^{1/2}$. A value for $\Delta E = 1$ or larger is considered visually detectable. This method is non-destructive and can measure time dependent change color.

Silicone elastomer rubber materials are composed of polymers of dimethyl siloxane, which is a viscous liquid cross-linked with good elastic properties. Silicone elastomer rubbers, in particular Molloplast-B, are especially resistant to initial water absorption. Clinically, the material became darker, possibly due to the addition of ingested colorants by water diffusion.[42]

6. Microbiological Interaction

The genus *Candida* contains approximately 200 species found in many environments, ranging from plants to the human gastrointestinal tract. *Candida* is a commensal yeast but under certain circumstances may become an opportunistic pathogen, where it can invade human tissues causing severe to life threatening pathologies.

Denture stomatitis is caused by fungal growth on dentures and is the most common form of *Candida* infection in humans, with roughly 50% of denture wearers being infected.[10,43–45] Several other factors promote oropharyngeal candidiasis, many associated with denture patients, including malignancies, diabetes, immunodeficiency, and malnutrition. *Candida albicans* is the main etiological agent of oropharyngeal candidiasis and denture stomatitis.

Candida glabrata is another common species present in the oral cavity, gastrointestinal tract, and respiratory tract. *C. glabrata* infections have been associated with endocarditis, meningitis, and multifocal disseminated disease.[46] Quantifying *Candida* type and prevalence on denture products is essential for the safety of denture-wearing patients. Due to the infectious tendencies of *Candida,* other species such as *C. tropicalis, Issatchenkia oreintalis* (formerly *C. krusei*), and *C. parapsilosis* could also be present.

Numerous clinical tests are used to identify *Candida* species such as carbohydrate assimilation, germ tube, and an assortment of media. These tests are specific to one species, labor intensive, and expensive. CHROMagarÔ Candida is a medium designed for isolating and identifying *Candida* species. CHROMagarÔ Candida identifies *Candida* species by colony characteristics, such as color and texture and can accurately identify *C. albicans, C. glabrata, C. tropicalis, Issatchenkia oreintalis, C. dubliniensis, C. neoformans*, and usually *C. parapsilosis,* and *C. guillermondii.*[47] The effectiveness of CHROMagarÔ specificity is 100% for *C. albicans, C. tropicalis,* and *Issatchenkia oreintalis* and 97% for *C. glabrata.*[48] The presence of fungal growth on Molloplast-B samples ranges from 65% to 85% of silicone elastomers liner samples.[10,43,49] Newer materials are being developed that only allow fungal growth on 45% of samples.[49]

The most abundant species found on silicone elastomeric resilient liners include *C. albicans* and *C. glabrata.*[10,43,49] Makila and Hopsu-Havu found *C. tropicalis* as the third most abundant *Candida* species on silicone elastomers liners,[10] while Wright *et al.* found *C. samata* and *C. parapsolosis* to be the next two most abundant species.[43]

7. Uses of Resilient Denture Liners

Resilient denture liners have multiple uses and come in various forms depending on the purpose for which they are intended.

Over-the-counter (OTC) dentures liners are temporary liners that also provide adhesive properties to aid in retention of the patients' dentures. They are sold in the form of preformed thermoplastic pads usually made of wax-impregnated gauze, resin gels, or strips. They only last a day or so and should not be used or recommended. As they are not customized to fit the patient's soft tissue contour, they tend to hide the ill-fitting dentures and result in damaged ridges and soft tissues. When patients use OTC denture liners over time, they also present with mucositis and *Candida albicans* infection.

Tissue conditioners are generally plasticized acrylic resin-based powder and liquid-based materials. The polymers have plasticizers that provide for the softest material with good elastic recovery properties. Although they do not undergo permanent deformation, they generally lose softness in days and must be replaced. The hardening of the material is due to the leaching and evaporation of the plasticizers. Tissue conditioners flow for hours during use making them ideal for use after surgical procedures or in cases where patients has sore ridges due to poorly fitting dentures. Patients with mucositis related to *Candida albicans* infection can be treated with a tissue conditioner with an antifungal medication incorporated into the material.

Functional impression materials are used in cases where there is difficulty in fitting the denture due to changes in the soft tissue supporting the denture. In situations where the dentures teeth are adequate and the vertical dimension of occlusion is at the desired height and the denture is to be relined, a functional impression can be made. The denture does not need to be remade, and polymers with plasticizers are used to obtain an impression under functional stresses. Functional impression material should have good flow with minimal elastic recovery. The flow allows for continual adaption of the material to the soft tissues in response to functional stresses. To allow for the functional impression and relining of the denture, the undercuts are removed from the denture and the functional impression material is added to the denture. The patient wears the denture for a week, removing the denture nightly. The denture is then sent to the laboratory for processing. As these materials deform plastically to record tissue, the functional impression results in a very well-fitting denture for the patient.

Short-term resilient denture liners are silicone elastomers or plasticized acrylic resin with plasticizers. These are most often fabricated in the patient's mouth. Silicone elastomers set is similar in principle to VPS impression materials. They are used in case where the patient is having issues with their current dentures and they are being assessed for future dentures or treatment of denture stomatitis. The denture relieved in areas that are causing trauma to the tissues and the periphery is trimmed to allow for at least a 2 mm bulk of material at the junction with the hard denture base. These will often last several months.

Long-term resilient denture liners are mostly silicone elastomer-based materials although there are few plasticized acrylic resin-based ones available. Long-term resilient denture liners are generally heat-cured laboratory-processed materials. The denture is fabricated using standard protocol with a modification to the processing procedure to allow for the processed resilient liner. A spacer is placed to allow for 3 mm of resilient denture material and the hard acrylic is initially processed to initiate the curing. The hard material is partially cured as the free ends of the polymer chains are needed to allow for the bonding of the silicone elastomers or the plasticized acrylic resin to the polymethyl methacrylate. The spacer is removed and the resilient denture liner is placed and the denture is fully cured. Denture is recovered, finished, and processed. A sealer is often placed over the resilient liner before the denture is delivered.

8. Maintenance of Resilient Denture Liners

All acrylics have porosities and micro-roughness that allow for the adhesion of a biofilm that results in the growth. *Candida albicans* is common to 50% of patients who wear removable prostheses. Due to the softness of resilient denture liners, cleaning must be done carefully. It is best to soak the dentures in a cleaning solution that does not contain alcohol or chlorine cleaners.[49]

9. Conclusions and Outlook

A good resilient liner is essential to reduce the impact of mastication on the supporting tissue of removable prosthesis. The thickness of the resilient denture liner should then be kept between 2.5 and 3.5 mm. Delamination is an issue with resilient denture materials. It is important to have a bulk of material at the junction of the materials and a chemical bond. Resilient denture liners change in all the color variables measured from baseline to the 6-month period of wear by the patients. *Candida* has the potential to become an opportunistic pathogen and should be investigated in the development of new denture materials.

References

1. Douglass, C. W.; Ostry, L.; Shih, A. *J. Dent. Res.* **1998**, *77* (Special Issue A), 209.
2. Marcus, S. E.; Drury, T. F.; Brown, L. J.; Zion G. R. *J. Dent. Res.* **1996**, *75*, 684–695.
3. Redford, M.; Drury, T. F.; Kingman. A.; Brown, L. J. *J. Dent. Res.* **1996**, *75*, 714–725.
4. Langer, A.; Michman, J.; Seifert, I. *J. Prosthet. Dent.* **1961**, *11*, 1019–1031.
5. Yoshizumi, D. T. *J. Prosthet. Dent.* **1964**, *14*, 866–878.
6. Von Fraunhofer, J. A.; Sichina, W. J. *Int. J. Prosthodont.* **1994**, *7* (2), 120–128.
7. Graham, B. S.; Jones, D. W.; Sutow, E. J. *J. Prosthet. Dent.* **1989**, *62* (4), 421–428.
8. Lewis, D. H.; Castleberry, D. J. *J. Prosthet. Dent.* **1980**, *43*, 426.
9. Bell, D. H. Jr. *J. Prosthet. Dent.* **1970**, *23* (4), 394–406.
10. Makila, E.; Hopsu-Havu, V. K. *Acta Odontol. Scand.* **1977**, *35* (4), 197–205.
11. Travaglini, E. A.; Gibbsons, P.; Craig, R. G. *J. Prosthet. Dent.* **1960**, *10* (4), 664–672.
12. Jepson, N. J.; McCabe, J. F.; Storer, R. *J. Dent* **1993**, *21* (3), 163–170.
13. Holt, R. A.; Zylinski, C. G.; Duncanson, M. G. Jr. *Int. J. Prosthdont.* **1991**, *4* (2), 164–168.
14. Jepson, N. J.; McCabe, J. F.; Storer, R. *Br. Dent. J.* **1994**, *177* (1), 11–16.
15. Makila, E.; Honka, O. *J. Oral Rehabil.* **1979**, *6* (2), 199–204.
16. Schmidt, W. F. Jr.; Smith, D. E. *J. Prosthet. Dent.* **1983**, *50* (3), 308–313.
17. Schmidt, W. F. Jr.; Smith, D. E.; *J. Prosthet. Dent.* **1983**, *50* (4), 459–465.
18. Wright, P. S. *J. Prosthet. Dent.* **1994**, *72* (4), 385–392.
19. Graham, B. S.; Jones. D.W.; Sutow, E. J. *J. Dent. Res.* **1991**, *70* (5), 870–873.
20. McCabe, J. F.; Basker, R. M.; Murata, H.; Wollwage, P.G. *Eur. J. Prosthodont. Restor. Dent.* **1996**, *4* (2), 77–81.
21. Jepson, N. J.; McCabe, J. F.; Storer, R. *J. Dent.* **1993**, *21* (3), 171–178.

22. Graham, B. S.; Jones, D. W.; Thomson, J. P.; Johnson, J. A. *J. Oral. Rehabil.* **1990**, *17* (2), 157–163.
23. Braden, M.; Wright, P. S.; Parker, S. *Eur. J. Prostho. Rest. Dent.* **1995**, *3* (4), 163–174.
24. Hekimoglu, C.; Anil, N. *J. Oral. Rehabil.* **1999**, *26*, 745–748.
25. Kawano, F.; Dootz, E. R.; Koran, A. 3rd; Craig, R. G., *J. Prosthet. Dent.* **1994**, *72* (4), 393–398.
26. Al-Athel, M. S.; Jagger, R. G. *J. Prosthet. Dent.* **1996**, *76* (5), 535–540.
27. Kawano, F.; Kon, M.; Koran, A.; Matsumoto, N. *J. Prosthet. Dent.* **1994**, *72* (6), 599–605.
27. Williams, K. R.; Jagger, R. G.; Sadamori, S.; Waters, M. G. *J. Dent.* **1996**, *24* (4), 301–308.
28. Dootz, E. R.; Koran. A.; Craig, R. G. *J. Prosthet. Dent.* **1993**, *69* (1), 114–119.
29. Hayakawa, I.; Hirano, S.; Takahashi, Y.; Sheng, K. E. *Int. J. Prosthodont.* **2000**, *13* (3), 227–231.
30. Sato, Y.; Abe, Y.; Okane, H.; Tsuga, K. *J. Oral. Rehabil.* **2000**, *27* (8), 660–663.
31. Waters, M. G. J.; Williams, D. W.; Jagger. R. G.; Lewis, M. A. O. *J. Prosthet. Dent.* **1997**, *77*, 306–312.
32. Waters, M.; Jagger, R.; Williams, K.; Jerolimov, V. *Biomat.* **1996**, *17*, 1627–1630.
33. Emmer, T. J. Jr.; Emmer, T. J. Sr.; Vaidynathan, J.; Vaidynathan, T. K., *J. Prosthet. Dent.* **1995**, *74* (6), 595–601.
34. Jepson, N. J.; McGill, J. T.; McCabe, J. F. *J. Prosthet. Dent.* **2000**, *83* (1), 25–31.
35. Farah, J.W.; Robinson, J. C.; Hood, J. A. A.; Koran, A.; Craig, R. G. *J. Oral Rehab.* **1988**, *15*, 277–283.
36. Kawano, F.; Koran, A.; Nuryanti, A.; Inoue, S. *Int. J. Prosthodont.* **1997**, *10*, 55–60.
37. Yoeli, Z.; Miller, V.; Zeltser, C. *J. Prosth. Dent.* **1996**, *75* (4), 412–418.
38. Koran, A.; Craig, R. G. *J. Dent. Res.* **1975**, *54* (6), 1216–1221.
39. Ko, C. C.; Delong, R.; Lai, J. H. *J. Dent. Res.* **1998**, *77* (Special Issue), 790.
40. Villar, A.; Pesun, I. J.; Brosky, M. E.; Fines, C.; Hodges, J. S.; DeLong, R.; Lai, J. H. *J. Prosthodont.* **2003**, *12* (2), 82–89.

41. Haug, S. P.; Andres, C. J.; Munoz, C. A.; Okamura, M. *J. Prosthet. Dent.* **1992**, *68* (5), 820–823.
42. Canay, S.; Hersek, N.; Tulunoglu, I. *J. Oral. Rehabil.* **1999**, *26*, 821–829.
43. Wright, P. S.; Clark, P.; Hardie, J. M. *J. Dent. Res.* **1985**, *64* (2), 122–125.
44. Zarb, G. A.; Bolender, C. L.; Carlsson, G. *Boucher's Prosthodontic Treatment for Edentulous Patients*, 11th ed. (St. Louis: CV Mosby, **1997**), p. 23.
45. McMullen-Vogel, C. G.; Jude, H. D.; Ollert, M. W.; Vogel, C. W. *Oral. Microbiol. Immunol.* **1999**, *14* (3), 183–189.
46. Murray, P. R.; Boron, E.; Pfaller, M.; Tenover, F.; Yolken, R. *Manual of Clinical Microbiology*, 7th ed. (Washington DC: ASM Press, **1999**), pp. 1184–1194.
47. Koehler, A. P.; Chu, K. C.; Houng, E. T.; Cheng, F. B. *J. Clin. Microbiol.* **1999**, *37* (2), 422–426.
48. Powell, H. L.; Sand, C. A.; Rennie, R. P. *Diagn. Microbiol. Infect. Dis.* **1998**, *32* (3), 201–204.
49. Brosky, M. E.; Pesun, I. J.; Morrison, B.; Hodges, J. S.; Lai, J. H.; Liljemark, W. *J. Prosthodont.* **2003**, *12* (3), 162–167.

Chapter 15

3D Printing — Additive Manufacturing of Dental Biomaterials

Rodrigo França*, Jeff Winkler, Helen H. Hsu, Maedeh Rahimnejad, and Zahra Abdali

Department of Restorative Dentistry and Department of Biomedical Engineering, University of Manitoba, 780 Bannatyne Avenue, Winnipeg, MB, R3E 0W2, Canada

**Rodrigo.franca@umanitoba.ca*

3D printing of dental devices is a new-age method of manufacturing using an additive process, which contrasts with the normal subtractive or molding processes used in traditional restorative dentistry. This chapter will serve as a review of the technology available as of present, and it is divided into two sections. In the first section, aspects such as the biostability and biocompatibility of 3D-printed dental devices will be examined, and this section will serve to provide an overview of the types of implants commonly produced via 3D printing. In addition, this first section describes the inherent risks and advantages for devices realized utilizing this methodology. The second section will be focused on the topic of bioprinting/3D printing of cells for organic tissue reconstruction. Fundamental concepts of bioprinting, common methods, biomaterials used, and other factors for a successful bioprintable structure will be discussed. Lastly, the properties of final bioprintable constructs (mechanical variations, permeability, and degradability) will be considered.

1. Introduction

3D biomaterial printing is considered as one of the foremost revolutionary technologies to date. As famously quoted by the previous President of the United States of America, Barack Obama, 3D printing technology has "the potential to revolutionize the way we make almost everything".[1] It is a methodology using 3D tooling for producing 3D models. Called *Additive Manufacturing*, it is also referred to as rapid prototyping, solid free-form, computer automated, or layered manufacturing depending on the kind of production method used.[2–4] In the recent years, the medical community has just begun to explore the many benefits of employing 3D printing technology to realize human bodily implants never before possible.

The process of generating a 3D-printed device for a patient begins with a patient's visit to a doctor. Computer-aided design software is utilized to generate a virtual model of the dental device that matches the patient's internal anatomy exactly. In collaboration with the design engineer, the doctor specifies the type of manufacturing technology, that is, the type of material and the structure that is to be desired for the end product. Once agreed upon, the device is printed and a physical dental appliance is produced in rough shape and form. Most devices require additional finishing, such as cleaning, coating, and most certainly always sterilization prior to being delivered to the operating room.

The most outstanding advantage of 3D-printed biomaterials is the ability to produce patient-specific devices that can be engineered to exactly match the requirements set forth by the patient's anatomy. Although a giant leap for the production of medical devices, 3D printing suffers from the major limitation arising from the printability of materials, in particular the lack of advancements relating to printability of a larger variety of biomaterials.[5,6]

2. Additive Manufacturing of Dental Devices

In Dentistry, additive manufacturing was introduced as a manufacturing technique early in the 1990s.[7] However, in that time, it was used mostly for prototyping study models, and for producing guides used in surgical procedures.[4] Recently, with the introduction of modern radiological tools in the dental field (i.e. computed tomography, cone-beam computed tomography, and optical surface scans), this has allowed for the use of additive manufacturing to be utilized in a larger variety of dental applications and implants.

2.1. *Additive Manufacturing in Restorative Dentistry*

Literature regarding indirect dental restorations manufactured by 3D-printing techniques is, as of now, rare. However, it is only a question of time before the technology of 3D printing becomes an everyday device at dental technician labs and at clinical offices around the globe. First, because the advantages of the digital impression would be from the computer-aided design computer-aided manufacturing (CAD-CAM) technique:[8]

- Patient comfort: eliminates the claustrophobic feeling that some patients have when the impression material is in their mouths.
- It is a clean procedure, avoiding the usual "chaos" of a typical dental impression.
- No risk of cross-infection.

Secondly, different from the CAD-CAM technique, additive manufacturing offers the possibility to design complex indirect restorations layer by layer. Parameters such as surface roughness, mechanical properties, and optical properties can be engineered to generate a dental prosthesis with high performance. Some examples of interim crowns, metallic crown and bridge copings, implants and abutments, chirurgical plates, and partial removable denture frameworks (Figure 1) are currently manufacturable.[4,7,9–12]

The limitations of rapid prototyping of indirect restorations at present are: the cost of the printing device, the time of learning a

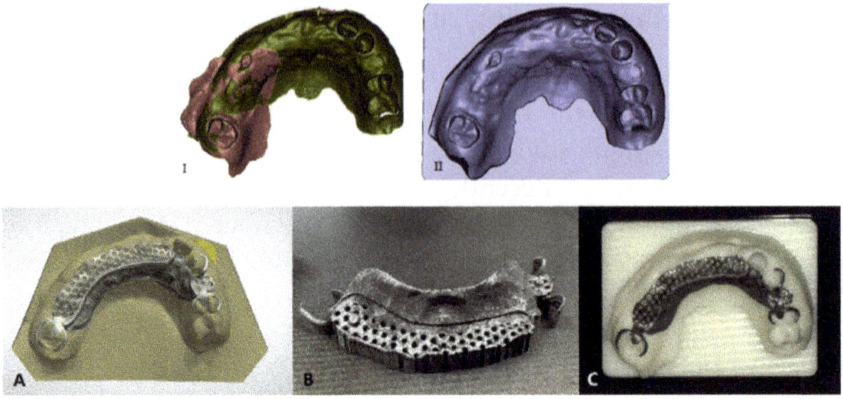

Figure 1. Partial removable denture framework manufactured by SLS technique. Adapted from Ref. [12]. Reprinted with the permission of Elsevier Science Publishers B.V

complex technology, and the lack of dental materials available for different 3D-printing techniques.

2.1.1. *Hard Tissue: Bone Reconstruction*

The principle of rapid prototyping is to use 3D computer models for the reconstruction of a 3D physical model by the addition of material layers.[13] Customized implants and prosthetics are one of the other widely explored areas for application of rapid prototyping.[14,15] Efforts have been made on the development of artificial organs and tissues using additive manufacturing.[14–16] Tissue engineering, particularly bone tissue, is rapidly expanding to become the most common type of application for 3D-printed medical/dental implants. Human bones are present in two different forms: cancellous, typically sponge-like in structure with a large degree of porosity (50–90%); or cortical, compact in structure having less than 10% porosity.[16] In developing a bone tissue implant, the porosity much match as closely as possible to the surrounding bone; too porous and the implant will easily collapse, too compact and the surrounding (human) bone tissue will be resorbed by the body leading to the eventual loss of attachment of the implant.

In the past, porous bone structures have been mimicked via techniques such as chemical/gas foaming, solvent casting, particle/salt leaching, freeze drying, foam gels, etc.; however, these techniques did not allow for the selection or control of pore size, shape, or scaffold interconnectivity.[16] 3D printing allows for the direct control of pore size, shape, or scaffold interconnectivity because it is an additive manufacturing technique, and extremely thin layers are printed one atop another, layer after layer, until an overall complete structure is formed. By this method, it is possible to design, slice by slice, the exact internal composition of each and every aspect of a bone tissue implant so as to match precisely with the surrounding tissues present in the individual's body. Internal channels or hanging features that often cause difficulty with traditional manufacturing techniques are realized with ease utilizing 3D printing since surrounding unbound powder material acts to support the structure until fabrication is complete.[2] Common techniques for 3D printing of bone tissue include extrusion (deformation and solidification), polymerization, laser-assisted sintering, and direct writing processes.[16]

3D printing of bone tissue can be done with a variety of different ceramic, metallic, polymeric, and other natural or synthetic composite materials. Powdered forms of tricalcium-phosphate (TCP), hydroxyapatite (HA), alumina (Al_2O_3), zirconia, polylactic acid (PLA), polypropylene (PP), and countless other types of high-strength, man-made synthetic substrates,[2,16] and any mixture of them can be used as a substrate for the 3D printing process, each of which has a long list of advantages and disadvantages relative to one another. Calcium phosphate-based ceramic materials stand out among the crowd and are widely used as substrate for bone-tissue implant production via 3D printing as these materials possess excellent bioactivity, osteoconductivity, and generally are very similar in composition to human bone structure.[16] Other tests have shown HA-printed materials to support the formation of capillaries and blood vessels within.[17]

As an aside from substrate selection, binder selection, that is, the choice of material used to bind and hence solidify powder material, is incredibly critical for successful implant fabrication as well.

Starch-based binders have shown good candidacy for producing bone tissue structures closely matching the properties of human trabecular bone.[16] Bone tissue implants printed with polyethylene using a starch-based binder have been shown to produce a porosity of 22.3–49.7%, resulting in a tensile strength of 4 MPa, and have not shown any toxicity to osteoblast cells, the primary bone extracellular matrix-producing cells of the human body.[16]

2.2. *Kinds of Additive Manufacturing Techniques: Advantages/Disadvantages*

Several different types of 3D-printing techniques have become popular in recent times, solid free-form fabrication (SFF), stereolithography (SLA), selective laser sintering (SLS), and 3D plotting/direct-write bioprinting are just to name a few.[3,5,6] Each of these techniques has its own inherent advantages/disadvantages, and most techniques specify the type of biomaterial that must be used to facilitate the fabrication process. The major disadvantage thus is the lack of selection of biomaterials available for each type of manufacturing/printing process. Commercially available devices are suitable for most patients. However, applications are generally very limited so far, and the issue is still in an early stage of research.

Rapid prototyping in general can only be applied to structures not exceeding certain dimensions as 3D printers are not able to produce extremely large products; this, however, is not a major concern for dental applications.[5] Even still, this limitation is currently overcome by producing a miniature version of a large structure by post-processing or by dividing the whole model into smaller parts which can be combined after printing. The major limitation of rapid prototyping lies within time and cost spent in generation of 3D objects.[18] For some authors, a widespread use of rapid prototyping for surgical planning or individual implant design does not seem to be justified because standard planning procedures or standard implants are sufficient.[18] However, in complicated cases, additional costs of rapid prototyping may be compensated by reduced operating times and higher success rates of the surgical procedure. The time needed for producing a 3D object also limits its use in surgery to elective cases and makes it unsuitable for emergency cases.[18,19]

2.2.1. *Solid Free-Form Fabrication (SFF)*

SFF is a type of rapid prototyping, which offers a method to control both the micro- and macroarchitecture to create complex biomedical devices. This technique allows for the design and fabrication of complex 3D structures which can be patient specific.[19] Some fabrication techniques use two materials in the course of constructing parts. The first material is the part material and the second is the support material, which is used to support overhanging features during construction.[19] The support material is later removed by heating or is dissolved with a solvent, commonly water. Depending on the fabrication technique, it is also possible to combine materials of different elasticity or color in one model. This can be useful to create more realistic models for educational or research purposes, or for naturally looking prosthetics. In addition, patient-specific imaging can be used to customize builds for individuals.[20,21] While conventional material processing techniques can be highly effective in scaffold engineering, SFF technologies offer exciting opportunities for tissue engineering of highly complex maxillofacial tissues. The selection of the fabrication technique depends upon the materials of interest, machine limitations, and the specific requirements of the final scaffold.[19,20]

2.2.2. *Selective Laser Sintering (SLS)*

SLS is based on small particles of thermoplastic, metal, ceramic, or glass powders that are fused by a high-power, focused laser.[6,22,23] Materials include polymers such as nylon, glass-filled nylon or polystyrene, or metals such as steel, stainless steel alloys, bronze alloys, or titanium. The key advantage of this technique is the ability to directly make metallic devices such as dental implants that promote bone ingrowth and regeneration for load-bearing applications in which high fracture toughness and mechanical strength are needed.[22,23] Even for non-load-bearing applications, polymers can be processed without

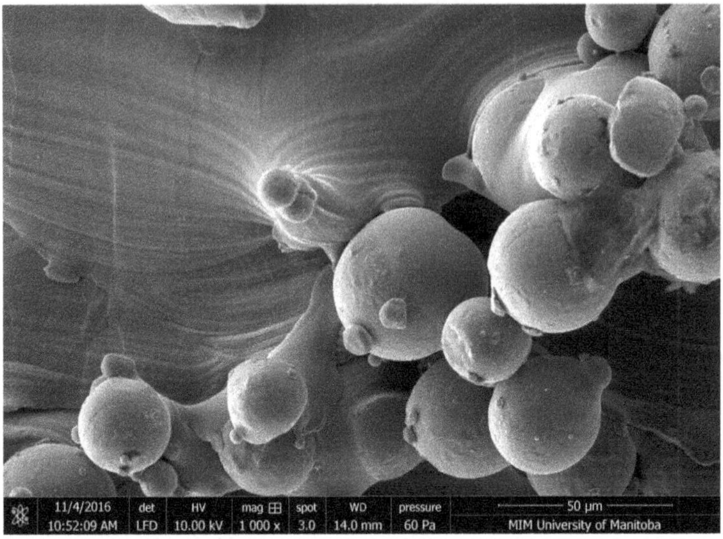

Figure 2. Raw stage of a 3D printed dental implant surface. Laser heat causes unwanted fusion of the neighboring powder particles

the use of an organic solvent. It is slightly easier to achieve compositional gradients in SLS than SLA by spreading different powder between different vertical layers, but compositional gradients in the horizontal plane is very limited. The main disadvantages are limited materials which fuse but do not decompose under the laser beam (high temperatures) and the post-processing needed to remove trapped powder.[22,23] Another limitation is the conduction and diffusion of laser heat that causes unwanted fusion of neighboring powder particles, thus limiting the resolution of final features (Figure 2). Lastly, smaller pore sizes are limited since the created pores depend on the particle size of the powder used. Powder particles that are too small cannot be used due to poor spreading from powder clumping.[22,23]

2.2.3. *Stereolithography (SLA)*

The advantages of SLA are the ability to create complex shapes with internal architecture, ease of removal of unpolymerized resin, and extremely high feature resolution.[5,6] The main disadvantage of SLA is the scarcity of biocompatible resins with proper SLA processing properties. Additional challenges are the use of photointiators and radicals which may prove cytotoxic with long processing times, entrapment of unreacted monomer and residual photoinitiator, and the inability to create compositional gradients along horizontal planes.[6,13] Photopolymerized resin also has poor mechanical properties that are needed for hard tissue engineering.[5,6] For these reasons, in dentistry SLA has a main role producing chairside devices like anatomic models for maxillofacial framework manufacturing.[4]

2.2.4. *Inkjet Printing Techniques*

Inkjet printing techniques are based on different kinds of fine powders such as plaster or starch.[3] After a layer of the powder has been dispensed by a piston, the parts of this layer belonging to the 3D object are bonded by an adhesive liquid, the binder, deposited by another piston.[20] Inkjet printing techniques can also be used to generate a 3D scaffold with different types of tissue by printing living cells and biomaterials simultaneously.[24] The first hurdle associated with these techniques is expanding upon the limited variety of available 3D printable biomaterials (biomaterial inks), which currently do not adequately represent the physical, chemical, and biological complexity and diversity of tissues and organs within the human body.[3] Newly developed biomaterial inks, and the resulting 3D-printed constructs, must meet numerous interdependent requirements, including those that lead to optimal printing, structural, and biological outcomes. The second challenge is developing and implementing comprehensive biomaterial ink and printed structure characterization combined with *in vitro* and *in vivo* tissue- and organ-specific evaluation.[3,24] This perspective outlines considerations for addressing these technical hurdles that, once overcome, will facilitate rapid advancement of 3D biomaterial printing as an indispensable tool for both investigating complex tissue and organ morphogenesis and for developing functional devices for a variety of diagnostic and regenerative medicine/dental applications.[20,24]

2.3. *Implants Suitable for 3D Printing*

Medical implants generated via the process of 3D printing are most often used in applications relating to the restoration of anatomic defects, the reconstruction of structural-based complex tissues (e.g. bone) with intricate 3D microarchitecture, and also for producing scaffolds atop which stem cells are typically deposited via traditional techniques. In the latter, designed surface properties and scaffold nanoarchitecture play roles in cell adhesion, proliferation, as well as differentiation.[2]

Examples with high success rates for 3D biomaterial printing applications are the cases involving large cranial defects. It has posed a significant challenge for neurosurgeons in the past, particularly owing to the high infection rate in the areas of the brain (33% by one study)[25] and significant bone resorption often seen around the graft region even when utilizing autologous bone for the graft. In the past, both titanium plates and mesh have been utilized to cover the cranial defect as titanium possesses the strength and biocompatibility properties desirable. However, such titanium grafts do not allow for the integration of human tissue and remain visible for the duration of the patient's life, sometimes causing severe psychological impacts.[25] Also, another common consequence arising from titanium graft is an increased sensitivity to temperature changes in the area around the graft, or foreign body sensation. A recent study presented the conclusions from the utilization of a 3D-printed bioceramic porous hydroxyapatite (HA) graft applied to the cranial defect. The study reports the results of 60 individuals, aged 17–75 years, who underwent complex cranial reconstructive surgery using customized 3D-printed grafts.[25] Cranial defects were located in the frontal–parietal–temporal, and frontal–occipital areas, respectively, and were greater that 25 cm^2 in size. Within the entire population, no incidence of infection was observed through the entire recovery time for the 51 patients who complied with attending all follow-up examinations within 2 years after the initial surgery. At the 2-year mark, the entire population also did not report any signs of rejection of the implant, neither were there any signs of foreign body reaction observed. Osteointegration of the implant was noted as normal for the majority of the patients, with 49 of the 51 patients reporting they were "very satisfied" with the implant, with the remaining 2 patients reporting as "moderately satisfied". One particular downside of the 3D-printed bioceramic porous hydroxyapatite (HA) implant is that, much like human bone, it is susceptible to fracture. Three patients reported implant fractures during their recovery periods, and each fracture was determined due to unrelated traumatic events sustained to the area of the graft.

Another case study involves a 3D-printed dental implant whereby the implant was realized by a form of SLS, namely direct-laser metal forming (DLMF). This study focused on a 50-year old female patient with a non-restorable second maxillary premolar.[26] In the past, surrounding bone resorption, infection, and implant fracture were common pitfalls of dental implants produced with traditional manufacturing techniques. With the use of DLMF-generated dental implants, the ability to design a porous surface with the desired control of pore size can be obtained. This allows for the highly desirable variability of density throughout the premolar implant. Put simply, it is desired that the implant has high density at the core for large load absorption, yet conversely it is desired that the outer surface be highly porous to promote anchorage via osteointegration. As a result, the implant produced is capable of lasting almost a life-time due to the high strength and favorable osteointegration properties resulting from the design of specific pore size. In addition, the healing timeframe is accelerated substantially from such a design. The patient returned for examination 1 year following implant of the premolar device. The implant was noted as stable, with no signs of infection, pain, or suppuration. Radiographic imaging displayed desirable osteointegration, and the crown complex was noted as "very similar to that of natural tooth". The implant showed exceptional aesthetic integration and had no associated prosthetic complications.[26]

3. Bioprinting

The shortage of replacement organs is still an ongoing issue in the medical and biomedical fields, and researchers are constantly investigating new methods to create new organs or replicate bodily organs. Bioprinting organs and tissues is one of the promising solutions that scientists have come out with in recent years. Its objective is to restore, support, or increase the human tissue functionality while maintaining the biocompatibility with and conformity of the tissues. However, many more studies are needed to first develop a successful technique for generating bioprinted organs with complex geometry and second to assess their biocompatibility in different patients. Thus, this leads to the rise of biological 3D printing which manufactures cell-encapsulated scaffolds.[27,28]

From a biomedical point of view, creating a cultured tissue and mimicking the surrounding environment which contains the extracellular matrix (ECM), various cells, and growth factors is admirable to replicate tissues functions *in vitro*. But, providing the cell and ECM interactions complexity and also multicellular construction properties with appropriate vascular systems is challenging in biomedical engineering.[29]

Bioprinting is a developing technology in the field of tissue engineering and regenerative medicine. This process includes simultaneous cell, biomaterial, and/or growth factor deposition under pressure via microscaled nozzles. 3D bioprinting is a procedure of controlling and managing the cell proliferation, attachment, and migration within 3D constructs. Moreover, as compared to solid scaffolds, the highly porous micro-/macroenvironment of bioprinted scaffolds is extremely beneficial for cell survival and differentiation, as metabolite, nutrient, and oxygen diffusion can be accomplished.[30,31]

The primary definition for biocompatibility is the compatibility with living tissues or biological systems without causing toxicity and immunological rejection. More generally, performance with a suitable host response in a particular condition and time could be a definition for biocompatibility.[32] Specifically, the artificial matrix must not only provide acceptable cell viability and growth but also provide suitable mechanical strength, ECM-like chemical and biological properties, signal transduction, and facilitate the exchange of nutrients, gases, and metabolic waste throughout the matrix. In the most recent years, organ transplantation or drug delivery systems have seen tremendous improvements due to bioprinted scaffolds in the form of hydrogels.[30,33,34]

To construct a bioprinted organ, many different factors that are interrelated and must be considered; their ability to work together affects their performance and subsequently the cell viability. The first consideration in the bioprinting process is the selection of an appropriate bioink; natural or synthetic, viscosity, printability, cross-linking and synthesis method, as well as degradability are just a few of the key factors to consider.

3.1. *Hydrogels as Bioinks*

Hydrogels are polymeric materials that are used as bioinks with the consistency similar to that of water-swollen gels. According to Peppas and Hoffman,[35] several mechanisms are used to form hydrogels:

(1) primary covalent cross-links;
(2) ionic forces;
(3) hydrogen bonds;
(4) affinity or "biorecognition" interactions;
(5) physical entanglements of individual polymer chains;
(6) a combination of two or more of the above interactions.[35]

Porosity and natural tissue resemblance are two main features of hydrogels that have made these 3D networks an amenable environment for cell survival and differentiation. Moreover, the hydrogel diffusivity enhances the exchange of nutrients and the elimination of cell metabolites.[36]

A wide range of natural and synthetic polymers have been used to construct hydrogels with different properties. The most commonly used natural polymers for biological 3D printing are based on collagen,[37–39] hyaluronic acid,[40] gelatin,[33,41] chondroitin sulfate,[42] fibrin,[43] alginate,[44] chitin,[33] and silk.[45] Among all these natural polymers, collagen and gelatin have been the most widely investigated since they are biocompatible, biodegradable, and are plentiful in nature. In some cases, natural polymers have presented issues that have lead to research involving a combination of natural polymers with other polymers or use with some modifications (Figure 3).[39]

For instance, pure gelatin solution has a low viscosity at physiological temperatures, which makes it tedious to be printed alone. Mixing gelatin with other viscous polymers, for example, alginate,[45] hyaluronic acid,[46,47] fibrin,[43] and silk,[45] is an approach to increase the viscosity for bioprinting. Another solution to enhance viscosity is partial cross-linking of polyethylene glycol polymer derivatives and gelatin blends before bioprinting.[48] Poor bioprinting resolution is another of the significant drawbacks associated with using gelatin as a bioink. To improve bioprinting resolution, gelatin should be mixed or blended with other polymers. It has been reported that blending gelatin methacrylamide with PEG to provide partial cross-linking improved the resolution significantly, as shown by the reduction of strut size from 1,100–1,300 μm to 350–450 μm, during bioprinting with a 200 μm diameter nozzle.[48]

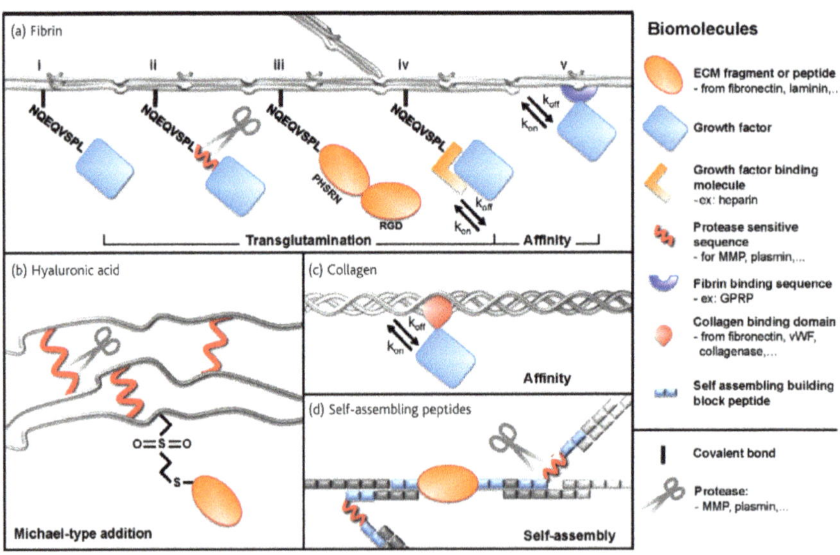

Figure 3. Types of chemically cross-linked hydrogels. According to Ref. [39]. Reprinted with the permission of Elsevier Science Publishers B.V

Klotz *et al.* focused on gelatin-based bioprinted hydrogels as injectable hydrogels for cell encapsulation in bioprinting. They mentioned that gelatin can cross-link with different types of polymers such as acrylamide, ferulic acid, furfurylamine, methacryloyl, etc., for cell encapsulation. So, the properties of gelatin could be easily manipulated in a cost-effective way, which also improves biocompatibility and biodegradability.[41] Wei Long Ng *et al.* developed a gelatin-based bioink for skin bioprinting consisting of chitosan and gelatin, in which polyelectrolyte complex was prepared for desirable wound healing properties. This bioprinted hydrogel showed constant mechanical properties under physiological condition in a week.[33,49]

Similar to gelatin, pure collagen has a low viscosity which makes it a difficult material to be printed. Many efforts have been focused on improving the viscosity using other polymers,[50] such as agarose,[51] chitosan,[52] fibrin,[53] as well as hyaluronic acid.[54] Blending with other polymers not only enhances the viscosity of collagen but also improves the shape fidelity. For instance, a collagen-based printed cylinder could be made 2 mm higher by adding 3% agarose and allowed to keep its shape for a day.[51] Also, collagen swelling capability has been improved (up to 85%) by combining collagen with phospholipid for cornea tissue repair application.[38] Furthermore, collagen-based biomaterials have the potential to provide cells with protection during bioprinting. Investigations demonstrated 86% viability of collagen-laden bovine aortic endothelial cells in which a 25 gauge nozzle was used. The scaffolds kept their viability and maintained their original spatial organization after 35 days of maintenance in culture.[55] In addition to cellular protection, collagen bioinks are able to preserve cell functionality and viability in printed cell-laden structures. Studies have shown that encapsulated human mesenchymal stromal cells in bioprintable type I collagen were induced to differentiate toward osteoblasts and adipocytes.[51]

Despite all the positive aspects of natural polymers, these products suffer from low mechanical properties and purity. Synthetic biodegradable polymers could solve this problem and have been utilized in scaffold construction, and these include common synthetic polymers including polyethylene glycol,[56] polylactic acid,[57] polyglycolic acid,[58] and their copolymers.[57] To achieve a broad range of suitable properties (biological, biophysical, and mechanical) for bioprinting, a combination of natural and synthetic hydrogels is a reasonable method. For instance, due to low viscosity, pure PEG is not appropriate for microextrusion bio 3D printing. However, integration of PEG derivatives into other bioinks as cross-linkers increases both mechanical properties of hydrogels and bioprinting resolution.[56]

3.1.1. *Hydrogel for Pulp-Regeneration*

Examples of a 3D-bioprinted dentin/pulp complex are not yet available in the literature. However, it will merely be a question of time because "the fundamental building blocks of this tissue" are already accessible.[59] Potential sites of stem cell for dentin/pulp regeneration are: postnatal dental pulp or exfoliated deciduous stem cells, as well as periodontal ligament stem cells among others.[60–62] Collagen, PEGylated fibrin, gelatin, and synthetic self-assembled nanofibrous peptide are some types of hydrogels already tested for injectable scaffolds for dentin/pulp regeneration.[61,63–65] In an interesting report,[66] heparin-conjugated gelatin was used to develop an injectable nanosphere system, which was in the form of nanofibrous biodegradable poly-L-lactic acid microsphere scaffold (Figure 4).

Dental pulp stem cells were seeded on these microspheres; the system was injected in a full-length human root canal (11 mm). Then the roots were implanted in an animal model (back of nude mice), for 9 weeks. The *in vitro* results showed complete regeneration of pulp tissue in the lower two-thirds of the root canal (Figure 5).[66]

Revascularization of the new tissue has been the major hitch for pulp regeneration techniques. Hydrogels with the controlled release of angiogenic growth factors have been proposed.[59,61] However, issues such as the duration of the angiogenic growth factor release and the place where this drug is delivered are still objectives to be accomplished.[61]

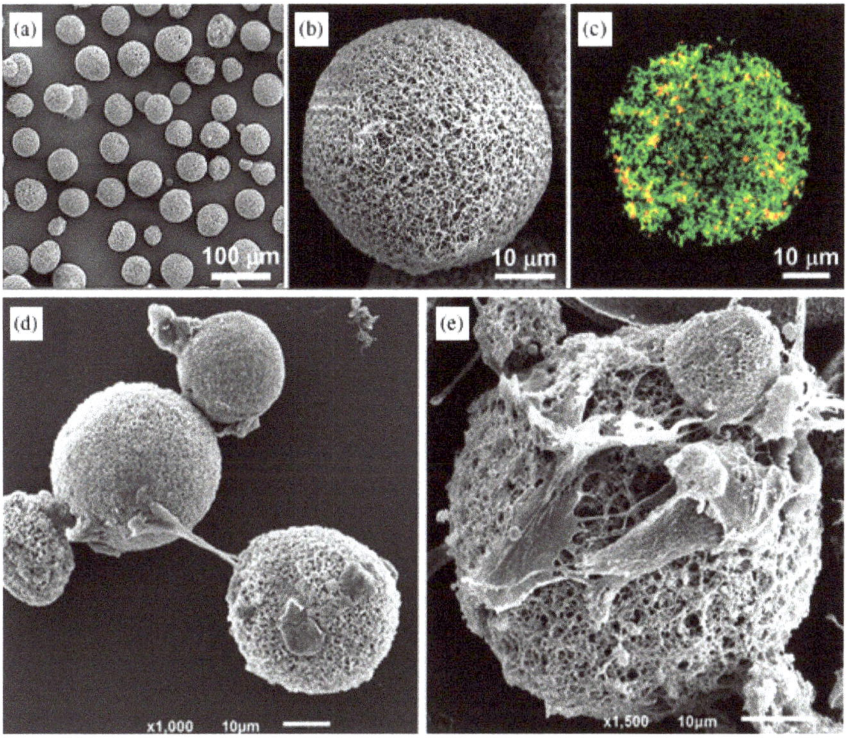

Figure 4. Overview of an SEM image that shows the dental pulp stem cells adhering to the surfaces of the hierarchical microspheres, expanding their processes and grasping the microspheres to form cell/microsphere aggregates. Adapted from Ref. [66]. Reprinted with the permission of Elsevier Science Publishers B.V

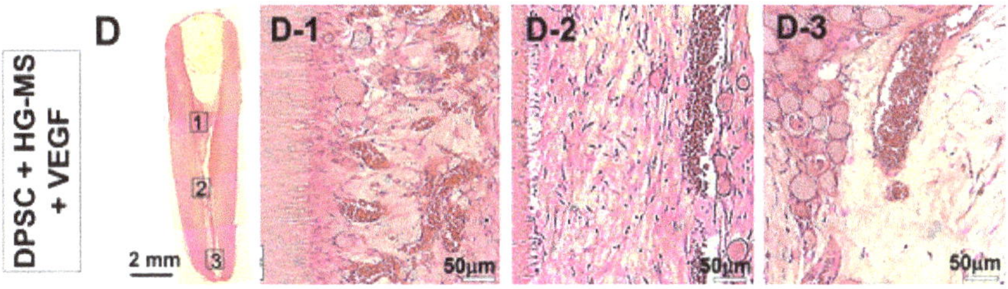

Figure 5. Regenerated pulp-like tissue filled both the apical and middle third regions and reached the coronal third of the canal. Adapted from Ref. [66]. Reprinted with the permission of Elsevier Science Publishers B.V

3.1.2. *Hydrogels for Periodontal Regeneration*

The periodontal system has a complex interaction among its anatomic features: cementum, periodontal ligament, and alveolar bone. This triphasic interphase brings an extra challenge for developing 3D bioprintable solutions for periodontal regeneration.[67] Multiphasic scaffolds with various compartments have been proposed for mimicking the architectural configuration of the periodontium.[59,67,68] Literature suggests several kinds of hydrogels as bioinks: N-(2-hydroxy) propyl-3-trimethyl ammonium chitosan chloride, quaternized chitosan with a-b glycerophosphate, poly(lactic-co-glycolic acid) (PLGA), and polycaprolactone.[61,67–69]

Hydrogels work as a scaffold for pluripotent cells, and they are frequently combined with calcium phosphate cements, hydroxyapatite, and beta-tricalcium phosphate to enhance periodontal healing.[67] Also, recombinant human bone morphogenetic proteins (rhBMP) are often added to the mix to promote periodontal regeneration. However, literature suggests that recombinant human growth/differentiation factor-5 (rhGDF-5) can have better performance in alveolar bone regeneration than rhBMP2 and rhBMP7.[70] Also, high doses of rhBMP2 and rhBMP7 were found to be associated with root resorption and ankylosis in an animal model.[61,70]

3.2. *Importance of Cross-Linking Process in Bioprinting Constructions*

The type of polymer selected for bioprinting mainly depends on the type of cross-linking technique employed to generate 3D networks. Various cross-linking mechanisms to obtain a structurally stable polymeric network include photo,- ion-, electrostatic, pH-, and temperature-based cross-linking mechanisms. Care must be taken when choosing the cross-linking method, as the viability of the encapsulated cells will be significantly affected by environmental conditions such as heat or pH. Similarly, the cross-linking technique influences construct outcomes with considerations of gelation via reversible or irreversible processes. To preserve the shape of hydrogels in bioprinting, gelation is an important and necessary factor which can be introduced physically, chemically, or via both procedures. The mentioned cross-linking methods modify the hydrogels mechanical properties, biocompatibility, and gelling time.

3.2.1. *Physical Cross-Linking*

Hydrogels that are cross-linked physically are the most popular category of hydrogels utilized in bioprinting. This mechanism of cross-linking involves polymer chain entanglements, hydrogen bonding, and hydrophobic as well as ionic interactions. Significant biocompatibility and good interaction with delicate molecules are the main properties of physically cross-linked hydrogels. Thermogelation and self-assembly are attractive as physical cross-linking systems due to their low cytotoxicity, for example, copolymers consisting of hydrophobic polylactic acid (PLA) and hydrophilic PEO moieties are commonly used for this reason.[36,71]

3.2.2. *Chemical Cross-Linking*

Low mechanical strength is the main weakness for physically cross-linked hydrogels. This flaw affects the bioprinted structure's stability significantly. Therefore, the chemical cross-linking method opens new horizons toward improvement of hydrogel stability, printability, and mechanical properties in order to be used in bioprinting constructs. Generally, gel precursors and a mixture of two solutions with low viscosity enable the chemical cross-linking process to achieve a hydrogel with higher viscosity. The reaction is initiated using radical polymerization and functional groups.

Free radical polymerization is a common way to achieve appropriate hydrogels for biomedical applications.[56,72] Hydrogels which are polymerized through vinyl functional groups are generated by redox, thermal, and photo initiators.[73,74] Among the natural and synthetic polymers, chitosan,[75,76] hyaluronic acid,[54] dextran,[44] PVA, and PEG,[77,78] respectively, are the most popular hydrogels in bioprinting. Photopolymerization provides a rapid rate of cross-linking; however, long exposure of cells to UV affects cell viability.[73,74] Furthermore, the heat released during the cross-linking procedure may lead to cellular necrosis. So, it is important to keep UV light intensity between 5 and 10 mW/cm^2 to prevent cell loss. Polymerization utilizing UV light *in vivo* is not efficient since the skin has low UV light penetration and absorption (>99%).[79] Polymerization through redox and thermal initiators like ammonium peroxydisulfate and N,N,N'N'-tetramethyl ethylene diamine (TEMED) are other alternatives. Enhancement of initiator concentration provides higher mechanical strength and lower gelation time. While increasing initiator concentration can be useful, it can incur negative effects as well, e.g. 10 mM may increase cytotoxicity and decrease cell viability to less than 30% after 4 days in cell culture.[80] Hence, free radical polymerization in hydrogels preparation needs further development to be used as a robust and suitable method.

The other type of chemically cross-linked hydrogels are those which are synthesized by reaction of their monomer functional groups. Schiff-based formation, peptide ligation, Michael-type additions, and "click" chemistry are the most common reactions in this category (Figure 3). In Schiff-based formation, an amine functional group reacts with an aldehyde group.[75] Glutaraldehyde is a frequent cross-linker which in spite of its high efficiency, results in toxicity, cell matrix degradation, and, consequently, prevents cell growth even if at low concentration. So, to remove unreacted reagents, hydrogels cross-linked by glutaraldehyde need to be extracted extensively. To reduce the toxicity effect of aldehyde groups, they can combined with other biocompatible polymers like hyaluronic acid.[81] Also, reactive aldehyde functional groups can be generated through oxidation of polysaccharides including alginate,[82] dextran,[44] and hyaluronic acid.[54] Aldehyde groups and PEG derivatives that create thiazolidine rings could be used to synthesize hydrogels through a peptide ligation method.[83,84] The reactions occur at moderate experimental conditions with a high rate of gelling (few minutes). Michael addition is the other method to prepare hydrogels via reaction of electrophilic functional groups such as vinyl, acrylate, or maleimide with nucleophiles like an amine or thiol group. So, polymers including dextran,[85] hyaluronic acid,[78] and PEG[78] are suitable for this kind of reaction. Peptides containing thiol groups have been used to create hydrogels with biofunctionality, which have improved cell adhesion and extracellular matrix production.[86] Generally, these types of hydrogels demonstrate good mechanical strength and mild gelling time between 0.5 and 60 min. The hydrogel's properties can be changed by alteration in functional group reactivity and cross-linker concentration which affects cross-linking density. Because of moderate circumstances in the Michael addition method, cells are not affected notably in hydrogel preparation and can normally sustain their viability for days to months.[87] However, excess concentration of thiol functional groups could lead to cell damage, which acts as restricting factor in their utilization.

Another strategy for chemical cross-linking is the reaction of azides and terminal alkynes using a copper catalyst.[88,89] Modified hyaluronic acid and gelatin have been used to synthesize biological hydrogels via click chemistry, mimicking the natural cartilage extracellular matrix.[90] Faster gelation, no by-products, and stability under physiological conditions are the most important advantages of this method. However, due to copper toxicity for mammalian cells, click chemistry catalyzed by copper may put end users in danger of death.[88] As removing the copper catalyst from the hydrogel is difficult and complicated, copper-free click polymerization methods have attracted researchers' attention as a new method in hydrogel preparation for biomedical applications. Table 1 summarizes the advantages and drawbacks of different cross-linking methods through the reaction of functional groups.

3.2.3. *Physical and Chemical Cross-Linking Combination*

Due to reversible interactions in physically cross-linked hydrogels, they have lower mechanical strength than chemically cross-linked hydrogels. On the other hand, biofavorable components in chemically cross-linked hydrogels could influence their biocompatibility. Although mechanical properties could be enhanced by increasing the molecular weight of polymers and cross-linkers concentration, it will

Table 1. Chemical cross-linking methods through functional groups

Chemical reaction	Functional groups involved	Advantages	Drawbacks
Schiff-based formation	Amine and aldehyde	❖ Applicable for incorporating and cross-linking proteins and amine-bearing peptides	❖ Possible side reaction by aldehyde ❖ Unstable Schiff-based linkages in acidic conditions
Peptide ligation	N-terminal cysteine and aldehyde	❖ Mild reaction conditions ❖ High substrate specificity ❖ High efficiency of cross-linking	❖ Complicated protection and de-protection steps in synthesis of peptides
Michael-type additions	Acrylate, vinyl, thiol, and amine	❖ Moderate reaction condition ❖ Adjustable properties appropriate for cell encapsulation	❖ Cell toxicity by unreacted thiol groups
Click chemistry	Azide and alkyne	❖ Fast gelation ❖ High reaction efficiency ❖ Stability	❖ Toxic copper from catalyst

be difficult then to control hydrogel viscosity. Mixing techniques of cross-linking both physically and chemically generate hydrogels with suitable biocompatibility and improved mechanical performance. For example, hydrogel development via the combination of photopolymerization and stereo complexation, an 8-arm PEG–PDLLA, and an 8-arm PEG–PLLA, stereo-complexed hydrogels functionalized with methacrylate groups (40%) are produced.[91] These hydrogels can be post-cross-linked using the application of UV light. The risk of cell damage and death from heat decreases because of the lower amount of initiator used for photopolymerization, which is approximately

0.003 wt.% in comparison with conventional photopolymerization and cross-linking methods that use 0.05 wt.%. The other combined systems consist of mixing different cross-linking methods involving inclusive complexation, stereo complexation, thermo-gelation, Michael addition reactions, and photopolymerization.[92,93] The combinations result in rapid gelling time, improved biocompatibility, and easier control of hydrogel properties.

3.3. *Properties of Bioink*

An appropriate bioink should fulfill biological requirements that include compatibility with cells and the ability to provide appropriate mechanical and physical features during the bioprinting process. From the physical perspective, the bioink should show gel-like behavior, having enough viscosity to stand freely. But, if the gel has higher stiffness with an associated high modulus, it will require a great shear force to inject the ink influencing cell viability and gel strength (fracture). From the mechanical perspective, the single-printed filaments need enough high strength and stiffness to keep the post-printing integrity of the structure.[94,95]

3.3.1. *Mechanical Properties*

Recently, there have been several studies undertaken on the initial mechanical properties of soft tissue structures and material characterization after printing.[96–98] To improve the mechanical strength of bioprinted structures, researchers have used a variety of different approaches: polymer concentration, cross-linking density, and the different methods for establishing cross-link structures can all act to improve the mechanical properties of final products.[99] For instance, a multi-cross-linking approach was used by Skardal *et al.* to produce extrudable bioinks and then a secondary cross-linking stabilized and increased the stiffness of the end products in order to match the desired tissue type. To modulate mechanical properties of hydrogel bioinks, they used combinations of polyethylene glycol cross-linkers with different molecular weights, geometries (linear, 4-arm, and 8-arm), and functional groups. This method enabled them to produce hydrogels with shear stiffness values ranging from approximately 100 Pa to 20 kPa and provided control over mechanical properties to mimic tissue stiffness.[53] In addition, hydrogels can be formed using natural or synthesized materials by chemical, physical, or biological cross-linking methods. For example, collagen can be chemically cross-linked by covalent bonding agents, which bind either free amine or carboxyl groups of collagen. Binding can occur via dehydrothermal treatment, UV radiation, or biologically by transglutaminase. Each of these methods have demonstrated different degrees of mechanical strength that depend on the mechanism, concentration, and exposure time.[95]

Mechanical properties of *in vitro* bioprinted hydrogels play an important role to mimic the *in vivo* mechanochemical microenvironment. In a study by Zhang *et al.*, a 3D *in vitro* soft tissue model with changing structures and porosity based on the 3D cell-assembly technique was constructed. Cells were embedded in a matrix of gelatin/alginate to examine mechanical characteristics and structural integrity, especially during the first 7 days of culture.[100] Based on the 3D soft tissue model results, it was seen that mechanical properties were affected by structural configuration. More importantly, it was observed that after 3 days of cell culture, the structural integrity and mechanical properties reduced drastically. This initial reduction could be due to the gelatin degradation during the first day under culture conditions as temperature changed. In addition, they observed the degradation of alginate in the 3D *in vitro* tissue models at the later stage, a possible explanation could be because of the effects of cellular activities and exposure to the culture conditions. Therefore, stability under both *in vitro* and *in vivo* conditions needs to be carefully considered before selecting an appropriate hydrogel.[100]

In an effort by Hunt *et al.*, rheological analysis was used to study the change in mechanical properties of alginate hydrogel during 28 days of *in vitro* culture. The results confirmed that despite the fact that at early-stage cellular activities influenced negatively encapsulating alginate mechanical characteristics, over a longer culture period, the hydrogels maintain acceptable mechanical integrity to show gel-like properties. In fact, as alginate degraded, encapsulated cells were released and started to proliferate and secrete extracellular matrix to facilitate tissue regeneration.[101]

3.3.2. *Permeability*

In 3D bioprinting, hydrogels not only serve as bioinks to deliver cells or support cell growth, but also provide cells with access to oxygen and nutrients which are essential for differentiation and proliferation. Therefore, hydrogels used in 3D printing should possess another important characteristic: a porous structure that allows filtration of oxygen and other such nutrients.[102] Besides, an interconnected pore network is essential for the effective mass transfer of gas, nutrients, and waste to achieve satisfactory cell viability.[103] When the engineered constructs are thicker than 1 mm, oxygen and nutrients perfuse with difficulty into the constructs, which may result in cell death.[36,104]

Additionally, it is undeniable that structures with enough porosity are proper to be used for functional tissues and organs with high thickness and metabolic activities because they have the ability to provide an integrated vascular network.[99] In fact, the internal architecture of tissue constructs plays a crucial role as it provides a porous environment for media exchange, vascularization, tissue growth, and engraftment. Recently, researchers have taken advantage of an innovation to prepare gel-like structure with hollow channel embedded arrays and utilized the resulting structure as a potential substitute for blood vessel networks. To fabricate several kinds of hollow nanofilaments, researchers have used a core–shell electrospinning technique. In this innovation, two immiscible solutions were electrospun through a coaxial, two-capillary spinneret.[105,106] Inspired by this concept, some researchers used a coaxial nozzle, which plays a key part in electrospinning equipment to fabricate microfluidic channels.[107–108] A commercially available, affordable, open-source 3D bioprinter modified with a microfluidic print-head was used by Attalla *et al.*[108] to create a system for generating a perfusable vascular network integrated with the cell. The print-head consisted of an integrated coaxial nozzle that provided the ability to fabricate hollow tubes based on calcium-polymerized alginate. By changing the flow rates or print-head speed, hollow channel diameter could be accurately controlled and varied. Hollow channel samples showed good cell viability after 24 h and 72 h, with about 81% and 70% viability, respectively. But, non-vascularized samples exhibited a significant decline in cell maintenance during this time period, from around 61% to 20%.[108]

3.3.3. *Degradation*

The main objective of bioprinted constructs is to allow the body's own cells, over time, to produce their own extracellular matrix and eventually replace the implanted scaffold. So, the first criterion for selecting an appropriate material for the bioprinted structure is their biodegradability, either by enzymes or hydrolysis.[109] Most synthetic biodegradable polymers are degraded by hydrolysis, which will lead to accumulation of acids in the local area, therefore altering the environment's pH and causing toxicity. Secondly, due to the body's immune response by macrophages, some hydrogels are destroyed by enzymes, which results in an inflammatory reaction around the implanted scaffold.[110]

The degradation properties of a hydrogel play a crucial role in the success of a bioprinted implant. Though, most of the by-products of polymers that are biodegradable are known to be non-toxic; there is limited data that shows acidic by-products depend on the rate of hydrogel degradation.[110] Kang *et al.* reported that the acidic by-product of PLGA can cause the degeneration of neocartilage tissue.[111]

Natural polymers are mostly biodegradable, and the degradation products are non-toxic. For example, metalloproteases normally degrade collagen, and hence cells in bioprinted hydrogels can control the procedure of degradation.[112] Gelatin has been modified to produce a photopolymerizable hydrogel via methylacrylate group addition to create methylacrylated gelatin (GelMA) for bioprinting applications.[46] Fibrin has been recently utilized within injectable hydrogels and cell delivery vehicles. Due to autologous cells derived from plasma, the degradation products of fibrin are biocompatible and the risk of inducing a foreign body reaction is low.[112] Alginate has low toxicity, and gels formed as a result of divalent cations such as Ba^+ or Ca^+ cooperatively interact with alginate to produce ionic links between chains of polymers. Studies show that the alginate hydrogel cross-linked by means of ions represents uncontrolled and slow dissolving behavior instead of demonstrating a particular trend of degradation.[113] Cao *et al.* studied the effect of Ca^+ concentration on cell viability and alginate hydrogel biocompatibility. Calcium ions can be used for cross-linking and improving printability; however, it has been demonstrated that higher Ca^+ concentrations have a higher probability of inducing cell death.[114] Chitosan can be degraded by human bodily enzymes and its structure is similar to glycosaminoglycan, hence it has good biocompatibility and non-toxic behavior. Chitosan is able to dissolve easily in diluted acids and form a gel like structure by pH enhancement, which are good features for chitosan. Lysozyme facilitates the degradation of chitosan, and the degradation kinetics proportionally depend on the degree of its crystallinity. Hyaluronic acid is a glycosaminoglycan and is present in most of the mammalian tissues. Its degradation process naturally takes place due to the presence of hyaluronidase, and it has been extensively applied for wound healing and skin regeneration and in various joint disorders such as osteoarthritis. Different methods like covalent cross-linking with hydrazide derivatives, annealing, and esterification have been used to prepare hyaluronic acid hydrogels. In addition, hyaluronic acid can be incorporated with other polymers like alginate, collagen, and gelatin to create composite hydrogels.[115,116]

Polyethylene glycol (PEG), a hydrophilic polymer, has a high water content, which can be incorporated into other polymer networks by cross-linking. By not eliciting a host immune response and being an easily modifiable polymer, PEG is a suitable polymer for biomedical applications. To achieve hydrogels which are able to degrade hydrolytically with physiologically acceptable degradation time scales, PEG is conjugated and functionalized with ester functional groups utilizing lactide or glycolide groups. As PEG chains have hydroxyl functional groups, they can be modified to form different PEG derivatives. PEG is not able to be adsorbed by the human body because of the lack of protein binding sites. These synthetic hydrogels successfully attract scientists for their use in bio 3D printing. For instance, photocurable PEG hydrogels are widely utilized in encapsulation of cells due to their naturally inert structure. Moreover, owing to its well structure, PEG can be employed as a mediator to immobilize the RGD sequence, a segment of protein which provides cell adhesion.[107,117]

Polylactic acid (PLA) is one of the popular synthetic polymers which has been used in bioprinting. Slow degradation rate, high tensile strength and modulus (~4.8 GPa), and low extension potentially make PLA an appropriate load-bearing alternative. However, the degradation rate is based on crystallinity degree and porosity of the construct. PLA is able to produce high-strength fibers that introduces the field of scaffold fabrication for replacement of ligaments. Polyglycolic acid (PGA) is highly crystalline and insoluble in most of the organic solvents. Although the degradation properties may change by utilizing different types of processing methods, PGA degradation products are natural metabolites. PGA degradation includes random hydrolysis of the ester bonds. In addition to hydrolysis, some enzymes, particularly those which have esterase activity, can decompose PGA structure. Various factors such as crystallinity, configuration of structure, molecular weight, and implantation site affect the degradation rate of PGA. Although desirable biocompatibility of PGA has been demonstrated by different *in vitro* and *in vivo* analyses[118]; two main problematic issues have been detected. One of them is related to orthopedic applications in which normally large size implants are required that leads to by-product release from PGA degradation producing a highly acidic environment. It was determined that toxic products can be produced by PGA acidic degradation.[118] The inflammatory response is the other concern, triggered via small released particles during degradation. Copolymer polylactic-glycolic acid (PLGA) shows high resistance behavior to be degraded hydrolytically.[58] Bulk erosion occurs in PLGA by hydrolyzing ester bonds. Different parameters affect the rate of degradation including molecular weight, the lactic acid/glycolic acid proportion, and matrix structure. Ease of processing makes PLGA a common copolymer, as it facilitates fabrication to develop several constructs.[58]

It is undeniable that cells must be subject to pressure and mechanical forces that occur through the bioprinting process. Therefore, there is an important question that must be answered. If cells are being compulsorily influenced by or subjected to external forces brought on by the bioink and biofabrication process, what will be the cell's fate? Investigations show that proliferation, motion, and differentiation of living cells, as dynamic compounds, will change under external forces and stimuli. Changes in cell geometry cause changes in mechanical signals, which consequently result in alteration of chemical signals and cellular regulations. The characteristics of the bioink are determined through its formalization and crucially affect the formed structure's delivery and integrity. More importantly, the bioink should possess some properties similar to the biological requirements that are essential for the cell system.[94,119]

3.3.4. *Viscosity*

Viscosity plays a key role in the properties of bioinks, and the ability of a hydrogel to be printed is partially controlled by its viscosity. Printability, or the hydrogel printing effectiveness, was studied by means of using compressed oxygen in order to drive hydrogels through a tube which delivered the bioink to print-head nozzles.[119] The software controlled the deposition by opening the print-head nozzles with precise timing while simultaneously configuring their movement over the printing surface. Bioinks in this system needed to have similar viscosity to be effectively steered via the tube and ejected from the nozzles.[110]

The viscosity of bioink is primarily influenced by the bioink concentration and is easily controllable. In addition, cross-linking processes can affect the viscosity of the bioink. It is important to control the extent of cross-linking within the biomaterials to obtain a suitable printing viscosity. Pre-cross-linked polymers could be too viscous to be used in the bioprinter. This issue has been addressed in the study by

Murphy *et al.*, who compared specific properties such as biocompatibility and printability of different hydrogels.[110] It was reported in this study that pre-cross-linked chitosan-based hydrogels showed highest cell death most likely because of the ammonium hydroxide vapor treatment utilized to pre-cross-link the hydrogel. Due to the high viscosity of certain hydrogels, they were not able to print the hydrogel using the bioprinting hardware. Therefore, these hydrogel solutions were printed utilizing a syringe deposition technique instead.

Long Ng *et al.*,[33] used a modification in the cross-linking method of chitosan-based hydrogels to increase the printability. The authors took advantage of the interaction between polyelectrolyte complexes, like positively charged chitosan and negatively charged gelatin to improve its printability. The positively charged ammonium ions from chitosan react with carboxylate groups from the ampholytic gelatin to form a polyelectrolyte complex. This method was much better than pre-cross-linking of the bioink, which increased the bioink viscosity undesirably.

The other strategy to control bioink viscosity and printability is to combine the ink with another component to modify the properties and form a gel that possesses proper biological features and satisfies the desired physical extrusion criteria. In the work done by Chung *et al.*, rheological properties of alginate–gelatin hydrogels were compared with pre-cross-linked alginate and alginate hydrogel to describe their printability.[120] Easy gelation, cell compatibility, and appropriate stability of alginate were presented as the convincing reasons to choose this polymer in the abovementioned study. By changing the concentration of alginate or by hydrogel pre-cross-linking prior to printing, rheological requirements for extrusion printing were obtained. The viscosity and storage modulus of alginate-based bioinks could be enhanced by employing the gelling characteristics at low temperatures, without the need for Ca^{2+} addition. Besides, this method made these gels more cell-friendly. According to live and dead cells assays, primary myoblasts maintained viability within the alginate–gelatin hydrogel, even after being printed at two or three times higher pressures than pressures that would normally provide good filament size and resolution.

3.4. *Methods of Bioprinting*

To assess the biocompatibility of bioprinting in microenvironment engineering, cell viability and functionality after the bioprinting process must be affirmed for different printing systems.[27,28,30] To exemplify, for the hamster ovary cells and rat primary embryonic motor neurons printing, a thermal inkjet printer was employed. During the cell suspension preparation, due to osmotic effects of phosphate-buffered saline, 15% of cells were lysed. During bioink printing, due to temperature enhancement in the ejector reservoir, 3% of cells were lysed. Furthermore, 74% viability was reported in primary rat embryonic hippocampal and cortical neuron printing.[30] Recently, various bio 3D-printing systems have gained 90% cell viability in comparison to control groups of non-printed cell cultures, which illustrate the explicit application of bio 3D-printing in future for several cell types ranging from neurons to stem cells. Additionally, for high-throughput single-cell isolation and pattering, valve-based bioprinting technology has been employed. Stem cell viabilities were stated around 97% and 94% in pre- and post-bioprinting procedures, respectively. Also, results demonstrated that functional genomic information of stem cells were maintained during bioprinting.[30]

Applications of tissue engineering and 3D bioprinting technology could involve various methods. The most common methods include the stereolithography apparatus (SLA) and digital light processing (DLP) techniques in which a vat of liquid photopolymer resin and a UV laser are used to provide the 3D structures. fused filament fabrication (FFF) utilizes material extrusion and creates a structure layer by layer. Selective laser sintering (SLS) fuses powder of a polymer by applying heat from a high-power laser, and the last is inkjet 3D printing, which consists of powder bed and binder jetting. Among the abovementioned common 3D bioprinting methods, FFF is not suitable for cell printing since it does not utilize any solvent. Inkjet 3D printing has been used for printing of cells and cell-encapsulated hydrogels, though it does not provide appropriate mechanical properties and may damage cell membrane and their functionalities during solution injection. Besides, SLA and DLP printing technologies increase cytotoxicity due to uncured photoinitiator in photopolymerization.[121]

From the laser power perspective, there is another category in 3D bioprinting, classified into the laser-assisted and laser-free bioprinting methods. In laser-assisted bioprinters, a laser beam, a focusing system, and a substrate are the main components. Living cells lead to determined positions on a substrate through a light trap created by the laser beam and focusing system. Excessive thermal energy exposure by the laser light onto the cell biolayer which overheats living cells can be one of the challenges in this method. Long exposure time and direct contact of the cell with the laser light causes low rates of cell survival. If the laser does not contact directly with living cells, the cells' survival rate will improve up to 95% cell viability. To overcome this important challenge, lights with near infrared wavelength (700–1,000 nm) have been utilized. However, DNA is not able to absorb near infrared photons, and free radical generation will be retarded too. Therefore, laser-guided direct bioprinting is defined as a system that does not cause mutation or trigger apoptosis, although optimization of wavelengths continues to exist as an open and unsolved issue. Laser-free bioprinters have been inspired by inkjet desktop printers. In these methods, printing pressure plays a pivotal role in cell viability. In this regard, some other factors such as needle shape and printing pressure affect cell viability and thus the biocompatibility of the bioink.[28]

Cell encapsulation technology that is based on picoliter droplet using an acoustic apparatus has been developed in recent times. Acoustic droplet formation rate can achieve up to 100,000 droplets per second with high cell viability. Droplets are formed from an open liquid reservoir and no nozzle is needed for the generation of a droplet. Complications regarding shear clogging will be avoided. In addition to these advantages, acoustic waves do not put living cells in danger because of low power droplet generation within only a few pulses, occurring within microseconds. In addition, acoustic ejectors can be combined in an adjustable array format as multiple ejectors, which would increase the printing rate and allow the deposition of several types of cells and ECM. Various biomaterials could be printed through the ejectors such as living cells, ECM proteins, nutrients, therapeutic drugs, and growth factors simultaneously from the same platform via integration of microfluidic systems into the ejectors. To gain reproducible outcomes for the cell-encapsulating droplet deposition, bioprinting spatial precision should be comparable to the cell size, for instance, around 10–20 μm in hydrogel or bioink. Acoustic techniques have been introduced as a method that can eject droplets in a broad size range from 3 μm in diameter to several hundred micrometers.[28]

3.4.1. *Bioprinting Parameter: Nozzle Diameter and Pressure*

Bioprinting methods which dispense the living cells by syringe affect various parameters with varied effects on living cells and the overall quality of the bioprinted construct. For example, nozzle diameter and the movement speed of nozzle head are parameters which could influence cell viability. Reduction in diameter of the dispensing nozzle will enhance the dispensing shear forces that living cells inside the nozzle experience. Also, changing the movement speed of the nozzle head could induce additional compressive or tensile forces on the dispensed strands.[122] For instance, at high speeds dispensed strands will be stretched and lead to higher tensile forces on the encapsulated cells, while, at lower speeds, the dispensing forces are lower and living cells experience less compression.[123]

The results obtained by Chang *et al.*[98] showed that cell recovery was dependent on procedure parameters. All dispensing pressures, 5, 10, 20, and 40 psi, demonstrated notable cell recovery of control values at the 7-day time endpoint with 94.67%, 91.07%, 90.02%, and 87.06% recovery values, respectively. Based on the calculation of the percentage of cell recovery, the smallest nozzle diameter group (i.e. 150 mm) represented meaningfully reduced cell viability and the larger nozzle diameter experimental groups between 250 and 400 mm exhibiting relatively higher cell recovery. From the information presented in abovementioned study, it can be concluded that cell recovery shows sensitivity to the parameters of the printing procedure. At higher pressures, cell recovery was higher and less for small nozzle tip diameter. A similar result was obtained by Nair *et al.*, which showed a more significant effect of dispensing pressure than the nozzle diameter on cell viability.[122]

Aside from the fact that viscosity affects the printability, it can influence other parameters like dispensing pressure within the nozzle.[124] A more viscous hydrogel would require a higher dispensing pressure, and this increment in dispensing pressure was shown to induce a significant decrease in cell viability. It is obvious that at higher dispensing pressure highly viscous bioinks can eject easily. However, the shear stress could be increased by higher viscosity, leading to reduced cell viability and increased cell damage. Referring to Yu *et al.*, the cell-laden conduits direct the fabrication ability utilizing an extrusion-based bioprinting technique.[100] They reported that due to variation in dispensing pressure, quantifiable cell death could be induced by the bioprinting procedure. In their study, most of the dead cells were distributed along the edge of the printed structure walls, where shear stresses were at the highest level. In another relevant effort by Tirella *et al.*, the shear stress influence on cell viability and functionality endured during the process of deposition were systematically investigated.[125] They employed a method that provided low shear stress extrusion of viscous hydrogel solutions consisting of cells. By process parameter optimization, like modifying the bioink concentration, nozzle diameter, pressure, and speed, they could overcome limitations created by viscous bioink.

4. Future Perspective

Additional progress for 3D printing technologies is needed for the ability to increase the resolution without sacrificing shape and the strength of the device. For both SLS and 3DP, there is a challenge with creating stronger structures without increasing dimensions.[126] To create small features which survive the fabrication process, powder particles must be bound together tightly. Additional work is needed to move to SLS and 3DP with smaller resolutions.[126,127] Advances of SLA have been made to synthesize new biodegradable moieties; however, these materials have not been FDA approved. Although macro- and microarchitecture has made great strides in the past 5 years, additional work should focus on the nano-architecture (e.g. biochemical molecules).[126,127]

Due to harsh processing conditions of SFF methods (e.g. heat, organic solvent), biochemical molecules are not generally incorporated directly into the scaffold. While biochemical molecules can be coated onto structures in post-processing, there is a need for sustained growth factor release over time.[23,126] Therefore, strategies to incorporate biochemical molecules directly into scaffolds for prolonged release will be needed. These systems unfortunately are not optimized for biomaterials of interest for *in vitro* and *in vivo* studies, and advances are still being made to improve the methods for biomaterials.

5. Conclusion

Although there has been recent progress in the field, medical research has already benefited from rapid prototyping providing a new vision into physiological and pathological processes. Several technical challenges have yet to be overcome. In cases where materials can be printed, 3D printing is particularly advantageous for one-of-a-kind, customized complex devices that are not cost-effective in conventional manufacturing methods. However, current biomaterial availability does not adequately represent the physical, chemical, and biological complexity and diversity of tissues and organs within the human body. The invention of a greater variety and complexity of printable materials is a key aspect that requires large developments for the more widespread acceptance and use of 3D printing to take place. Still, for the materials currently available for bioprinting applications, biocompatibility is an essential factor that poses many challenges yet to be overcome. The dream of printing a complete living tissue that can be readily implanted into the body and can replace damaged bodily organs with complex functions, sadly, is still a distant dream. Nevertheless, at least some of the limitations presented within this chapter might be overcome by future technological developments.

References

1. Gross, D. Obama's speech highlights rise of 3-D printing. https://www.cnn.com/2013/02/13/tech/innovation/obama-3d-printing/index.html (Accessed December 2, 2016).
2. Chia, H. N.; Wu, B. M. *J. Biol. Eng.* **2015**, *9* (1), 4.
3. Jakus, A. E.; Rutz, A. L.; Shah, R. N. *Biomed. Mater.* **2016**, *11* (1), 014102.
4. van Noort, R. *Dent. Mater.* **2012**, *28* (1), 3–12.
5. Chia, H. N.; Wu, B. M. *J. Biol. Eng.* **2015**, *9* (1), 1.
6. Eshraghi, S.; Das, S. *Acta Biomater.* **2012**, *8* (8), 3138–3143.
7. Dawood, A.; Marti Marti, B.; Sauret-Jackson, V.; Darwood, A. *Br. Dent. J.* **2015**, *219* (11), 521–529.
8. Christensen, G. J. *J. Am. Dent. Assoc.* **2014**, *145* (8), 862–864.
9. Joo, H. S.; Park, S. W.; Yun, K. D.; Lim, H. P. *J. Prosthet. Dent.* **2016**, *116* (1), 3–7.
10. Mai, H. N.; Lee, K. B.; Lee, D. H. *J. Prosthet. Dent.* **2017**.
11. Mangano, F.; Chambrone, L.; van Noort, R.; Miller, C.; Hatton, P.; Mangano, C. *Int. J. Biomater.* **2014**, *2014*, 461534.
12. Wu, J.; Li, Y.; Zhang, Y. *J. Am. Dent. Assoc.* **2017**, *148* (5), 338–341.
13. Billiet, T.; Vandenhaute, M.; Schelfhout, J.; Van Vlierberghe, S.; Dubruel, P. *Biomaterials* **2012**, *33* (26), 6020–6041.
14. Inzana, J. A.; Olvera, D.; Fuller, S. M.; Kelly, J. P.; Graeve, O. A.; Schwarz, E. M.; Kates, S. L.; Awad, H. A. *Biomaterials* **2014**, *35* (13), 4026–4034.
15. Lee, J.-Y.; Choi, B.; Wu, B.; Lee, M. *Biofabrication* **2013**, *5* (4), 045003.
16. Bandyopadhyay, A.; Bose, S. *Characterization of Biomaterials* (Amsterdam: Elsevier, **2013**).
17. Becker, S. T.; Bolte, H.; Schünemann, K.; Seitz, H.; Bara, J.; Beck-Broichsitter, B.; Russo, P.; Wiltfang, J.; Warnke, P. H. *Int. J. Oral Maxillofac. Surg.* **2012**, *41* (9), 1153–1160.
18. Lohfeld, S.; Tyndyk, M.; Cahill, S.; Flaherty, N.; Barron, V.; McHugh, P. *J. Biomed. Sci. Eng.* **2010**, *3* (02), 138.
19. Lee, J.-S.; Hong, J. M.; Jung, J. W.; Shim, J.-H.; Oh, J.-H.; Cho, D.-W. *Biofabrication* **2014**, *6* (2), 024103.

20. Park, J. H.; Jung, J. W.; Kang, H.-W.; Cho, D.-W. *Biofabrication* **2014**, *6* (2), 025003.
21. Shim, J.-H.; Lee, J.-S.; Kim, J. Y.; Cho, D.-W. *J. Micromechanics Microengineering* **2012**, *22* (8), 085014.
22. Shuai, C.-j.; Mao, Z.-z.; Han, Z.-k.; Peng, S.-p. *J. Bioact. Compat. Polym.* **2014**, *29* (2), 110–120.
23. Giannitelli, S.; Accoto, D.; Trombetta, M.; Rainer, A. *Acta Biomater.* **2014**, *10* (2), 580–594.
24. Olszewski, R. *Proceedings of the Belgian Royal Academies of Medicine* **2013**, *2*, 43–77.
25. Staffa, G.; Barbanera, A.; Faiola, A.; Fricia, M.; Limoni, P.; Mottaran, R.; Zanotti, B.; Stefini, R. *J. Craniomaxillofac. Surg.* **2012**, *40* (3), e65–e70.
26. Figliuzzi, M.; Mangano, F.; Mangano, C. *Int. J. Oral Maxillofac. Surg.* **2012**, *41* (7), 858–862.
27. Ozbolat, I. T.; Peng, W.; Ozbolat, V. *Drug Discov. Today* **2016**, *21*, 1257–1271.
28. Mandrycky, C.; Wang, Z.; Kim, K.; Kim, D. H. *Biotechnol. Adv.* **2016**, *34*, 422–434.
29. Khatiwala, C.; Law, R; Shepherd, B.; Dorfman, S; Csete, M. *Gene Ther. Reg.* **2012**, *07*, 1230004.
30. Zhu, W.; Ma, X.; Gou, M.; Mei, D.; Zhang, K.; Chen, S. *Curr. Opin. Biotechnol.* **2016**, *40*, 103–112.
31. Mehrban, N.; Teoh, G. Z.; Birchall, M. A. *IJB* **2016**, *2*.
32. Williams, D. F. *Biomaterials* **2008**, *29*, 2941–2953.
33. Ng, W. L.; Yeong, W. Y.; Naing, M. W. *Procedia CIRP* **2016**, *49*, 105–112.
34. Visscher, D. O.; Farré-Guasch, E.; Helder, M. N.; Gibbs, S.; Forouzanfar, T.; van Zuijlen, P. P.; Wolff, J. *Trends Biotechnol.* **2016**, *34*, 700.
35. Buddy D. Ratner; Allan S. Hoffman; Frederick J. Schoen; Lemons, J. E. *Biomaterials Science — An Introduction to Material in Medicine.* 3rd ed. (Amstersam: Elsevier, **2012**).
36. Wang, M.; He, J.; Liu, Y.; Li, M.; Li, D.; Jin, Z. *IJB* **2015**, *1*, 15–26.
37. Lee, W.; Debasitis, J. C.; Lee, V. K.; Lee, J. H.; Fischer, K.; Edminster, K.; Park, J. K.; Yoo, S. S. *Biomaterials* **2009**, *30*, 1587–1595.

38. Islam, M. M.; Cepla, V.; He, C.; Edin, J.; Rakickas, T.; Kobuch, K.; Ružele, Ž.; Jackson, W. B.; Rafat, M.; Lohmann, C. P.; Valiokas, R.; Griffith, M. *Acta Biomater.* **2015**, *12*, 70–80.
39. Patterson, J.; Martino, M. M.; Hubbell, J. A., *Mater. Today* **2010**, (Jan–Feb).
40. Wüst, S.; Godla, M. E.; Müller, R.; Hofmann, S. *Acta Biomater.* **2014**, *10*, 630–640.
41. Klotz, B. J.; Gawlitta, D.; Rosenberg, A. J. W. P.; Malda, J.; Melchels, F. P. W. *Trends Biotechnol.* **2016**, *34*, 394–407.
42. Wang, S.; Lee, J. M.; Yeong, W. Y., *Int. J. Bioprinting*, **2015**, *1*, 3.
43. Zhao, X.; Wang, X. *J. Bioact. Compat. Polym.* **2013**, *28*, 191–203.
44. Khalil, S.; Sun, W. *J. Biomech. Eng.* **2009**, *131*, 111002.
45. Das, S.; Pati, F.; Choi, Y. J.; Rijal, G.; Shim, J. H.; Kim, S. W.; Ray, A. R.; Cho, D. W.; Ghosh, S. *Acta Biomater.* **2015**, *11*, 233–246.
46. Schuurman, W.; Levett, P. A.; Pot, M. W.; van Weeren, P. R.; Dhert, W. J. A.; Hutmacher, D. W.; Melchels, F. P. W.; Klein, T. J.; Malda, J. *Macromol. Biosci.* **2013**, *13*, 551–561.
47. Gaetani, R.; Feyen, D. A. M.; Verhage, V.; Slaats, R.; Messina, E.; Christman, K. L.; Giacomello, A.; Doevendans, P. A. F. M.; Sluijter, J. P. G. *Biomaterials* **2015**, *61*, 339–348.
48. Rutz, A. L.; Hyland, K. E.; Jakus, A. E.; Burghardt, W. R.; Shah, R. N. *Adv. Mater.* **2015**, *27*, 1607–1614.
49. M. Rahimnejad, S. D. a. W. Z. *Burn. Trauma* **2017**, *5* (4).
50. Inzana, J. A.; Olvera, D.; Fuller, S. M.; Kelly, J. P.; Graeve, O. A.; Schwarz, E. M.; Kates, S. L.; Awad, H. A. *Biomaterials* **2014**, *35*, 4026–4034.
51. Duarte Campos, D. F.; Blaeser, A.; Korsten, A.; Neuss, S.; Jäkel, J.; Vogt, M.; Fischer, H. *Tissue Eng. A* **2015**, *21*, 740–756.
52. Zhang, Y.; Fan, W.; Nothdurft, L.; Wu, C.; Zhou, Y.; Crawford, R.; Xiao, Y. *Tissue Eng. C Meth.* **2011**, *17*, 789–797.
53. Skardal, A.; Devarasetty, M.; Kang, H. W.; Mead, I.; Bishop, C.; Shupe, T.; Lee, S. J.; Jackson, J.; Yoo, J.; Soker, S.; Atala, A. *Acta Biomater.* **2015**, *25*, 24–34.
54. Park, H.; Choi, B.; Hu, J.; Lee, M. *Acta Biomater.* **2013**, *9*, 4779–4786.

55. Smith, C. M.; S. A.; Parkhill, R. L.; Stewart, R. L.; Simpkins, M. W.; Kachurin, A. M.; Warren, W. L.; Williams, S. K. *Tissue Eng. Part A* **2004**, *10* (9–10), 1566–1576.
56. Zhu, J. *Biomaterials* **2010**, *31*, 4639–4656.
57. Nicodemus, G. D.; Bryant, S. J. *Tissue Eng. Part B Rev.* **2008**, *14*, 149–165.
58. Hsieh, F. Y.; Lin, H. H.; Hsu, S. H. *Biomaterials* **2015**, *71*, 48–57.
59. Obregon, F.; Vaquette, C.; Ivanovski, S.; Hutmacher, D. W.; Bertassoni, L. E. *J. Dent. Res.* **2015**, *94* (9 Suppl), 143S–52S.
60. Gronthos, S.; Brahim, J.; Li, W.; Fisher, L. W.; Cherman, N.; Boyde, A.; DenBesten, P.; Robey, P. G.; Shi, S. *J. Dent. Res.* **2002**, *81* (8), 531–535.
61. Chang, B.; Ahuja, N.; Ma, C.; Liu, X. *Mater. Sci. Eng. R: Reports* **2017**, *111*, 1–26.
62. Seo, B.-M.; Miura, M.; Gronthos, S.; Mark Bartold, P.; Batouli, S.; Brahim, J.; Young, M.; Gehron Robey, P.; Wang, C. Y.; Shi, S. *The Lancet* **2004**, *364* (9429), 149–155.
63. Huang, G. T. *Regen. Med.* **2009**, *4* (5), 697–707.
64. Luo, Z.; Wang, S.; Zhang, S. *Biomaterials* **2011**, *32* (8), 2013–2020.
65. Poh, P. S.; Chhaya, M. P.; Wunner, F. M.; De-Juan-Pardo, E. M.; Schilling, A. F.; Schantz, J. T.; van Griensven, M.; Hutmacher, D. W. *Adv. Drug Deliv. Rev.* **2016**, *107*, 228–246.
66. Li, X.; Ma, C.; Xie, X.; Sun, H.; Liu, X. *Acta Biomater.* **2016**, *35*, 57–67.
67. Park, C. H.; Rios, H. F.; Jin, Q.; Sugai, J. V.; Padial-Molina, M.; Taut, A. D.; Flanagan, C. L.; Hollister, S. J.; Giannobile, W. V. *Biomaterials* **2012**, *33* (1), 137–145.
68. Lee, C. H.; Hajibandeh, J.; Suzuki, T.; Fan, A.; Shang, P.; Mao, J. J. *Tissue Eng. Part A* **2014**, *20* (7–8), 1342–1351.
69. Ji, Q. X.; Chen, X. G.; Zhao, Q. S.; Liu, C. S.; Cheng, X. J.; Wang, L. C. *J. Mater. Sci. Mater. Med.* **2009**, *20* (8), 1603–1610.
70. Kwon, D. H.; Bennett, W.; Herberg, S.; Bastone, P.; Pippig, S.; Rodriguez, N. A.; Susin, C.; Wikesjo, U. M. *J. Clin. Periodontol.* **2010**, *37* (4), 390–397.
71. Klouda, L. *Eur. J. Pharm. Biopharm.* **2015**, *97*, 338–349.
72. Tan, H.; Marra, K. G. *Materials* **2010**, *3*, 1746–1767.

73. Chan, V.; Zorlutuna, P.; Jeong, J. H.; Kong, H.; Bashir, R. *Lab. Chip* **2010**, *10*, 2062–2070.
74. Galperin, A.; Long, T. J.; Ratner, B. D. *Biomacromolecules* **2011**, *11*, 2583–2592.
75. Hennink, W. E.; van Nostrum, C. F. *Adv. Drug Deliv. Rev.* **2012**, *64*, 223–236.
76. Moura, M. J.; Faneca, H.; Lima, M. P.; Gil, M. H.; Figueiredo, M. M. *Biomacromolecules* **2011**, *12*, 3275–3284.
77. Zustiak, S. P.; Leach, J. B. *Biomacromolecules* **2010**, *11*, 1348–1357.
78. Jin, R.; Teixeira, L. S. M.; Krouwels, A.; Dijkstra, P. J.; Van Blitterswijk, C. A.; Karperien, M.; Feijen, J. *Acta Biomater.* **2010**, *6*, 1968–1977.
79. Wu, D. C.; Loh, X. J.; Wu, Y. L.; Lay, C. L.; Liu, Y. *J Am. Chem. Soc.* **2010**, *132*, 15140–15143.
80. Malda, J.; Visser, J.; Melchels, F. P.; Jüngst, T.; Hennink, W. E.; Dhert, W. J. A.; Groll, J.; Hutmacher, D. W. *Adv. Mater.* **2013**, *25*, 5011–5028.
81. Schanté, C. E.; Zuber, G.; Herlin, C.; Vandamme, T. F. *Carbohydr. Polym.* **2011**, *85*, 469–489.
82. Sun, J.; Tan, H. *Materials* **2013**, *6*, 1285–1309.
83. Takaoka, Y.; Ojida, A.; Hamachi, I. *Ang. Chem. Int. Ed.* **2013**, *52*, 4088–4106.
84. Kaga, S.; Arslan, M.; Sanyal, R.; Sanyal, A. *Molecules* **2016**, *21*.
85. Lin, C.; Zhao, P.; Li, F.; Guo, F.; Li, Z.; Wen, X. *Mater. Sci. Eng. C* **2010**, *30*, 1236–1244.
86. Park, J.; Lim, E.; Back, S.; Na, H.; Park, Y.; Sun, K. *J. Biomed. Mater. Res. Part A* **2010**, *93*, 1091–1099.
87. Liu, Z.; Lin, Q.; Sun, Y.; Liu, T.; Bao, C.; Li, F.; Zhu, L. *Adv. Mater.* **2014**, *26*, 3912–3917.
88. Chang, P. V.; Prescher, J. A.; Sletten, E. M.; Baskin, J. M.; Miller, I. A.; Agard, N. J.; Lo, A.; Bertozzi, C. R. *Proceedings of the National Academy of Sciences of the United States of America* **2010**, *107*, 1821–1826.
89. Van Dijk, M.; Van Nostrum, C. F.; Hennink, W. E.; Rijkers, D. T. S.; Liskamp, R. M. J. *Biomacromolecules* **2010**, *11*, 1608–1614.
90. Hu, X.; Li, D.; Zhou, F.; Gao, C. *Acta Biomater.* **2011**, *7*, 1618–1626.
91. Hiemstra, C.; Zhou, W.; Zhong, Z.; Wouters, M.; Feijen, J. *J. Am. Chem. Soc.* **2007**, *129*, 9918–9926.

92. Bearat, H. H.; Lee, B. H.; Vernon, B. L. *Acta Biomater.* **2012**, *8*, 3629–3642.
93. Niu, G.; Zhang, H.; Song, L.; Cui, X.; Cao, H.; Zheng, Y.; Zhu, S.; Yang, Z.; Yang, H. *Biomacromolecules* **2008**, *9*, 2621–2628.
94. Ouyang, L.; Yao, R.; Zhao, Y.; Sun, W. *Biofabrication* **2016**, *8*, 035020.
95. Holzl, K.; Lin, S.; Tytgat, L.; Van Vlierberghe, S.; Gu, L.; Ovsianikov, A. *Biofabrication* **2016**, *8* (3), 032002.
96. Zhang, T.; Yan, K. C.; Ouyang, L.; Sun, W. *Biofabrication* **2013**, *5*, 45010.
97. Fedorovich, N. E.; Schuurman, W.; Wijnberg, H. M.; Prins, H.-J.; van Weeren, P. R.; Malda, J.; Alblas, J.; Dhert, W. J. A. *Tissue Eng. Part C Meth.* **2012**, *18*, 33–44.
98. Yan, K. C.; Nair, K.; Sun, W. *J. Biomech.* **2010**, *43* (6), 1031-8.
99. Zhang, H.-B.; Xing, T.-L.; Yin, R.-X.; Shi, Y.; Yang, S.-M.; Zhang, W.-J. *CJT* **2016**, *19*, 187–192.
100. Yu, Y.; Zhang, Y.; Martin, J. A.; Ozbolat, I. T. *J. Biomech. Eng.* **2013**, *135*, 91011.
101. Hunt, N. C.; Smith, A. M.; Gbureck, U.; Shelton, R. M.; Grover, L. M. *Acta Biomater.* **2010**, *6*, 3649–3656.
102. Korpela, J.; Kokkari, A.; Korhonen, H.; Malin, M.; Narhi, T.; Seppalea, J. *J. Biomed. Mater. Res. Part B Appl. Biomater.* **2013**, *101*, 610–619.
103. Peng, X. F.; Mi, H. Y.; Jing, X.; Yu, P.; Qu, J. P.; Chen, B. Y. *Mater. Des.* **2016**, *101*, 285–293.
104. Visser, J.; Melchels, F. P. W.; Jeon, J. E.; van Bussel, E. M.; Kimpton, L. S.; Byrne, H. M.; Dhert, W. J. a.; Dalton, P. D.; Hutmacher, D. W.; Malda, J. *Nat. Commun.* **2015**, *6*, 6933.
105. Sperling, L. E.; Reis, K. P.; Pranke, P.; Wendorff, J. H. *Drug Discov. Today* **2016**, *21*, 1243–1256.
106. Duan, N.; Geng, X.; Ye, L.; Zhang, A.; Feng, Z.; Guo, L.; Gu, Y. *Biomed. Mater.* **2016**, *11* (3), 035007.
107. Gao, Q.; He, Y.; Fu, J.-z.; Liu, A.; Ma, L. *Biomaterials* **2015**, *61*, 203–215.
108. Attalla, R.; Ling, C.; Selvaganapathy, P. *Biomed. Microdevices* **2016**, *18*, 1–12.
109. Kirchmajer, D. M.; Gorkin III, R.; in het Panhuis, M. *J. Mater. Chem. B* **2015**, *3*, 4105–4117.

110. Murphy, S. V.; Skardal, A.; Atala, A. *J. Biomed. Mater. Res. Part A* **2013**, *101 A*, 272–284.
111. Kang, S. W.; Lee, S. J.; Kim, J. S.; Choi, E. H.; Cha, B. H.; Shim, J. H.; Cho, D. W.; Lee, S. H. *Macromol. Biosci.* **2011**, *11*, 267–274.
112. Gasperini, L.; Mano, J. F,; Reis,. R. L. *J. R. Soc. Interface.* **2014**, *11*, 20140817.
113. Duan, B.; Hockaday, L. A.; Kang, K. H.; Butcher, J. T. *J. Biomed. Mater. Res. Part A* **2013**, *101 A*, 1255–1264.
114. Cao, N.; Chen, X. B.; Schreyer, D. J. *ISRN Chem. Eng.* **2012**, *2012*, 1–9.
115. Burdick, J. A.; Prestwich, G. D. *Adv. Mater.* **2011**, *23*, 41–56.
116. Skardal, A.; Zhang, J.; McCoard, L.; Xu, X.; Oottamasathien, S.; Prestwich, G. D. *Tissue Eng. Part A* **2010**, *16*, 2675–2685.
117. Cui, X.; Britenkamp, K.; Finn, M. G.; Lotz, M.; D'Lima, D. D. *Tissue Eng. Part A* **2012**, *18*, 1304–1312.
118. Di Bella, C.; Fosang, A.; Donati, D. M.; Wallace, G. G.; Choong, P. F. M. *Front. Surg.* **2015**, *2*, 39.
119. Dababneh, A. B.; Ozbolat, I. T. *J. Manufact. Sci. Eng.* **2014**, *136*, 061016.
120. Chung, J. H. Y.; Kapsa, R.; Quigley, A., **2013**, *1*.
121. Gu, B. K.; Choi, D. J.; Park, S. J.; Kim, M. S.; Kang, C. M.; Kim, C.-H. *Biomaterial. Res.* **2016**, *20*, 12.
122. Nair, K.; Gandhi, M.; Khalil, S.; Yan, K. C.; Marcolongo, M.; Barbee, K.; Sun, W. *Biotechnol. J.* **2009**, *4*, 1168–1177.
123. Chang, R.; Nam, J.; Sun, W. *Tissue Eng. Part A* **2008**, *14*, 41–48.
124. Billiet, T.; Gevaert, E.; De Schryver, T.; Cornelissen, M.; Dubruel, P. *Biomaterials* **2014**, *35*, 49–62.
125. Tirella, A.; Vozzi, F.; Vozzi, G.; Ahluwalia, A. *Tissue Eng. Part C* **2011**, *17*, 229–237.
126. Parthasarathy, J. *Ann. Maxillofac. Surg.* **2014**, *4* (1), 9.
127. Duan, B.; Wang, M. *MRS Bull.* **2011**, *36* (12), 998–1005.

Index

Lightning Source UK Ltd.
Milton Keynes UK
UKHW022158231218
334474UK00002B/14/P

9 789813 225671